Pocket Guide to
Diagnostic
Tests

fifth edition

Diana Nicoll, MD, PhD, MPA
Clinical Professor and Vice Chair
Department of Laboratory Medicine
University of California, San Francisco
Associate Dean
University of California, San Francisco
Chief of Staff and Chief, Laboratory Medicine Service
Veterans Affairs Medical Center, San Francisco

Stephen J. McPhee, MD
Professor of Medicine
Division of General Internal Medicine
Department of Medicine
University of California, San Francisco

Michael Pignone, MD, MPH
Assistant Professor of Medicine
Division of General Internal Medicine
Department of Medicine
University of North Carolina, Chapel Hill

Chuanyi Mark Lu, MD
Assistant Professor of Clinical Laboratory Medicine
University of California, San Francisco
Chief, Hematology and Hematopathology
Laboratory Medicine Service
Veterans Affairs Medical Center, San Francisco

With Associate Authors

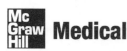 **Medical**

New York Chicago San Francisco Lisbon London Madrid Mexico City
Milan New Delhi San Juan Seoul Singapore Sydney Toronto

The McGraw·Hill Companies

Pocket Guide to Diagnostic Tests, Fifth Edition

5 6 7 8 9 0   DOC/DOC   0

ISBN: 978-0-07-148968-3
MHID: 0-07-148968-1
ISSN: 1061-3463

Notice

Medicine is an ever-changing science. As new research and clinical experience broaden our knowledge, changes in treatment and drug therapy are required. The authors and the publisher of this work have checked with sources believed to be reliable in their efforts to provide information that is complete and generally in accord with the standards accepted at the time of publication. However, in view of the possibility of human error or changes in medical sciences, neither the authors nor the publisher nor any other party who has been involved in the preparation or publication of this work warrants that the information contained herein is in every respect accurate or complete, and they disclaim all responsibility for any errors or omissions or for the results obtained from use of the information contained in this work. Readers are encouraged to confirm the information contained herein with other sources. For example and in particular, readers are advised to check the product information sheet included in the package of each drug they plan to administer to be certain that the information contained in this work is accurate and that changes have not been made in the recommended dose or in the contraindications for administration. This recommendation is of particular importance in connection with new or infrequently used drugs.

This book was set in Times Roman by International Typesetting and Composition.
The editors were Ruth W. Weinberg and Robert Pancotti.
The production supervisor was Catherine Saggese.
Project management was provided by International Typesetting and Composition.
RR Donnelley was printer and binder.

This book was printed on acid-free paper.

Contents

Associate Authors

Jane Jang, BS, MT (ASCP) SM
Laboratory Medicine Service
Veterans Affairs Medical Center, San Francisco
Microbiology: Test Selection

Fred Kusumoto, MD
Associate Professor of Medicine
Department of Medicine
Division of Cardiovascular Diseases
Director of Electrophysiology and Pacing
Mayo Clinic Jacksonville, FL
Basic Electrocardiography

Susan D. Wall, MD
Professor of Radiology
University of California, San Francisco
Diagnostic Imaging: Test Selection and Interpretation

Benjamin M. Yeh, MD
Associate Professor of Radiology
Department of Radiology
University of California, San Francisco
Diagnostic Imaging: Test Selection and Interpretation

Preface

Purpose

The *Pocket Guide to Diagnostic Tests, fifth edition,* is intended to serve as a pocket reference manual for medical, nursing, and other health professional students, house officers, and practicing physicians and nurses. It is a quick reference guide to the selection and interpretation of commonly used diagnostic tests, including laboratory procedures in the clinical setting, laboratory tests (chemistry, hematology, immunology, microbiology, and molecular and genetic testing), diagnostic imaging tests (plain radiography, CT, MRI, and ultrasonography), electrocardiography, and the use of tests in differential diagnosis, including helpful algorithms.

This book will enable readers to understand commonly used diagnostic tests and diagnostic approaches to common disease states.

Outstanding Features

- Over 350 tests are presented in a concise, consistent, and readable format.
- Expanded content regarding molecular and genetic tests.
- Added microbiologic coverage of emerging (new) and reemerging pathogens and infectious agents.
- Fields covered include internal medicine, pediatrics, surgery, neurology, and obstetrics and gynecology.
- Costs and risks of various procedures and tests are noted.
- Literature references with PubMed (PMID) numbers are included for each entry.
- An index for quick reference is included on the back cover.

Organization

This pocket reference manual is not intended to include all diagnostic tests or disease states. The authors have selected those tests and diseases that are most common and relevant to the general practice of medicine.

The *Guide* is divided into nine sections:
1. Basic Principles of Diagnostic Test Use and Interpretation
2. Laboratory Procedures in the Clinical Setting
3. Common Laboratory Tests: Selection and Interpretation
4. Therapeutic Drug Monitoring: Principles and Test Interpretation

New to This Edition

1. More than two dozen new clinical laboratory test entries, including: Bcr/abl, t(9;22) translocation by RT-PCR, qualitative; Bcr/abl mutation analysis (Bcr/Abl genotyping); C-reactive protein, high sensitivity (hs-CRP); factor assays: Factor II (prothrombin); G20210A mutation; heparin anti-Xa assay; heparin-associated anti-body detection (HIT work-up); hepatitis B virus DNA quantitative (HBV-DNA) (viral load); hepatitis C RNA, quantitative (viral load); hepatitis C virus genotyping; HIV RNA, quantitative (viral load); HIV resistance testing; homocysteine; *Jak2* (V617F) mutation; leukemia/lymphoma phenotyping by flow cytometry; methylenetetrahydrofolate reductase (MTHFR) mutation; platelet function (PFA-100 closure time); sirolimus; tacrolimus; and transferrin receptor, soluble (sTfR).

2. Microbiological tests for emerging (new) and reemerging pathogens and infectious agents.

3. More than a dozen new tables and algorithms concerning diagnostic approaches to: anemia work-up; acid-base disturbances; bleeding disorders; coagulation cascade; hypocalcemia; hyperlipidemia; female infertility; immunophenotyping and genetics of leukemias and lymphomas; polycythemia; prolongation of activated partial thromboplastin time; sleep disturbance; thrombocytopenia; thrombocytosis; venous thrombosis; and transfusion: preparation and use of blood components for transfusion.

Intended Audience

Medical students will find the concise summary of diagnostic laboratory, microbiologic, and imaging studies, and of electrocardiography in this pocket-sized book of great help during clinical ward rotations.

Busy house officers and practitioners will find the clear organization and current literature references useful in devising proper patient management.

Nurses and other health practitioners will find the format and scope of the *Guide* valuable for understanding the use of laboratory tests in patient management.

Acknowledgments

The editors acknowledge the invaluable editorial contributions of William M. Detmer, MD, and Tony M. Chou, MD, to the first three editions of this book.

In addition, the late G. Thomas Evans, Jr., MD, contributed the electrocardiography chapter for the second and third editions. In the fourth and this fifth edition, the chapter has been revised by Fred M. Kusumoto, MD.

We thank our associate authors for their contributions to this book and are grateful to the many physicians, residents, and students who have made useful suggestions.

We welcome comments and recommendations from our readers for future editions.

Diana Nicoll, MD, PhD, MPA
Stephen J. McPhee, MD
Michael Pignone, MD, MPH
Chuanyi Mark Lu, MD

San Francisco
September 2007

Basic Principles of Diagnostic Test Use and Interpretation

Diana Nicoll, MD, PhD, MPA, and Michael Pignone, MD, MPH

The clinician's main task is to make reasoned decisions about patient care despite incomplete clinical information and uncertainty about clinical outcomes. Although data elicited from the history and physical examination are often sufficient for making a diagnosis or for guiding therapy, more information may be required. In these situations, clinicians often turn to diagnostic tests for help.

BENEFITS, COSTS, AND RISKS

When used appropriately, diagnostic tests can be of great assistance to the clinician. Tests can be helpful for **screening,** that is to identify risk factors for disease and to detect occult disease in asymptomatic persons. Identification of risk factors may allow early intervention to prevent disease occurrence, and early detection of occult disease may reduce disease morbidity and mortality through early treatment. Screening tests recommended for preventive care of asymptomatic low-risk adults include measurement of blood pressure and serum lipids. Screening for breast, cervix, and colon cancer is also recommended, whereas prostate cancer screening remains controversial. Optimal screening tests meet the criteria listed in Table 1–1.

Tests can also be helpful for **diagnosis,** to help establish or exclude the presence of disease in symptomatic persons. Some tests assist in early diagnosis after onset of symptoms and signs; others assist in developing a differential diagnosis; others help determine the stage or activity of disease.

Tests can be helpful in **patient management.** Tests can help: (1) evaluate the severity of disease, (2) estimate prognosis, (3) monitor the course of disease (progression, stability, or resolution), (4) detect disease recurrence, and (5) select drugs and adjust therapy.

When ordering diagnostic tests, clinicians should weigh the potential benefits against the potential costs and disadvantages. Some tests carry

TABLE 1–1. CRITERIA FOR USE OF SCREENING PROCEDURES.

Characteristics of population
  1. Sufficiently high prevalence of disease.
  2. Likely to be compliant with subsequent tests and treatments.

Characteristics of disease
  1. Significant morbidity and mortality.
  2. Effective and acceptable treatment available.
  3. Presymptomatic period detectable.
  4. Improved outcome from early treatment.

Characteristics of test
  1. Good sensitivity and specificity.
  2. Low cost and risk.
  3. Confirmatory test available and practical.

a risk of morbidity or mortality—for example, cerebral angiogram leads to stroke in 0.5% of cases. The potential discomfort associated with tests such as colonoscopy may deter some patients from completing a diagnostic workup. The result of a diagnostic test may mandate further testing or frequent follow-up—for example, a patient with a positive fecal occult blood test may incur significant cost, risk, and discomfort during follow-up colonoscopy.

Furthermore, a false-positive test may lead to incorrect diagnosis or further unnecessary testing. Classifying a healthy patient as diseased based on a falsely positive diagnostic test can cause psychological distress and may lead to risks from unnecessary or inappropriate therapy. A diagnostic or screening test may identify disease that would not otherwise have been recognized and that would not have affected the patient. For example, early-stage low-grade prostate cancer detected by prostate-specific antigen (PSA) screening in an 84-year-old man with known severe congestive heart failure will probably not become symptomatic or require treatment during his lifetime.

The costs of diagnostic testing must always be understood and considered. Total costs may be high, or cost-effectiveness may be unfavorable. An individual test such as MRI of the head can cost more than $1400, and diagnostic tests as a whole account for approximately 20% of health care expenditures in the United States. Even relatively inexpensive tests may have poor cost-effectiveness if they produce very small health benefits.

Genetic testing is becoming more readily available. Diagnostic genetic testing based on symptoms (eg, testing for fragile X in a boy with mental retardation) differs from predictive genetic testing (eg, evaluating a healthy person with a family history of Huntington disease) and from predisposition genetic testing, which may indicate relative susceptibility to certain conditions (eg, *BRCA-1* testing for breast cancer). Carrier testing (eg, for cystic fibrosis) and prenatal fetal testing (eg, for Down syndrome) are other uses of genetic testing. All such testing requires extensive counseling of patients so that there is adequate understanding of the clinical and emotional impact of the results.

PERFORMANCE OF DIAGNOSTIC TESTS

Test Preparation

Factors affecting both the patient and the specimen are important. The most crucial element in a properly conducted laboratory test is an appropriate specimen.

Patient Preparation

Preparation of the patient is important for certain tests—for example, a fasting state is needed for optimal glucose and triglyceride measurements; posture and sodium intake must be strictly controlled when measuring renin and aldosterone levels; and strenuous exercise should be avoided before taking samples for creatine kinase determinations, since vigorous muscle activity can lead to falsely abnormal results.

Specimen Collection

Careful attention must be paid to patient identification and specimen labeling. Knowing when the specimen was collected may be important. For instance, aminoglycoside levels cannot be interpreted appropriately without knowing whether the specimen was drawn just before ("trough" level) or after ("peak" level) drug administration. Drug levels cannot be interpreted if they are drawn during the drug's distribution phase (eg, digoxin levels drawn during the first 6 hours after an oral dose). Substances that have a circadian variation (eg, cortisol) can be interpreted only in the context of the time of day the sample was drawn.

During specimen collection, other principles should be remembered. Specimens should not be drawn above an intravenous line, as this may contaminate the sample with intravenous fluid. Excessive tourniquet time will lead to hemoconcentration and an increased concentration of protein-bound substances such as calcium. Lysis of cells during collection of a blood specimen will result in spuriously increased serum levels of substances concentrated in cells (eg, lactate dehydrogenase and potassium). Certain test specimens may require special handling or storage (eg, blood gas specimens). Delay in delivery of specimens to the laboratory can result in ongoing cellular metabolism and therefore spurious results for some studies (eg, low serum glucose).

TEST CHARACTERISTICS

Table 1–2 lists the general characteristics of useful diagnostic tests. Most of the principles detailed below can be applied not only to laboratory and radiologic tests but also to elements of the history and physical examination.

Accuracy

The accuracy of a laboratory test is its correspondence with the true value. An inaccurate test is one that differs from the true value even though the results may be reproducible (Figure 1–1A). In the clinical laboratory, accuracy of tests is maximized by calibrating laboratory equipment with reference material and by participation in external quality control programs.

Precision

Test precision is a measure of a test's reproducibility when repeated on the same sample. An imprecise test is one that yields widely varying results on repeated measurements (Figure 1–1B). The precision of diagnostic tests, which is monitored in clinical laboratories by using control material, must be good enough to distinguish clinically relevant changes in a patient's status from the analytic variability of the test. For instance, the manual white blood cell differential count is not precise enough to detect important changes in the distribution of cell types, because it is calculated by subjective evaluation of a small sample (100 cells). Repeated measurements by different technicians on the same sample result in widely different results. Automated differential counts are more precise because they are obtained from machines that use objective physical characteristics to classify a much larger sample (10,000 cells).

TABLE 1–2. PROPERTIES OF USEFUL DIAGNOSTIC TESTS.

1. Test methodology has been described in detail so that it can be accurately and reliably reproduced.
2. Test accuracy and precision have been determined.
3. The reference range has been established appropriately.
4. Sensitivity and specificity have been reliably established by comparison with a gold standard. The evaluation has used a range of patients, including those who have different but commonly confused disorders and those with a spectrum of mild and severe, treated and untreated disease. The patient selection process has been adequately described so that results will not be generalized inappropriately.
5. Independent contribution to overall performance of a test panel has been confirmed if a test is advocated as part of a panel of tests.

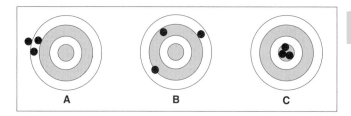

Figure 1–1. Relationship between accuracy and precision in diagnostic tests. The center of the target represents the true value of the substance being tested. **(A)** A diagnostic test that is precise but inaccurate; on repeated measurement, the test yields very similar results, but all results are far from the true value. **(B)** A test that is imprecise and inaccurate; repeated measurement yields widely different results, and the results are far from the true value. **(C)** An ideal test that is both precise and accurate.

Reference Range

Reference ranges are method- and laboratory-specific. In practice, they often represent test results found in 95% of a small population presumed to be healthy; by definition, then, 5% of healthy patients will have an abnormal test result (Figure 1–2). Slightly abnormal results should be interpreted critically—they may be either truly abnormal or falsely abnormal. The practitioner should also be aware that the more tests ordered, the greater the chance of obtaining a falsely abnormal result. For a healthy person subjected to 20 independent tests, there is a 64% chance that one test result will

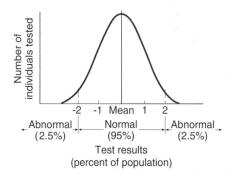

Figure 1–2. The reference range is usually defined as within 2 SD of the mean test result (shown as −2 and 2) in a small population of healthy volunteers. Note that in this example, test results are normally distributed; however, many biologic substances will have distributions that are skewed.

TABLE 1–3. RELATIONSHIP BETWEEN THE NUMBER OF TESTS AND THE PROBABILITY THAT A HEALTHY PERSON WILL HAVE ONE OR MORE ABNORMAL RESULTS.

Number of Tests	Probability That One or More Results Will Be Abnormal
1	5%
6	26%
12	46%
20	64%

lie outside the reference range (Table 1–3). Conversely, values within the reference range may not rule out the actual presence of disease since the reference range does not establish the distribution of results in patients with disease.

It is important to consider also whether published reference ranges are appropriate for the patient being evaluated, since some ranges depend on age, sex, weight, diet, time of day, activity status, or posture. For instance, the reference ranges for hemoglobin concentration are age- and sex- dependent. Some diagnostic tests are simply reported as positive or negative. This dichotomization involves an inherent information loss. Test performance characteristics such as sensitivity and specificity are needed to interpret results and are discussed below.

Interfering Factors

The results of diagnostic tests can be altered by external factors, such as ingestion of drugs; and internal factors, such as abnormal physiologic states.

External interferences can affect test results in vivo or in vitro. In vivo, alcohol increases γ-glutamyl transpeptidase, and diuretics can affect sodium and potassium concentrations. Cigarette smoking can induce hepatic enzymes and thus reduce levels of substances such as theophylline that are metabolized by the liver. In vitro, cephalosporins may produce spurious serum creatinine levels due to interference with a common laboratory method of analysis.

Internal interferences result from abnormal physiologic states interfering with the test measurement. As an example, patients with gross lipemia may have spuriously low serum sodium levels if the test methodology used includes a step in which serum is diluted before sodium is measured. Because of the potential for test interference, clinicians should be wary of unexpected test results and should investigate reasons other than disease that may explain abnormal results, including laboratory error.

Sensitivity and Specificity

Clinicians should use measures of test performance such as sensitivity and specificity to judge the quality of a diagnostic test for a particular disease. Test **sensitivity** is the likelihood that a test result will be positive in a patient with a given disease. If *all* patients with a given disease have a positive test result, the test sensitivity is 100%. Generally, a test with high sensitivity is useful to exclude a diagnosis because a highly sensitive test will render few results that are falsely negative. To exclude infection with the virus that causes AIDS, for example, a clinician might choose a highly sensitive test, such as the HIV antibody test.

A test's **specificity** is the likelihood that a healthy patient has a negative test. If *all* patients who do not have a given disease have negative test results, the test specificity is 100%. A test with high specificity is useful to confirm a diagnosis, because a highly specific test will have few results that are falsely positive. For instance, to make the diagnosis of gouty arthritis, a clinician might choose a highly specific test, such as the presence of negatively birefringent needle-shaped crystals within leukocytes on microscopic evaluation of joint fluid.

To determine test sensitivity and specificity for a particular disease, the test must be compared against an independent "gold standard" test that defines the true disease state of the patient. For instance, the sensitivity and specificity of the ventilation-perfusion scan for pulmonary emboli are obtained by comparing the results of scans with the gold standard, pulmonary arteriography. Application of the gold standard examination to patients with positive scans establishes specificity. Failure to apply the gold standard examination following negative scans may result in an overestimation of sensitivity, since false negatives will not be identified. However, for many disease states (eg, pancreatitis), an independent gold standard test either does not exist or is very difficult or expensive to apply—and in such cases reliable estimates of test sensitivity and specificity are sometimes difficult to obtain.

Sensitivity and specificity can also be affected by the population from which these values are derived. For instance, many diagnostic tests are evaluated first using patients who have severe disease and control groups who are young and well. Compared with the general population, this study group will have more results that are truly positive (because patients have more advanced disease) and more results that are truly negative (because the control group is healthy). Thus, test sensitivity and specificity will be higher than would be expected in the general population, where more of a spectrum of health and disease is found. Clinicians should be aware of this **spectrum bias** when generalizing published test results to their own practice. Other biases, including spectrum composition, population recruitment, absent or inappropriate reference standard, and verification bias, are discussed in the references.

Test sensitivity and specificity depend on the threshold above which a test is interpreted to be abnormal (Figure 1–3). If the threshold is lowered, sensitivity is increased at the expense of decreased specificity. If the threshold is raised, sensitivity is decreased while specificity is increased.

Figure 1–4 shows how test sensitivity and specificity can be calculated using test results from patients previously classified by the gold standard as diseased or nondiseased.

The performance of two different tests can be compared by plotting the sensitivity and (1 minus the specificity) of each test at various reference range cutoff values. The resulting **receiver operator characteristic (ROC) curve** often shows which test is better; a clearly superior test will have an ROC curve that always lies above and to the left of the inferior test curve, and, in general, the better test has a larger area under the ROC curve. For instance, Figure 1–5 shows the ROC curves for PSA and prostatic acid phosphatase (PAP) in the diagnosis of prostate cancer. PSA is a superior test because it has higher sensitivity and specificity for all cutoff values.

USE OF TESTS IN DIAGNOSIS AND MANAGEMENT

The value of a test in a particular clinical situation depends not only on the test's sensitivity and specificity but also on the probability that the patient has the disease before the test result is known **(pretest probability).** The results of a useful test will substantially change the probability that the

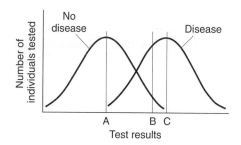

Figure 1–3. Hypothetical distribution of test results for healthy and diseased individuals. The position of the "cutoff point" between "normal" and "abnormal" (or "negative" and "positive") test results determines the test's sensitivity and specificity. If point A is the cutoff point, the test would have 100% sensitivity but low specificity. If point C is the cutoff point, the test would have 100% specificity but low sensitivity. For many tests, the cutoff point is determined by the reference range, ie, the range of test results that is within 2 SD of the mean of test results for healthy individuals (point B). In some situations, the cutoff is altered to enhance either sensitivity or specificity.

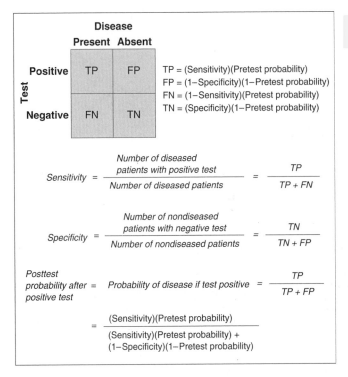

Figure 1–4. Calculation of sensitivity, specificity, and probability of disease after a positive test (posttest probability). **TP** = true positive; **FP** = false positive; **FN** = false negative; **TN** = true negative.

patient has the disease **(posttest probability).** Figure 1–4 shows how posttest probability can be calculated from the known sensitivity and specificity of the test and the estimated pretest probability of disease (or disease prevalence).

The pretest probability of disease has a profound effect on the posttest probability of disease. As demonstrated in Table 1–4, when a test with 90% sensitivity and specificity is used, the posttest probability can vary from 8% to 99% depending on the pretest probability of disease. Furthermore, as the pretest probability of disease decreases, it becomes more likely that a positive test result represents a false positive.

As an example, suppose the clinician wishes to calculate the posttest probability of prostate cancer using the PSA test and a cutoff value of

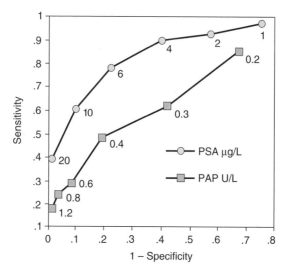

Figure 1–5. Receiver operator characteristic (ROC) curves for prostate-specific antigen (PSA) and prostatic acid phosphatase (PAP) in the diagnosis of prostate cancer. For all cutoff values, PSA has higher sensitivity and specificity; therefore, it is a better test based on these performance characteristics. *(Modified and reproduced with permission from Nicoll D et al. Routine acid phosphatase testing for screening and monitoring prostate cancer no longer justified. Clin Chem 1993;39(12):2540.)*

4 mcg/L. Using the data shown in Figure 1–5, sensitivity is 90% and specificity is 60%. The clinician estimates the pretest probability of disease given all the evidence and then calculates the posttest probability using the approach shown in Figure 1–4. The pretest probability that an otherwise healthy 50-year-old man has prostate cancer is equal to the prevalence of prostate cancer in that age group (probability = 10%), and the posttest

TABLE 1–4. INFLUENCE OF PRETEST PROBABILITY ON THE POSTTEST PROBABILITY OF DISEASE WHEN A TEST WITH 90% SENSITIVITY AND 90% SPECIFICITY IS USED.

Pretest Probability	Posttest Probability
0.01	0.08
0.50	0.90
0.99	0.999

probability after a positive test is only 20%—that is even though the test is positive, there is still an 80% chance that the patient does not have prostate cancer (Figure 1–6A). If the clinician finds a prostate nodule on rectal examination, the pretest probability of prostate cancer rises to 50% and the posttest probability using the same test is 69% (Figure 1–6B). Finally, if the clinician estimates the pretest probability to be 98% based on a prostate nodule, bone pain, and lytic lesions on spine radiographs, the posttest probability using PSA is 99% (Figure 1–6C). This example illustrates that pretest probability has a profound effect on posttest probability and that tests provide more information when the diagnosis is truly uncertain (pretest probability about 50%) than when the diagnosis is either unlikely or nearly certain.

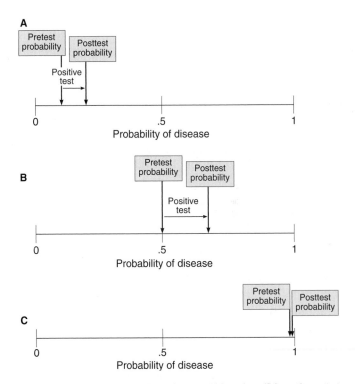

Figure 1–6. Effect of pretest probability and test sensitivity and specificity on the posttest probability of disease. (See text for explanation.)

ODDS-LIKELIHOOD RATIOS

Another way to calculate the posttest probability of disease is to use the odds-likelihood approach. Sensitivity and specificity are combined into one entity called the likelihood ratio (LR).

$$LR = \frac{\text{Probability of result in diseased persons}}{\text{Probability of result in nondiseased persons}}$$

When test results are dichotomized, every test has two likelihood ratios, one corresponding to a positive test (LR^+) and one corresponding to a negative test (LR^-):

$$LR^+ = \frac{\text{Probability that test is positive in diseased persons}}{\text{Probability that test is positive in nondiseased persons}}$$

$$= \frac{\text{Sensitivity}}{1 - \text{Specificity}}$$

$$LR^- = \frac{\text{Probability that test is negative in diseased persons}}{\text{Probability that test is negative in nondiseased persons}}$$

$$= \frac{1 - \text{Sensitivity}}{\text{Specificity}}$$

For continuous measures, multiple likelihood ratios can be defined to correspond to ranges of results. (See Table 1–5 for an example.)

TABLE 1–5. LIKELIHOOD RATIOS OF SERUM FERRITIN IN THE DIAGNOSIS OF IRON DEFICIENCY ANEMIA.

Serum Ferritin (mcg/L)	Likelihood Ratios for Iron Deficiency Anemia
≥100	0.08
45–99	0.54
35–44	1.83
25–34	2.54
15–24	8.83
<15	51.85

From Guyatt G et al: Laboratory diagnosis of iron deficiency anemia. J Gen Intern Med 1992;7(2):145.

Lists of likelihood ratios can be found in some textbooks, journal articles, and computer programs (see Table 1–6 for sample values). Likelihood ratios can be used to make quick estimates of the usefulness of contemplated diagnostic tests in particular situations. The simplest method for calculating posttest probability from pretest probability and likelihood ratios is to use a nomogram (Figure 1–7). The clinician places a straightedge through the points that represent the pretest probability and the likelihood ratio and then reads the posttest probability where the straightedge crosses the posttest probability line.

A more formal way of calculating posttest probabilities uses the likelihood ratio as follows:

$$\text{Pretest odds} \times \text{Likelihood ratio} = \text{Posttest odds}$$

To use this formulation, probabilities must be converted to odds, where the odds of having a disease are expressed as the chance of having the disease divided by the chance of not having the disease. For instance, a probability of 0.75 is the same as 3:1 odds (Figure 1–8).

To estimate the potential benefit of a diagnostic test, the clinician first estimates the pretest odds of disease given all available clinical information and then multiplies the pretest odds by the positive and negative likelihood ratios. The results are the **posttest odds,** or the odds that the patient has the disease if the test is positive or negative. To obtain the posttest probability, the odds are converted to a probability (Figure 1–8).

For example, if the clinician believes that the patient has a 60% chance of having a myocardial infarction (pretest odds of 3:2) and the troponin

TABLE 1–6. EXAMPLES OF LIKELIHOOD RATIOS (LR).

Target Disease	Test	LR⁺	LR⁻
Abscess	Abdominal CT scanning	9.5	0.06
Coronary artery disease	Exercise electrocardiogram (1 mm depression)	3.5	0.45
Lung cancer	Chest radiograph	15	0.42
Left ventricular hypertrophy	Echocardiography	18.4	0.08
Myocardial infarction	Troponin I	24	0.01
Prostate cancer	Digital rectal examination	21.3	0.37

From http://www.med.unc.edu/medicine/edursrc/lrmain.htm

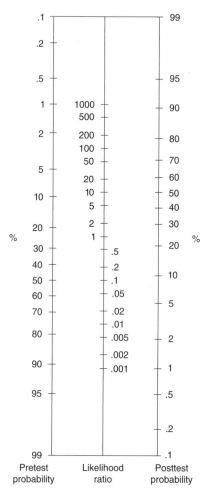

Figure 1–7. Nomogram for determining posttest probability from pretest probability and likelihood ratios. To figure the posttest probability, place a straightedge between the pretest probability and the likelihood ratio for the particular test. The posttest probability will be where the straightedge crosses the posttest probability line. *(Adapted and reproduced, with permission, from Fagan TJ. Nomogram for Bayes theorem. [Letter.] N Engl J Med 1975;293(5):257.)*

$$\text{Odds} = \frac{\textbf{Probability}}{\textbf{1 − Probability}}$$

Example: If probability = 0.75, then

$$\text{Odds} = \frac{0.75}{1 − 0.75} = \frac{0.75}{0.25} = \frac{3}{1} = 3\!:\!1$$

$$\textbf{Probability} = \frac{\textbf{Odds}}{\textbf{Odds + 1}}$$

Example: If odds = 3:1, then

$$\text{Probability} = \frac{3/1}{3/1 + 1} = \frac{3}{3 + 1} = 0.75$$

Figure 1–8. Formulas for converting between probability and odds.

I test is positive ($LR^+ = 24$), then the posttest odds of having a myocardial infarction are

$$\frac{3}{2} \times 24 = \frac{72}{2} \text{ or } 36\!:\!1 \text{ odds} \left(\frac{36/1}{36/1+1} = \frac{36}{37} = 97\% \text{ probability} \right)$$

If the troponin I test is negative ($LR^- = 0.01$), then the posttest odds of having a myocardial infarction are

$$\frac{3}{2} \times 0.01 = \frac{0.03}{2} \text{ odds} \left(\frac{0.03/2}{(0.03/2)+1} = \frac{0.15}{0.015+2} = 1.5\% \text{ probability} \right)$$

Sequential Testing

To this point, the impact of only one test on the probability of disease has been discussed, whereas during most diagnostic workups, clinicians obtain clinical information in a sequential fashion. To calculate the posttest odds after three tests, for example, the clinician might estimate the pretest odds and use the appropriate likelihood ratio for each test:

$$\text{Pretest odds} \times LR_1 \times LR_2 \times LR_3 = \text{Posttest odds}$$

When using this approach, however, the clinician should be aware of a major assumption: the chosen tests or findings must be **conditionally independent**. For instance, with liver cell damage, the aspartate aminotransferase (AST) and alanine aminotransferase (ALT) enzymes may be released by the same process and are thus not conditionally independent. If conditionally dependent tests are used in this sequential approach, an inaccurate posttest probability will result.

Threshold Approach to Decision Making

A key aspect of medical decision making is the selection of a treatment threshold, that is the probability of disease at which treatment is indicated. Figure 1–9 shows a possible way of identifying a treatment threshold by considering the value (utility) of the four possible outcomes of the treat/don't treat decision.

Use of a diagnostic test is warranted when its result could shift the probability of disease across the treatment threshold. For example, a clinician might decide to treat with antibiotics if the probability of streptococcal pharyngitis in a patient with a sore throat is greater than 25% (Figure 1–10A). If, after reviewing evidence from the history and physical examination, the clinician estimates the pretest probability of strep throat to be 15%, then a diagnostic test such as throat culture (LR$^+$ = 7) would be useful only if a positive test would shift the posttest probability above 25%. Use of the nomogram shown in Figure 1–7 indicates that the posttest probability would be 55% (Figure 1–10B); thus, ordering the test would be justified as it affects patient management. On the other hand, if the history and physical

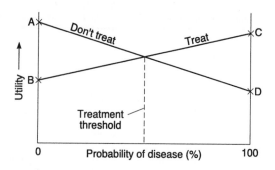

Figure 1–9. The "treat/don't treat" threshold. **(A)** Patient does not have disease and is not treated (highest utility). **(B)** Patient does not have disease and is treated (lower utility than A). **(C)** Patient has disease and is treated (lower utility than A). **(D)** Patient has disease and is not treated (lower utility than C).

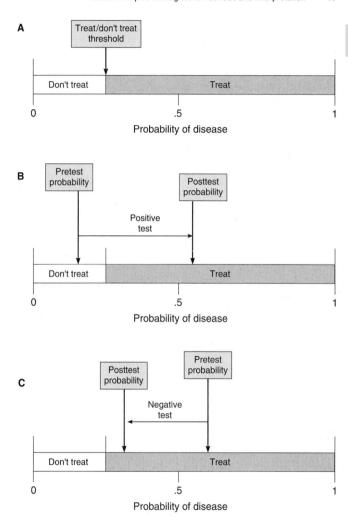

Figure 1–10. Threshold approach applied to test ordering. If the contemplated test will not change patient management, the test should not be ordered. (See text for explanation.)

examination had suggested that the pretest probability of strep throat was 60%, the throat culture ($LR^- = 0.33$) would be indicated only if a negative test would lower the posttest probability below 25%. Using the same nomogram, the posttest probability after a negative test would be 33% (Figure 1–10C). Therefore, ordering the throat culture would not be justified as it does not affect patient management.

This approach to decision making is now being applied in the clinical literature.

Decision Analysis

Up to this point, the discussion of diagnostic testing has focused on test characteristics and methods for using these characteristics to calculate the probability of disease in different clinical situations. Although useful, these methods are limited because they do not incorporate the many outcomes that may occur in clinical medicine or the values that patients and clinicians place on those outcomes. To incorporate outcomes and values with characteristics of tests, decision analysis can be used.

The basic idea of decision analysis is to model the options in a medical decision, assign probabilities to the alternative actions, assign values (utilities) to the various outcomes, and then calculate which decision gives the greatest expected value (expected utility). To complete a decision analysis, the clinician would proceed as follows: (1) Draw a decision tree showing the elements of the medical decision. (2) Assign probabilities to the various branches. (3) Assign values (utilities) to the outcomes. (4) Determine the expected value (expected utility) (the product of probability and value [utility]) of each branch. (5) And select the decision with the highest expected value (expected utility).

Figure 1–11 shows a decision tree in which the decision to be made is whether to treat without testing, perform a test and then treat based on the test result, or perform no tests and give no treatment. The clinician begins the analysis by building a decision tree showing the important elements of the decision. Once the tree is built, the clinician assigns probabilities to all the branches. In this case, all the branch probabilities can be calculated from (1) the probability of disease before the test (pretest probability), (2) the chance of a positive test if the disease is present (sensitivity), and (3) the chance of a negative test if the disease is absent (specificity). Next, the clinician assigns value (utility) to each of the outcomes.

After the expected value (expected utility) is calculated for each branch of the decision tree, by multiplying the value (utility) of the outcome by the probability of the outcome, the clinician can identify the alternative with the highest expected value (expected utility).

Although time-consuming, decision analysis can help structure complex clinical problems and make difficult clinical decisions. Currently there

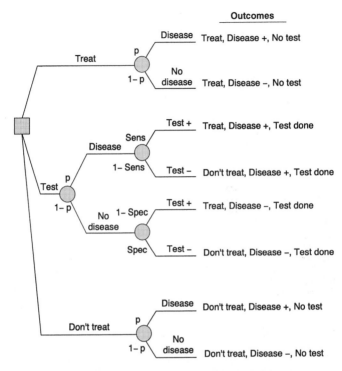

Figure 1–11. Generic tree for a clinical decision where the choices are (1) to treat the patient empirically, (2) to do the test and then treat only if the test is positive, or (3) to withhold therapy. The square node is called a decision node, and the circular nodes are called chance nodes. **p** = pretest probability of disease; **Sens** = sensitivity; **Spec** = specificity.

is interest in how evidence-based information is communicated to patients in the process of shared decision making.

Evidence-Based Medicine

Evidence-based medicine stresses the use of evidence from clinical research—rather than intuition and pathophysiologic reasoning—as a basis for clinical decision making. Evidence-based medicine relies on the identification of methodologically sound evidence, critical appraisal of research studies, and the dissemination of accurate and useful summaries of evidence to inform clinical decision making. Systematic reviews can be used to summarize evidence for dissemination, as can evidence-based synopses of current research. Systematic reviews often use meta-analysis—statistical techniques to combine evidence from different studies to produce a more precise estimate of the effect of an intervention or the accuracy of a test.

Clinical practice guidelines are systematically developed statements intended to assist practitioners and patients in making decisions about health care. Clinical algorithms and practice guidelines are now ubiquitous in medicine. Their utility and validity depend on the quality of the evidence that shaped the recommendations, on their being kept current, and on their acceptance and appropriate application by clinicians. Although some clinicians are concerned about the effect of guidelines on professional autonomy and individual decision making, many organizations are trying to use compliance with practice guidelines as a measure of quality of care.

REFERENCES

Genetic Testing

Kroese M et al: Genetic tests and their evaluation: Can we answer the key questions? Genet Med 2004;6:5. [PMID: 15545742]

McPherson E: Genetic diagnosis and testing in clinical practice. Clin Med Res 2006;4(2):123. [PMID: 16809405]

Pignone M et al: Challenges in systematic reviews of economic analyses. Ann Intern Med 2005;142(12 Pt 2):1073. [PMID 15968032]

Test Characteristics

Bewick V et al: Statistics review 13: Receiver operating characteristic curves. Crit Care 2004;8:508. [PMID: 15566624]

Obuchowski NA et al: ROC curves in clinical chemistry: Uses, misuses, and possible solutions. Clin Chem 2004;50:1118. [PMID: 15142978]

Whiting P et al: Development and validation of methods for assessing the quality of diagnostic accuracy studies. Health Technol Assess 2004;8:iii, 1. [PMID: 15193208]

Whiting P et al: Sources of variation and bias in studies of diagnostic accuracy: A systematic review. Ann Intern Med 2004;140:189. [PMID: 14757617]

Diagnosis & Management

de Graaf I et al: Diagnosis of lumbar spinal stenosis: A systematic review of the accuracy of diagnostic tests. Spine 2006;31:1168. [PMID: 16648755]

Hogg K et al: The emergency department utility of Simplify D-dimer to exclude pulmonary embolism in patients with pleuritic chest pain. Ann Emerg Med 2005;46:305. [PMID: 16187460]

Roy PM et al: Systematic review and meta-analysis of strategies for the diagnosis of suspected pulmonary embolism. BMJ 2005;331:259. [PMID: 16052017]

Sequential Testing

Gisbert JP et al: Accuracy of *Helicobacter pylori* diagnostic tests in patients with bleeding peptic ulcer: A systematic review and meta-analysis. Am J Gastroenterol 2006;101:848. [PMID: 16494583]

Hellmich M et al: A ruler for interpreting diagnostic test results. Methods Inf Med 2005;44:124. [PMID: 15778803]

Puhan MA et al: A randomized trial of ways to describe test accuracy: The effect on physicians' post-test probability estimates. Ann Intern Med 2005;143:184. [PMID: 16061916]

Wells PS et al: Does this patient have deep vein thrombosis? JAMA 2006;295:1997. [PMID: 16403932]

Decision Analysis

Gazelle GS et al: Cost-effectiveness analysis in the assessment of diagnostic imaging technologies. Radiology 2005;235:361. [PMID: 15858079]

Inadomi JM: Decision analysis and economic modelling: A primer. Eur J Gastroenterol Hepatol 2004;16:535. [PMID: 15167154]

Evidence-Based Medicine

Ghosh AK et al: Translating evidence-based information into effective risk communication: Current challenges and opportunities. J Lab Clin Med 2005;145:171. [PMID: 15962835]

Hess DR: What is evidence-based medicine and why should I care? Respir Care 2004;49:730. [PMID: 15222906]

Torpy JM et al: JAMA patient page. Evidence-based medicine. JAMA 2006;296:1192. [PMID: 16954497] http://jama.ama-assn.org/cgi/content/full/296/9/1192

2

Laboratory Procedures in the Clinical Setting

Stephen J. McPhee, MD, and Chuanyi Mark Lu, MD

This chapter presents information on how to perform common bedside laboratory tests and procedures.

In the United States, test results can be used for patient care only if the tests have been performed according to the requirements of the Clinical Laboratory Improvement Amendments of 1988 (CLIA '88). These include personnel training and competence assessment before performing any test or procedure, and performance and documentation of quality control for all tests. Physician interpretation of certain microscopic findings (eg, Gram stain smear and Wright-stained peripheral blood smear) requires appropriate clinical privileges.

Contents

1. OBTAINING AND PROCESSING BODY FLUIDS

A. Safety Considerations

General Safety Considerations

Because all patient specimens are potentially infectious, the following precautions should be observed:

  a. Universal body fluid and needle stick precautions must be observed at all times. The use of safety needle devices is recommended and/or required as established by institutional policy.
  b. Disposable gloves and sometimes gown, mask, and goggles should be worn when collecting specimens.
  c. Gloves must be changed and hands washed after contact with each patient. Dispose of gloves in an appropriate biohazard waste container.
  d. Care should be taken not to spill or splash blood. Any spills should be cleaned up with freshly made 10% bleach solution.

Handling and Disposing of Needles and Gloves

  a. Do not resheathe needles.
  b. Discard needles and gloves only into designated containers.
  c. Do not remove a used needle from a syringe by hand. The needle may be removed using a specially designed waste collection system, or the entire assembly may (if disposable) be discarded as a unit into a designated container.
  d. When obtaining blood cultures, it is hazardous and unnecessary to change needles.
  e. Do not place phlebotomy or other equipment on the patient's bed.

B. Specimen Handling

Identification of Specimens

  a. Identify the patient by verifying two identifiers (eg, full name, date of birth, social security number) before obtaining any specimen.
  b. Label each specimen container with the patient's name and identification number.

Specimen Tubes: Standard specimen tubes that contain a vacuum (called evacuated tubes) are now widely available and are easily identified by the color of the stopper (see also p 41):

  a. Red-top tubes contain no anticoagulants or preservatives and are used for chemistry tests.
  b. Serum separator tubes (SST) contain material that allows ready separation of serum and clot by centrifugation.
  c. Lavender-top (purple) tubes contain EDTA and are used for hematology tests (eg, blood or cell counts, differentials) and molecular diagnostic tests.
  d. Green-top tubes contain heparin and are used for tests that require plasma or anticoagulation.

  e. Blue-top tubes contain citrate and are used for coagulation tests.
  f. Gray-top tubes contain sodium fluoride and are used for some chemistry tests (eg, glucose or alcohol requiring inhibition of glycolysis) if the specimen cannot be analyzed immediately.
  g. Yellow-top tubes contain acid citrate dextrose (ACD) and are used for flow cytometric immunophenotyping.

Procedure

  a. When collecting multiple specimens, fill sterile tubes used for bacteriologic tests, then tubes without additives (ie, red-, marbled-, or gold-top tubes) before filling those with additives to avoid the potential for bacterial contamination, transfer of anticoagulants, etc. However, be certain to fill tubes containing anticoagulants before the blood specimen clots.
  b. The recommended order of filling evacuated tubes is (by type and color): (1) blood culture, (2) red top, (3) blue top, (4) tube with gel separator, (5) green top, (6) lavender (purple) top, (7) gray top.
  c. Fill each tube completely. Tilt each tube containing anticoagulant or preservative to mix thoroughly. Place any specimens on ice as required (eg, arterial blood). Deliver specimens to the laboratory promptly.
  d. For each of the major body fluids, Table 2–1 summarizes commonly requested tests and requirements for specimen handling and provides cross-references to tables and figures elsewhere in this book for help in interpretation of the results.

2. BASIC STAINING METHODS
A. Gram Stain
Preparation of Smear

  a. Obtain a fresh specimen of the material to be stained (eg, sputum) and smear a small amount on a glass slide using a sterile applicator. Thin smears give the best results (eg, press a sputum sample between two glass slides).
  b. Let the smear air dry before heat fixing, because heating a wet smear will usually distort cells and organisms.
  c. Heat-fix the smear by using slide warmer (45–55 °C) or by passing the clean side of the slide quickly through a Bunsen burner or other flame source (no more than three or four times). The slide should be warm, not hot.
  d. Let the slide cool before staining.

Staining Technique

  a. Put on gloves.
  b. Stain with crystal violet (15 seconds).
  c. Rinse with gently running water (5 seconds).

TABLE 2–1. BODY FLUID TESTS, HANDLING, AND INTERPRETATION.

Body Fluid	Commonly Requested Tests	Specimen Tube and Handling	Interpretation Guide
Arterial blood	pH, P_{O_2}, P_{CO_2}	Glass syringe. Evacuate air bubbles; remove needle; position rubber cap; place sample on ice; deliver immediately.	See acid–base nomogram, Figure 8–1.
Ascitic fluid	Cell count, differential Protein, amylase Gram stain, culture Cytology (if neoplasm suspected)	Lavender top Red top Sterile Cytology	See ascitic fluid profiles, Table 8–5.
Cerebrospinal fluid	Cell count, differential Gram stain, culture Protein, glucose VDRL or other studies (oligoclonal bands) Cytology (if neoplasm suspected)	Tube #1 Tube #2 Tube #3 Tube #4 Cytology	See cerebrospinal fluid profiles, Table 8–8.
Pleural fluid	Cell count, differential Protein, glucose, amylase Gram stain, culture Cytology (if neoplasm suspected)	Lavender top Red top Sterile Cytology	See pleural fluid profiles, Table 8–16.
Synovial fluid	Cell count, differential Protein, glucose Gram stain, culture Microscopic examination for crystals Cytology (if neoplasm [villonodular synovitis, metastatic disease] suspected)	Lavender top Red top Sterile Green top Cytology	See synovial fluid profiles, Table 8–4, and Figure 2–6.

Urine	Urinalysis
	  Dipstick
	  Microscopic examination
	  Gram stain, culture
	Cytology (if neoplasm suspected)
		
		Clean tube
		Centrifuge tube
		Sterile
		Cytology
			See Table 8–26.
			See Table 2–2.
			See Figure 2–3.

    d. Flood with Gram iodine solution (10–30 seconds).
    e. Rinse with gently running water (5 seconds).
    f. Decolorize with acetone-alcohol solution until no more blue color leaches from the slide (5 seconds).
    g. Rinse immediately with water (5 seconds).

h. Counterstain with safranin O (10 seconds).

i. Rinse with water (5 seconds).

j. Let the slide air-dry (or carefully blot with filter paper), then examine it under the microscope.

k. Label positive slides with the patient's name and identification number and save them for review.

Microscopic Examination

a. Examine the smear first using the low-power lens for leukocytes and fungi. Screen for the number and color of polymorphonuclear cells (cell nuclei should be pink, not blue).

b. Examine using the high-power oil-immersion lens for microbial forms. Screen for intracellular organisms. Review the slide systematically for: (1) fungi (mycelia, then yeast), (2) small gram-negative rods (bacteroides, haemophilus, etc), (3) gram-negative cocci (neisseria, etc), (4) gram-positive rods (listeria, etc), and (5) gram-positive cocci (streptococcus, staphylococcus, etc).

c. Figure 2–1 illustrates typical findings on a Gram-stained smear of sputum.

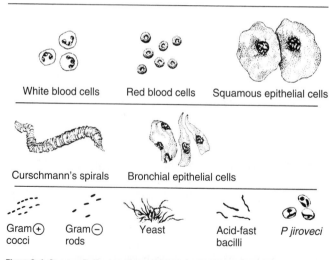

White blood cells   Red blood cells   Squamous epithelial cells

Curschmann's spirals   Bronchial epithelial cells

Gram ⊕ cocci   Gram ⊖ rods   Yeast   Acid-fast bacilli   P jiroveci

Figure 2–1. Common findings on microscopic examination of sputum. Most elements can be seen on Gram-stained smears except for acid-fast bacilli (auramine-rhodamine stain) and *Pneumocystis carinii* (Giemsa stain). *(Modified and reproduced, with permission from Krupp MA et al: Physician's Handbook, 21st ed. Originally published by Lange Medical Publications. Copyright © 1985 by The McGraw-Hill Companies, Inc.)*

B. Wright Stain of Peripheral Blood Smear
Preparation of Smear
   a. Obtain a fresh specimen of blood by pricking the patient's finger with a lancet. If alcohol is used to clean the fingertip, wipe it off first with a gauze pad.
   b. Place a single drop of blood on a glass slide. Lay a second glass slide over the first one and rapidly pull it away lengthwise to leave a thin smear.
   c. Let the smear air-dry. Do not heat-fix.
Manual Staining Technique
   a. Stain with fresh Wright stain (1 minute).
   b. Gently add an equal amount of water and gently mix the stain and water. Repeat by adding more water and mix. Look for formation of a shiny surface scum. Then allow the stain to set (3–4 minutes).
   c. Rinse with gently running water (5 seconds).
   d. Clean the back of the slide with an alcohol pad if necessary.
   e. Label slides with the patient's name and identification number and save them for review.
   Note: An automated slide stainer is available in most clinical laboratories.
Microscopic Examination
   a. Examine the smear first using the low-power lens to select a good area for study (red and white cells separated from one another).
   b. Then move to the high-power oil-immersion lens. Review the slide systematically for: (1) platelet morphology (size, granulations, clumping, satellitism, etc), (2) white cells (differential types, morphology, toxic granulations, and vacuoles, etc), and (3) red cells (size, shape, color, stippling, nucleation, etc).
   c. See Figure 2–2 for examples of common peripheral blood smear abnormalities.

3. OTHER BEDSIDE LABORATORY PROCEDURES
A. Urinalysis
Collection and Preparation of Specimen
   a. Obtain a midstream urine specimen from the patient. The sample must be free of skin epithelium or bacteria, secretions, hair, lint, etc.
   b. Examine the specimen while fresh (still warm). Otherwise, bacteria may proliferate, casts and crystals may dissolve, and particulate matter may settle out. (Occasionally, amorphous crystals precipitate out, obscuring formed elements. In cold urine, they are amorphous urate crystals; these may be dissolved by gently rewarming the urine. In alkaline urine, they are amorphous

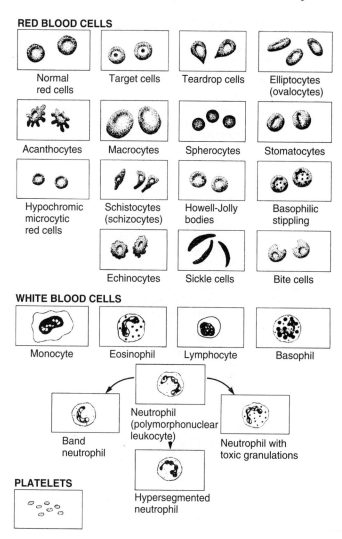

RED BLOOD CELLS

Normal red cells

Target cells

Teardrop cells

Elliptocytes (ovalocytes)

Acanthocytes

Macrocytes

Spherocytes

Stomatocytes

Hypochromic microcytic red cells

Schistocytes (schizocytes)

Howell-Jolly bodies

Basophilic stippling

Echinocytes

Sickle cells

Bite cells

WHITE BLOOD CELLS

Monocyte

Eosinophil

Lymphocyte

Basophil

Neutrophil (polymorphonuclear leukocyte)

Band neutrophil

Neutrophil with toxic granulations

Hypersegmented neutrophil

PLATELETS

Figure 2–2. Common peripheral blood smear findings.

phosphate crystals; these may be dissolved by adding 1 mL of acetic acid.)

c. Place 10 mL in a tube and centrifuge at 2000–3000 rpm for 3–5 minutes.

d. Discard the supernatant. Resuspend the sediment in the few drops that remain by gently tilting the tube.

e. Place a drop on a glass slide, cover it with a coverslip, and examine under the microscope; no stain is needed. If bacterial infection is present, a single drop of methylene blue applied to the edge of the coverslip, or a Gram-stained smear of an air-dried, heat-fixed specimen, can assist in distinguishing gram-negative rods (eg, *Escherichia coli,* proteus, klebsiella) from gram-positive cocci (eg, enterococcus, *Staphylococcus saprophyticus*).

Procedural Technique

a. While the urine is being centrifuged, examine the remainder of the specimen by inspection and reagent strip ("dipstick") testing.

b. Inspect the specimen for color and clarity. Normally, urine is yellow or light orange. Dark orange urine is caused by ingestion of the urinary tract analgesic phenazopyridine (Pyridium, others); red urine, by erythrocytes, hemoglobinuria, myoglobinuria, beets, senna, or rifampin therapy; green urine, by *Pseudomonas* infection or iodochlorhydroxyquin or amitriptyline therapy; brown urine, by bilirubinuria or fecal contamination; black urine, by intravascular hemolysis, alkaptonuria, melanoma, or methyldopa therapy; purplish urine, by porphyria; and milky white urine, by pus, chyluria, or amorphous crystals (urates or phosphates). Turbidity of urine is caused by pus, red blood cells, or crystals.

c. Reagent strips provide information about specific gravity, pH, protein, glucose, ketones, bilirubin, heme, nitrite, and esterase (Table 2–2). Dip a reagent strip in the urine and compare it with the chart on the bottle. Follow the timing instructions carefully. *Note:* Reagent strips cannot be relied on to detect some proteins (eg, globulins, light chains) or reducing sugars (other than glucose). Falsely positive protein results may be obtained with alkaline urine (eg, urine pH > 8.0). Substances that cause abnormal urine color may affect the readability of test pads on reagent strips (eg, visible levels of blood or bilirubin and drugs containing dyes, nitrofurantoin, or rifampicin).

d. Record the results.

Manual Microscopic Examination

a. Examine the area under the coverslip under the low-power and high-dry lenses for cells, casts, crystals, and bacteria. (If a Gram stain is done, examine under the oil immersion lens.)

TABLE 2–2. COMPONENTS OF THE URINE DIPSTICK.[1]

Test	Normal Values	Sensitivity	Comments
Specific gravity	1.001–1.035	1.000–1.030[4]	Highly buffered alkaline urine may cause low specific gravity readings. Moderate proteinuria (100–750 mg/dL) may cause high readings. Loss of concentrating or diluting capacity indicates renal dysfunction. If the specific gravity of a random urine specimen is 1.023 or greater, the concentrating ability of the kidneys can be considered normal.
pH	4.6–8.0	5.0–8.5[4]	Excessive urine on strip may cause protein reagent to run over onto pH area, yielding falsely low pH reading. Bacterial growth by certain organisms (eg, proteus) in a specimen may cause a marked alkaline shift (pH >8), usually because of urea conversion to ammonia.
Protein	Negative <15 mg/dL	15–30 mg/dL albumin	False-positive readings can be caused by highly buffered alkaline urine. Reagent more sensitive to albumin than other proteins. A negative result does not rule out the presence of globulins, hemoglobin, Bence Jones proteins, or mucoprotein. 1+ = 30 mg/dL 3+ = 300 mg/dL 2+ = 100 mg/dL 4+ = ≥2000 mg/dL
Glucose	Negative <15 mg/dL	75–125 mg/dL	Test is specific for glucose. False-negative results occur with urinary ascorbic acid concentrations ≥50 mg/dL and with ketone body levels ≥40 mg/dL. Test reagent reactivity also varies with specific gravity and temperature. Trace = 100 mg/dL 1 = 1000 mg/dL $1/4$ = 250 mg/dL 2 = ≥2000 mg/dL $1/2$ = 500 mg/dL
Ketone	Negative	5–10 mg/dL acetoacetate	Test does not react with acetone or β-hydroxybutyric acid. (Trace) false-positive results may occur with highly pigmented urines or those containing levodopa metabolites or sulfhydryl-containing compounds (eg, mesna). Trace = 5 mg/dL Moderate = 40 mg/dL Small = 15 mg/dL Large = 80–160 mg/dL

(continued)

TABLE 2–2 COMPONENTS OF THE URINE DIPSTICK.[1] (*CONTINUED*).

Test	Normal Values	Sensitivity	Comments
Bilirubin	Negative (0.02 mg/dL or less)	0.4–0.8 mg/dL	Indicates hepatitis (conjugated bilirubin). False-negative readings can be caused by ascorbic acid concentrations ≥25 mg/dL. False-positive readings can be caused by metabolites of etodolac. Test is less specific than Ictotest Reagent Tablets. A positive test should be confirmed by Ictotest Reagent Tablets.
Blood	Negative (<0.010 mg/dL hemoglobin or <3 RBC/mcL)[2]	0.015–0.062 mg/dL hemoglobin or 5–20 RBC/mcL	Test is equally sensitive to myoglobin and hemoglobin (including both intact RBC and free hemoglobin). False-positive results can be caused by oxidizing contaminants (hypochlorite) and microbial peroxidase (urinary tract infection). Test sensitivity is reduced in urines with high specific gravity, captopril, or heavy proteinuria.
Nitrite	Negative	0.06–0.10 mg/dL nitrite ion	Test depends on the conversion of nitrate (derived from the diet) to nitrite by gram-negative bacteria in urine when their number is >10[5]/mcL (≥0.075 mg/dL nitrite ion). Test specific for nitrite. False-negative readings can be caused by ascorbic acid. Test sensitivity is reduced in urines with high specific gravity. A negative result does not rule out significant bacteriuria.
Leukocytes (esterase)	Negative[3]	5–15 WBCs/hpf in clinical urine	Indicator of urinary tract infection. Test detects esterases contained in granulocytic leukocytes. Test sensitivity is reduced in urines with elevated glucose concentrations ≥3 g/dL), or presence of cephalexin, cephalothin, tetracycline, or high concentrations of oxalate.

[1] *Package insert, revised 11/05. Bayer Diagnostics Reagent Strips for Urinalysis, Bayer Corporation.*
[2] *Except in menstruating females.*
[3] *Except in females with vaginitis.*
[4] *Analytical measurement range (AMR) of the reagent strips.*

   b. Cells may be red cells, white cells, squamous cells, transitional (bladder) or tubular epithelial cells, or atypical (tumor) cells. Red cells suggest upper or lower urinary tract infections (cystitis, prostatitis, pyelonephritis), glomerulonephritis, collagen vascular disease, trauma, renal calculi, tumors, drug reactions, and structural abnormalities (polycystic kidneys). White cells suggest inflammatory processes such as urinary tract infection (most common), collagen vascular disease, or interstitial nephritis. Red cell casts are considered pathognomonic of glomerulonephritis; white cell casts, of pyelonephritis; and fatty (lipid) casts, of nephrotic syndrome.

c. The finding on a Gram-stained smear of unspun, clean, fresh urine of even one bacterium per field under the oil-immersion lens correlates fairly well with bacterial culture colony counts of greater than 100,000 organisms per mcL.

d. See Table 8–26 for a guide to interpretation of urinalysis; and Figure 2–3 for a guide to microscopic findings in urine.

Note: Fully automated urinalysis systems are now available in most clinical laboratories.

B. Vaginal Fluid Wet-Mount Preparation

Preparation of Smear and Staining Technique

a. Place a small amount of vaginal discharge on a glass slide.

b. Add 2 drops of sterile saline solution.

c. Place a coverslip over the area to be examined.

Microscopic Examination

a. Examine under the microscope, using the high-dry lens and a low light source.

b. Look for motile trichomonads (undulating protozoa propelled by four flagella). Look for clue cells (vaginal epithelial cells with large numbers of organisms attached to them, obscuring cell borders), pathognomonic of *Gardnerella vaginalis*-associated vaginosis.

c. See Figure 2–4 for an example of a positive wet prep (trichomonads, clue cells) and Table 8–27 for the differential diagnosis of vaginal discharge.

C. Skin or Vaginal Fluid KOH Preparation

Preparation of Smear and Staining Technique

a. Obtain a skin specimen by using a No. 15 scalpel blade to scrape scales from the skin lesion onto a glass slide or to remove the top of a vesicle onto the slide. Or place a single drop of vaginal discharge on the slide.

b. Label the slides with patient name and identification number.

c. Place 1 or 2 drops of potassium hydroxide (10–20%) on top of the specimen on the slide. Lay a coverslip over the area to be examined.

d. Heat the slide from beneath with a match or Bunsen burner flame until the slide contents begin to bubble.

e. Clean carbon off the back side of the slide with an alcohol pad if necessary.

Note: A fishy amine odor upon addition of KOH to a vaginal discharge is typical of bacterial vaginosis caused by *Gardnerella vaginalis.*

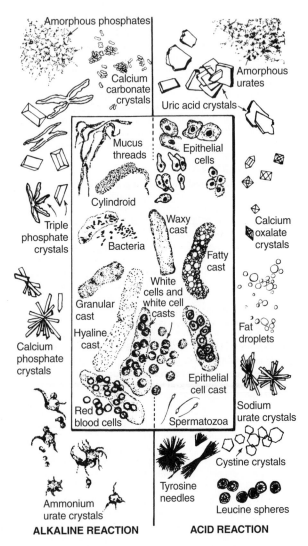

Amorphous phosphates

Calcium carbonate crystals

Amorphous urates

Uric acid crystals

Mucus threads

Epithelial cells

Cylindroid

Triple phosphate crystals

Waxy cast

Bacteria

Calcium oxalate crystals

Fatty cast

White cells and white cell casts

Granular cast

Hyaline cast

Fat droplets

Calcium phosphate crystals

Epithelial cell cast

Red blood cells

Spermatozoa

Sodium urate crystals

Cystine crystals

Tyrosine needles

Leucine spheres

Ammonium urate crystals

ALKALINE REACTION

ACID REACTION

Figure 2–3. Microscopic findings on examination of the urine. *(Modified and reproduced, with permission from Krupp MA et al: Physician's Handbook, 21st ed. Originally published by Lange Medical Publications. Copyright © 1985 by The McGraw-Hill Companies, Inc.)*

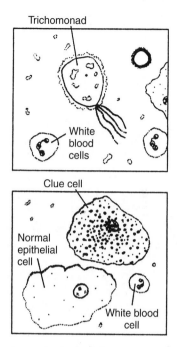

Figure 2–4. Wet-mount preparation showing trichomonads, white blood cells, and clue cells.

Microscopic Examination
    a. Examine the smear under the high-dry lens for mycelial forms. Branched, septate hyphae are typical of dermatophytosis (eg, trichophyton, epidermophyton, microsporum species); branched, septate pseudohyphae with or without budding yeast forms are seen with candidiasis (candida species); and short, curved hyphae plus clumps of spores ("spaghetti and meatballs") are seen with tinea versicolor *(Malassezia furfur)*.

    b. See Figure 2–5 for an example of a positive KOH prep.

D. Synovial Fluid Examination for Crystals
Preparation of Smear
    a. No stain is necessary.
    b. Place a small amount of synovial fluid on a glass slide.
    c. Place a coverslip over the area to be examined.

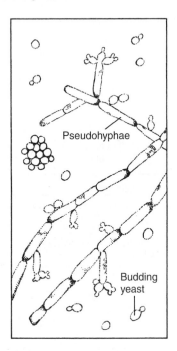

Figure 2–5. KOH preparation showing mycelial forms (pseudohyphae) and budding yeast typical of *Candida albicans*.

Microscopic Examination

    a. Examine under a polarized light microscope with a red compensator, using the high-dry lens and a moderately bright light source.

    b. Look for needle-shaped, negatively birefringent urate crystals (crystals parallel to the axis of the compensator appear yellow) in gout or rhomboidal, positively birefringent calcium pyrophosphate crystals (crystals parallel to the axis of the compensator appear blue) in pseudogout.

    c. See Figure 2–6 for examples of positive synovial fluid examinations for these two types of crystals.

E. Pulse Oximetry

Indications

To measure oxygen saturation in a noninvasive and often continuous fashion.

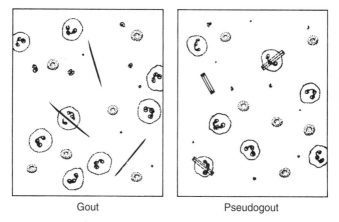

Gout   Pseudogout

Figure 2–6. Examination of synovial fluid for crystals using a compensated, polarized microscope. In gout, crystals are needle shaped, negatively birefringent, and composed of monosodium urate. In pseudogout, crystals are rhomboidal, positively birefringent, and composed of calcium pyrophosphate dihydrate. In both diseases, crystals can be found free-floating or within polymorphonuclear cells.

Contraindications
   a. Hypotension, hypothermia, low perfusion states, severe or rapid desaturation, and severe anemia (hemoglobin <5 g/dL) cause inaccurate readings.
   b. Hyperbilirubinemia, methemoglobinemia, fetal hemoglobinemia, and carboxyhemoglobinemia can falsely elevate oxygen saturation measurements.
   c. Excessive ambient light, simultaneous use of a blood pressure cuff, the presence of intravascular dyes (eg, methylene blue), and electrical interference (eg, MRI scanners, electrosurgery) can also cause erroneous readings.

Approach to the Patient
   The patient should be positioned close to the pulse oximeter and should hold the probe site still. The sampling area should have good circulation and be free of skin irritation.

Procedural Technique
   a. Plug the pulse oximeter into a grounded AC power outlet or make sure that sufficient battery power is available. Turn the oximeter on and wait until self-calibration is complete.
   b. Select the probe to be used and connect it to the pulse oximeter. The probe consists of a light source (a red light-emitting device

in most cases) and a photodetector. Probes are available for the ear, finger, and, in neonates, the foot, ankle, palm, calf, and forearm.

c. Attach the probe to the patient after cleansing the surrounding skin with an alcohol swab. Some probes come with double-sided adhesive disks that improve probe signal.

d. Watch the waveform and pulse indicators to assess the quality of the signal. Readjust if a poor signal is present.

e. Set alarm warnings on the device.

f. Check the probe site at least every 4 hours. Care should be taken not to apply tension to the probe cables.

Possible Complications

Allergic reaction to adhesives.

Comments

Because of the curvilinear nature of the oxygen-hemoglobin dissociation curve, oxygen saturation (SaO_2) is not directly proportionate to oxygen partial pressure (PaO_2). Therefore, a relatively small change in SaO_2 (eg, from 94% to 83%) can represent a large change in (PaO_2) (eg, from 80 mm Hg to 50 mm Hg). In addition, the dissociation curve varies markedly from patient to patient and with pH, temperature, and altitude. To ensure accurate assessment of oxygenation, one should correlate pulse oximetry with arterial blood gas analysis.

REFERENCES

Gram Stain

Bartlett JG: Diagnostic test for etiologic agents of community-acquired pneumonia. Infect Dis Clin North Am 2004;18:809. [PMID: 15555826]

Fournier AM: The Gram stain. Ann Intern Med 1998;128:776. [PMID: 9556475]

Popescu A, Doyle RJ: The Gram stain after more than a century. Biotech Histochem 1996;71:145. [PMID: 8724440]

Urinalysis

Patel HP: The abnormal urinalysis. Pediatr Clin North Am 2006;53:325. [PMID: 16716783]

Simerville JA et al: Urinalysis: A comprehensive review. Am Fam Physician 2005;71:1153. [PMID: 15791892]

Wilson LA: Urinalysis. Nurs Stand 2005;19:51. [PMID: 1591598]

Vaginal Wet-Mount Preparation

ACOG Committee on Practice Bulletins—Gynecology: ACOG Practice Bulletin. Clinical management guidelines for obstetrician-gynecologists. Vaginitis. Obstet Gynecol 2006;107:1195. [PMID: 16648432]

Anderson MR et al: Evaluation of vaginal complaints. JAMA 2004; 291:1368. [PMID: 15026404]

French L et al: Abnormal vaginal discharge: Using office diagnostic testing more effectively. J Fam Pract 2004;53:805. [PMID: 15469777]

Owen MK, Clenney TL: Management of vaginitis. Am Fam Physician 2004;70:2125. [PMID: 15606061]

Sheeley A: Sorting out common causes of abnormal vaginal discharge. JAAPA 2004;17:15. [PMID: 15532320]

Synovial Fluid Examination

Li SF et al: Laboratory tests in adults with monoarticular arthritis: Can they rule out a septic joint? Acad Emerg Med 2004;11:276. [PMID: 15001408]

Siva C et al: Diagnosing acute monoarthritis in adults: A practical approach for the family physician. Am Fam Physician 2003;68:83. [PMID: 12887114]

Tercic D, Bozic B: The basis of the synovial fluid analysis. Clin Chem Lab Med 2001;39:1221. [PMID: 11798081]

Pulse Oximetry

Allen K: Principles and limitations of pulse oximetry in patient monitoring. Nurs Times 2004;100:34. [PMID: 15517733]

Considine J: The reliability of clinical indicators of oxygenation: A literature review. Contemp Nurse 2005;18:258. [PMID: 15918255]

Giuliano KK, Higgins TL: New-generation pulse oximetry in the care of critically ill patients. Am J Crit Care 2005;14:26. [PMID: 15608106]

Pedersen T et al: Pulse oximetry for perioperative monitoring. Cochrane Database Syst Rev 2003;(3):CD002013. [PMID: 12917918]

Salyer JW: Neonatal and pediatric pulse oximetry. Respir Care 2003; 48:386. [PMID: 12667266]

3

Common Laboratory Tests: Selection and Interpretation

Diana Nicoll, MD, PhD, MPA, Stephen J. McPhee, MD,
Michael Pignone, MD, MPH, and Chuanyi Mark Lu, MD

HOW TO USE THIS SECTION

This section contains information about commonly used laboratory tests. It includes most of the blood, urine, and cerebrospinal fluid tests found in this book, with the exception of drug levels. Entries are in outline format and are arranged alphabetically.

Test/Reference Range/Collection

This first outline listing begins with the common test name, the specimen analyzed, and any test name abbreviation (in parentheses).

Below this in the first outline listing is the reference range for each test. The first entry is in conventional units, and the second entry (in [brackets]) is in SI units (Système International d'Unités). Any panic values for a particular test are placed here after the word *Panic*. The reference ranges provided are from several large medical centers; consult your own clinical laboratory for those used in your institution.

This outline listing also shows which tube to use for collecting blood and other body fluids, how much the test costs (in relative symbolism; see below), and how to collect the specimen. Listed below are the common collection tubes and their contents:

Tube Top Color	Tube Contents	Typically Used In
Lavender	EDTA	Complete blood count; molecular testing
Serum separator tube (SST)	Clot activator and serum separator gel	Serum chemistry tests

(continued)

Tube Top Color	Tube Contents	Typically Used In
Red	None	Blood banking (serum)
Blue	Citrate	Coagulation studies
Green	Heparin	Plasma studies
Yellow	Acid citrate	HLA typing
Navy	Trace metal free	Trace metals (eg, lead)
Gray	Inhibitor of glycolysis (sodium fluoride)	Lactic acid

The scale used for the cost of each test is:

Approximate Cost	Symbol Used in Tables
$1–20	$
$21–50	$$
$51–100	$$$
>$100	$$$$

Physiologic Basis

This outline listing contains physiologic information about the substance being tested. Information on classification and biologic importance, as well as interactions with other biologic substances and processes, is included.

Interpretation

This outline lists clinical conditions that affect the substance being tested. Generally, conditions with higher prevalence are listed first. When the sensitivity of the test for a particular disease is known, that information follows the disease name in parentheses, for example, "rheumatoid arthritis (83%)." Some of the common drugs that can affect the test substance in vivo are also included in this outline listing.

Comments

This outline listing sets forth general information pertinent to the use and interpretation of the test and important in vitro interferences with the test procedure. Appropriate general references are also listed.

Test Name

The test name is placed as a header to the rest of the outline list to allow for quick referencing.

Test/Range/Collection	Physiologic Basis	Interpretation	Comments
ABO typing, serum or plasma and red cells (ABO) Red or lavender $ Properly identified and labeled blood specimens are critical.	The ABO antigen and antibodies remain the most significant for transfusion practice. The four blood groups A, B, O, and AB are determined by the presence or absence of antigens A and B or their absence (O) on a patient's red blood cells. Individuals possess antibodies directed toward the A or B antigen absent from their own red cells.	In the US white population, 45% are type O, 40% A, 11% B, 4% AB. In the US Hispanic population, 57% are type O, 30% A, 10% B, 3% AB. In the African American population, 49% are type O, 27% A, 20% B, 4% AB. In the US Asian population, 40% are type O, 28% A, 27% B, 5% AB. In the Native American Indian population, 55% are type O, 35% A, 8% B, 2% AB.	For both blood donors and recipients, routine ABO typing includes both red cell and serum testing, as checks on each other. Tube testing is as follows: patient's red cells are tested with anti-A and anti-B for the presence or absence of agglutination (forward or cell type), and patient's serum or plasma is tested against known A and B cells (reverse or serum type). *Technical Manual of the American Association of Blood Banks,* 15th ed. American Association of Blood Banks, 2005. Transfusion 2004;44:703. [PMID: 15104651]
Acetaminophen, serum (Tylenol; others) 10–20 mg/L [66–132 mcmol/L] ***Panic:*** >50 mg/L SST $$ For suspected overdose, draw two samples at least 4 hours apart, at least 4 hours after ingestion. Note time of ingestion, if known. Order test stat.	In overdose, liver and renal toxicity are produced by the hydroxylated metabolite if it is not conjugated with glutathione in the liver.	**Increased in:** Acetaminophen overdose. Interpretation of serum acetaminophen level depends on time since ingestion. Levels drawn <4 hours after ingestion cannot be interpreted since the drug is still in the absorption and distribution phase. Use nomogram (Figure 9–1) to evaluate possible toxicity. Levels >150 mg/L at 4 hours or >50 mg/L at 12 hours after ingestion suggest toxicity. Nomogram inaccurate for chronic ingestions.	Do not delay acetylcysteine (Mucomyst) treatment (140 mg/kg orally) if stat levels are unavailable. Crit Care 2002;6(2):108. [PMID: 11983032] Ann Emerg Med 2005;46:263. [PMID: 16126138]

Test/Range/Collection	Physiologic Basis	Interpretation	Comments
Acetoacetate			
Acetoacetate, serum or urine 0 mg/dL [mcmol/L] SST or urine container $ Urine sample should be fresh.	Acetoacetate, acetone, and β-hydroxybutyrate contribute to ketoacidosis when oxidative hepatic metabolism of fatty acids is impaired. Proportions in serum vary but are generally 20% acetoacetate, 78% β-hydroxybutyrate, and 2% acetone.	**Present in:** Diabetic ketoacidosis, alcoholic ketoacidosis, prolonged fasting, severe carbohydrate restriction with normal fat intake.	Nitroprusside test is semiquantitative; it detects acetoacetate and is sensitive down to 5–10 mg/dL. Trace = 5 mg/dL, small = 15 mg/dL, moderate = 40 mg/dL, large = 80 mg/dL [1 mg/dL = 100 mcmol/L]. β-Hydroxybutyrate is not a ketone and is not detected by the nitroprusside test. Acetone is also not reliably detected by this method. Failure of test to detect β-hydroxybutyrate in ketoacidosis may produce a seemingly paradoxical increase in ketones with clinical improvement as nondetectable β-hydroxybutyrate is replaced by detectable acetoacetate. Pediatr Diabetes 2006;7:223. [PMID: 16911010]
Acetylcholine receptor antibody			
Acetylcholine receptor antibody, serum Negative SST $$	Acetylcholine receptor antibodies are involved in the pathogenesis of myasthenia gravis. Sensitive radioassay or ELISA is available based on inhibition of binding of ^{125}I α-bungarotoxin to the acetylcholine receptor.	**Positive in:** Myasthenia gravis (sensitivity 87–98%, specificity 98–100%)	Titer has been found to correlate with clinical severity. Neuromuscul Disord 2006;16:459. [PMID: 16793269]

Activated clotting time		
Activated clotting time, whole blood (ACT) 70–180 sec (method-specific) $$ Obtain blood in a plastic syringe without antico-agulant. Test should be performed immediately at patient bedside. A clean venipuncture is required. A special vacutainer tube containing activator (eg, celite, kaolin) is also available.	ACT is a point-of-care test used to monitor high-dose heparin as an anticoagulant during cardiac surgery (extracorporeal circulation), angioplasty, and hemodialysis. It is also used to determine the dose of protamine sulfate to reverse the heparin effect upon completion of the procedure. ACT may also be used to monitor heparin or direct thrombin inhibitor in patients with documented lupus anticoagulant.	**Prolonged in:** Heparin therapy, direct thrombin inhibitor therapy, severe deficiency of clotting factors (except factors VII and XIII), functional platelet disorders, afibrinogenemia. In general, the accepted goal during cardiopulmonary bypass surgery is 400–500 sec. For carotid artery stenting, the optimal ACT is 250–300 sec.	ACT is the choice of test when heparin levels are too high (eg, >1.0 U/mL heparin) to allow monitoring with PTT and/or when a rapid result is necessary to monitor treatment. Because different methodologies and a number of variables (eg, platelet count and function, hypothermia, hemodilution and certain drugs like aprotinin) may affect the ACT, the ACT test is not standardized. Reproducibility of prolonged ACTs may be poor. Catheter Cardiovasc Interv 2005;65:330. [PMID: 15864806] Acta Anaesthesiol Scand 2006;50:461. [PMID: 16548858] Am J Cardiol 2006;97:1657. [PMID: 16728233] Perfusion 2006;21:27. [PMID: 16485696]

Test/Range/Collection	Physiologic Basis	Interpretation	Comments
Adrenocorticotropic hormone, plasma (ACTH) 20–100 pg/mL [4–22 pmol/L] Heparinized plastic container $$$$ Send promptly to laboratory on ice. ACTH is unstable in plasma, is inactivated at room temperature, and adheres strongly to glass. Avoid all contact with glass.	Pituitary ACTH (release stimulated by hypothalamic corticotropin-releasing factor) stimulates cortisol release from the adrenal gland. There is feedback regulation of the system by cortisol. ACTH is secreted episodically and shows circadian variation, with highest levels at 6:00–8:00 AM; lowest levels at 9:00–10:00 PM.	**Increased in:** Pituitary (40–200 pg/mL) and ectopic (200–71,000 pg/mL) Cushing syndrome, primary adrenal insufficiency (>250 pg/mL), adrenogenital syndrome with impaired cortisol production. **Decreased in:** Adrenal Cushing syndrome (<20 pg/mL), pituitary ACTH (secondary adrenal) insufficiency (<50 pg/mL).	ACTH levels (RIA) can only be interpreted when measured with cortisol after standardized stimulation or suppression tests (see Adrenocortical insufficiency algorithm, Figure 8–3, and Cushing syndrome algorithm, Figure 8–8). J Clin Endocrinol Metab 2006;91:3746. [PMID: 16860050] Am J Med 2005;118:1340. [PMID: 16378774]
Alanine aminotransferase, serum (ALT, SGPT, GPT) 0–35 U/L [0–0.58 mckat/L] (laboratory-specific) SST $	Intracellular enzyme involved in amino acid metabolism. Present in large concentrations in liver, kidney; in smaller amounts, in skeletal muscle and heart. Released with tissue damage, particularly liver injury.	**Increased in:** Acute viral hepatitis (ALT > AST), biliary tract obstruction (cholangitis, choledocholithiasis), alcoholic hepatitis and cirrhosis (AST > ALT), liver abscess, metastatic or primary liver cancer; nonalcoholic steatohepatitis; right heart failure, ischemia or hypoxia, injury to liver ("shock liver"), extensive trauma. Drugs that cause cholestasis or hepatotoxicity. **Decreased in:** Pyridoxine (vitamin B_6) deficiency.	ALT is the preferred enzyme for evaluation of liver injury. Screening ALT in low-risk populations has a low (12%) positive predictive value. See Liver function tests (Tables 8–12 & 8–13) Am J Gastroenterol 2006;101:76. [PMID: 16405534]

	Adrenocorticotropic hormone	Alanine aminotransferase

Albumin		
Albumin, serum 3.4–4.7 g/dL [34–47 g/L] SST $	Major component of plasma proteins; influenced by nutritional state, hepatic function, renal function, and various diseases. Major binding protein. Although there are more than 50 different genetic variants (alloalbumins), only occasionally does a mutation cause abnormal binding (eg, in familial dysalbuminemic hyperthyroxinemia).	**Increased in:** Dehydration, shock, hemoconcentration. **Decreased in:** Decreased hepatic synthesis (chronic liver disease, malnutrition, malabsorption, malignancy, congenital analbuminemia [rare]). Increased losses (nephrotic syndrome, burns, trauma, hemorrhage with fluid replacement, fistulas, enteropathy, acute or chronic glomerulonephritis). Hemodilution (pregnancy, CHF). Drugs: estrogens.	Serum albumin indicates severity in chronic liver disease. Useful in nutritional assessment if there is no impairment in production or increased loss of albumin. Independent risk factor for all-cause mortality in the elderly (age >70) and for complications in hospitalized patients. There is a 10% reduction in serum albumin level in late pregnancy (related to hemodilution). See liver function tests (Table 8–13) Clin Nutr 2001;20:477. [PMID: 11883995] J Am Diet Assoc 2004;104:1258. [PMID: 15281044]

Aldosterone, plasma

Test/Range/Collection	Physiologic Basis	Interpretation	Comments
Aldosterone, plasma *Salt-loaded* (120 meq Na+/d for 3–4 days): Supine: 3–10 ng/dL Upright: 5–30 ng/dL *Salt-depleted* (10 meq Na+/d for 3–4 days): Supine: 12–36 ng/dL Upright: 17–137 ng/dL Lavender or green $$$$ Early AM fasting specimen. Separate immediately and freeze.	Aldosterone is the major mineralocorticoid hormone and is a major regulator of extracellular volume and serum potassium concentration. For evaluation of hypoaldosteronism (associated with hyperkalemia), patients should be salt-depleted and upright when specimen is drawn.	**Increased in:** Primary hyperaldosteronism (2/3 from adrenal hyperplasia, 1/3 from adrenal adenomas) may account for 5–10% of hypertension. **Aldosterone / PRA ratio >15** (mL/dL/h) (sensitivity 73–87%, specificity 74–75%) **Decreased in:** Primary or secondary hypoaldosteronism.	Screening for hyperaldosteronism should use simultaneous determination of plasma aldosterone and plasma plasma renin activity (PRA) (see Figure 8–11). In primary aldosteronism, plasma aldosterone is usually elevated while PRA is low; in secondary hyperaldosteronism, both plasma aldosterone and PRA are usually elevated. The aldosterone/PRA ratio is often used for diagnosis of hyperaldosteronism, but the cut-off value has not been well established and the specificity is low. Endocrinol Metab Clin North Am 2002;31:619. [PMID: 12227124] Semin Nephrol 2002;22:44. [PMID: 11785068] Clin Chem 2005;51:386. [PMID: 15681560] Curr Cardiol Rep 2005;7:412. [PMID: 16256009] Nat Clin Pract Nephrol 2006;2:198. [PMID: 16932426]

Aldosterone, urine		
Aldosterone, urine* *Salt-loaded* (120 meq Na+/d for 3–4 days): 1.5–12.5 mcg/24 hours *Salt-depleted* (20 meq Na+/d for 3–4 days): 18–85 mcg/24 hours [1 mcg/24 h = 2.77 nmol/d] Bottle containing boric acid $$$$	Secretion of aldosterone is controlled by the renin-angiotensin system. Renin (synthesized and stored in juxtaglomerular cells of kidney) is released in response to both decreased perfusion pressure at the juxtaglomerular apparatus and negative sodium balance. Renin then hydrolyzes angiotensinogen to angiotensin I, which is converted to angiotensin II, which then stimulates the adrenal gland to produce aldosterone.	**Increased in:** Primary and secondary hyperaldosteronism, some patients with essential hypertension. **Decreased in:** Primary hypoaldosteronism (eg, 18-hydroxylase deficiency), secondary hypoaldosteronism (hyporeninemic hypoaldosteronism).	Urinary aldosterone is the most sensitive test for primary hyperaldosteronism. Levels >14 mcg/24 h after 3 days of salt-loading have a 96% sensitivity and 93% specificity for primary hyperaldosteronism: 7% of patients with essential hypertension have urinary aldosterone levels >14 mcg/24 h after salt-loading. J Hypertens 2006;24:737. [PMID: 16531803]

*To evaluate hyperaldosteronism, patient is salt-loaded and recumbent. Obtain 24-hour urine for aldosterone (and for sodium to check that sodium excretion is >250 meq/d).
To evaluate hypoaldosteronism, patient is salt-depleted and upright; check patient for hypotension before 24-hour urine is collected.

Test/Range/Collection	Physiologic Basis	Interpretation	Comments
Alkaline phosphatase, serum 41–133 IU/L [0.7–2.2 mckat/L] (method- and age-dependent) SST $	Alkaline phosphatases are found in liver, bone, intestine, and placenta.	**Increased in:** Obstructive hepatobiliary disease, bone disease (physiologic bone growth, Paget disease, osteomalacia, osteogenic sarcoma, bone metastases), hyperparathyroidism, rickets, benign familial hyperphosphatasemia, pregnancy (third trimester), GI disease (perforated ulcer or bowel infarct), hepatotoxic drugs. **Decreased in:** Hypophosphatasia.	Alkaline phosphatase performs well in measuring the extent of bone metastases in prostate cancer. Normal in osteoporosis. Alkaline phosphatase isoenzyme separation by electrophoresis or differential heat inactivation is unreliable. Use γ-glutamyl transpeptidase, which increases in hepatobiliary disease but not in bone disease, to infer origin of increased alkaline phosphatase (ie, liver rather than bone). Clin Lab Med 2002;22:377. [PMID: 12134466] Endocr Pract 2006;12:676. [PMID: 17229666] Pediatr Rev 2006;27:382. [PMID: 17012488]
Amebic serology, serum <1:64 titer SST $$	Test for presence of *Entamoeba histolytica* by detection of antibodies that develop 2–4 weeks after infection. Tissue invasion by the organism may be necessary for antibody production.	**Increased in:** Current or past infection with *E histolytica.* Amebic abscess (91%), amebic dysentery (84%), asymptomatic cyst carriers (9%), patients with other diseases, and healthy people (2%).	In some endemic areas, as many as 44% of those tested have positive serologies. Precipitin or indirect hemagglutination and recombinant antigen-based ELISA tests are available. J Clin Microbiol 2005;43:4801. [PMID: 16145144]

Ammonia		
Ammonia, plasma (NH$_3$) 18–60 mcg/dL [11–35 mcmol/L] Green $$ Separate plasma from cells immediately. Avoid hemolysis. Analyze immediately. Place on ice.	Ammonia is liberated by bacteria in the large intestine or by protein metabolism and is rapidly converted to urea in the liver. In liver disease or portal-systemic shunting, the blood ammonia concentration increases. In acute liver failure, elevation of blood ammonia may cause brain edema; in chronic liver failure, it may be responsible for hepatic encephalopathy.	**Increased in:** Liver failure, hepatic encephalopathy (especially if protein consumption is high or if there is GI bleeding), fulminant hepatic failure, Reye syndrome, portacaval shunting, cirrhosis, urea cycle metabolic defects, urea-splitting urinary tract infection with urinary diversion, and organic acidemias. Drugs: diuretics, acetazolamide, asparaginase, fluorouracil (transient), others. Spuriously increased by any ammonia-containing detergent on laboratory glassware. **Decreased in:** Decreased production by gut bacteria (kanamycin, neomycin). Decreased gut absorption (lactulose).	Correlates poorly with degree of hepatic encephalopathy in chronic liver disease. Test not useful in adults with known liver disease. Clin Biochem 2005;38:696. [PMID: 15963970]

Test/Range/Collection	Physiologic Basis	Interpretation	Comments
Amylase, serum 20–110 U/L [0.33–1.83 mckat/L] (laboratory-specific) SST $	Amylase hydrolyzes complex carbohydrates. Serum amylase is derived primarily from pancreas and salivary glands and is increased with inflammation or obstruction of these glands. Other tissues have some amylase activity, including ovaries, small and large intestine, and skeletal muscle.	**Increased in:** Acute pancreatitis (70–95%), pancreatic pseudocyst, pancreatic duct obstruction (cholecystitis, choledocholithiasis, pancreatic carcinoma, stone, stricture, duct sphincter spasm), bowel obstruction and infarction, mumps, parotitis, diabetic ketoacidosis, penetrating peptic ulcer, peritonitis, ruptured ectopic pregnancy, macroamylasemia. Drugs: azathioprine, hydrochlorothiazide. **Decreased in:** Pancreatic insufficiency, cystic fibrosis. Usually normal or low in chronic pancreatitis.	Macroamylasemia is indicated by high serum but low urine amylase. Serum lipase is an alternative test for acute pancreatitis. Amylase isoenzymes are not of practical use because of technical problems. J Clin Gastroenterol 2002;34:459. [PMID: 11907364] Clin Chim Acta 2005;362:26. [PMID: 16024009]
Angiotensin-converting enzyme, serum (ACE) 12–35 U/L [<590 nkat/L] (method-dependent) SST $$	ACE is a dipeptidyl carboxypeptidase that converts angiotensin I to the vasopressor, angiotensin II. ACE is normally present in the kidneys and other peripheral tissues. In granulomatous disease, ACE levels increase, derived from epithelioid cells within granulomas.	**Increased in:** Sarcoidosis (sensitivity 63%, specificity 93%, LR+ = 9.0) (when upper limit of normal is 50), hyperthyroidism, acute hepatitis, primary biliary cirrhosis, diabetes mellitus, multiple myeloma, osteoarthritis, amyloidosis, Gaucher disease, pneumoconiosis, histoplasmosis, miliary tuberculosis. Drugs: dexamethasone. **Decreased in:** Renal disease, obstructive pulmonary disease, hypothyroidism.	Test is not useful as a screening test for sarcoidosis (low sensitivity). Specificity is compromised by positive tests in diseases more common than sarcoidosis. Some advocate measurement of ACE to follow disease activity in sarcoidosis. Ann Clin Biochem 2002;39:436. [PMID: 12227849] Semin Ophthalmol 2005;20:177. [PMID: 16282152]

Antibody screen		
Antibody screen, serum or plasma Red or lavender $ Properly identified and labeled blood specimens are critical.	Detects antibodies to non-ABO red blood cell antigens in recipient's serum, using reagent red cells selected to possess antigens against which common antibodies can be produced. Further identification of the specificity of any antibody detected (using panels of red cells of known antigenicity) makes it possible to test donor blood for the absence of the corresponding antigen. Primary response to first antigen exposure requires 20–120 days; antibody is largely IgM with a small quantity of IgG. Secondary response requires 1–14 days; antibody is mostly IgG.	**Positive in:** Presence of alloantibody, autoantibodies.	In practice, a type and screen (ABO and Rh grouping and antibody screen) is adequate work-up for patients undergoing operative procedures unlikely to require transfusion. A negative antibody screen implies that a recipient can receive type-specific (ABO-Rh identical) blood with minimal risk. Some antibody activity (eg, anti-Jkᵃ, anti-E) may become so weak as to be undetectable but increase rapidly after secondary stimulation with the same antigen. *Technical Manual of the American Association of Blood Banks*, 15th ed. American Association of Blood Banks, 2005.

	Antidiuretic hormon

Test/Range/Collection	Physiologic Basis	Interpretation	Comments
Antidiuretic hormone, plasma (ADH) If serum osmolality >290 mosm/kg H_2O: 2–12 pg/mL If serum osmolality <290 mosm/kg H_2O: <2 pg/mL Lavender $$$$ Draw in two chilled tubes and deliver to lab on ice. Specimen for serum osmolality must be drawn at same time.	Antidiuretic hormone (vasopressin) is a hormone secreted from the posterior pituitary that acts on the distal nephron to conserve water and regulate the tonicity of body fluids. Water deprivation provides both an osmotic and a volume stimulus for ADH release by increasing plasma osmolality and decreasing plasma volume. Water administration lowers plasma osmolality and expands blood volume, inhibiting the release of ADH by the osmoreceptor and the atrial volume receptor mechanisms.	**Increased in:** Nephrogenic diabetes insipidus, syndrome of inappropriate antidiuretic hormone (SIADH). Drugs: nicotine, morphine, chlorpropamide, clofibrate, cyclophosphamide. **Normal relative to plasma osmolality in:** Primary polydipsia. **Decreased in:** Central (neurogenic) diabetes insipidus. Drugs: ethanol, phenytoin.	Test very rarely indicated. Measurement of serum and urine osmolality usually suffices. Test not indicated in diagnosis of SIADH. Patients with SIADH show decreased plasma sodium and decreased plasma osmolality, usually with high urine osmolality relative to plasma. These findings in a normovolemic patient with normal thyroid and adrenal function are sufficient to make the diagnosis of SIADH without measuring ADH itself. Crit Care Clin 2001;17:11. [PMID: 11219224] Ann Intern Med 2006;144:186. [PMID: 16461963]

Antiglobulin test, direct

Antiglobulin test, direct, red cells (direct Coombs, DAT)	Direct antiglobulin test is used to demonstrate in vivo coating of red cells with globulins, in particular IgG and C3d.	Positive in: Autoimmune hemolytic anemia, hemolytic disease of the newborn, alloimmune reactions to recently transfused cells, and drug-induced hemolysis.	A positive DAT implies in vivo red cell coating by immunoglobulins or complement. Such red cell coating may or may not be associated with immune hemolytic anemia.
Negative	Washed red cells from a patient or donor are tested directly with antihuman globulin (AHG, Coombs) reagents. DAT is positive (shows agglutination) immediately when IgG coats red cells. Complement or IgA coating may only be demonstrated after incubation at room temperature.	Drugs may induce the formation of antibodies, either against the drug itself or against intrinsic red cell antigens, that may result in a positive DAT, immune red cell destruction, or both. Some of the antibodies produced appear to be dependent on the presence of the drug (eg, penicillin, quinidine, ceftriaxone), whereas others are independent of the continued presence of the inciting drug (eg, methyldopa, levodopa, procainamide, cephalosporins, fludarabine).	The DAT can detect a level of 100–500 molecules of IgG per red cell and 400–1100 molecules of C3d per red cell, depending on the reagent and technique used. Positive DATs without clinical manifestations of immune-mediated red cell destruction are reported in the range of 1 in 1000 up to 1 in 14,000 blood donors and 1–15% of hospital patients.
$			A false-positive DAT is often seen in patients with hypergammaglobulinemia, eg, in some HIV-positive patients.
Blood anticoagulated with EDTA is used to prevent in vitro uptake of complement components. A red top tube may be used, if necessary.			*Technical Manual of the American Association of Blood Banks*, 15th ed. American Association of Blood Banks, 2005.

Test/Range/Collection	Physiologic Basis	Interpretation	Comments
	Antiglobulin test, indirect		**Anti-streptolysin O**
Antiglobulin test, indirect, serum (indirect Coombs) Negative Red or lavender $	Indirect antiglobulin test is used to demonstrate the presence in patients' serum of unexpected antibody to ABO and Rh-compatible reagent red blood cells. In the procedure, patient's serum or plasma is incubated in vitro with reagent red cells, which are then washed to remove unbound globulins. Agglutination that occurs when antihuman globulin (AHG, Coombs) reagent is added indicates that antibody has bound to a specific antigen present on the red cells.	**Positive in:** Presence of alloantibody or autoantibody. Drugs: methyldopa.	The technique is used in antibody detection and identification and in the major cross-match prior to transfusion (see Type and Cross-Match). *Technical Manual of the American Association of Blood Banks,* 15th ed. American Association of Blood Banks, 2005.
Anti-streptolysin O, serum (ASO) 0–1 year: <200 IU/mL; 2–12 years: <240 IU/mL 13 years or older: <330 IU/mL (laboratory-specific) SST $$	Detects the presence of antibody to the antigen streptolysin O produced by group A streptococci. Streptococcal antibodies appear about 2 weeks after infection. Titer rises to a peak at 4–6 weeks and may remain elevated for 6 months to 1 year. Test is based on the neutralization of hemolytic activity of streptolysin O toxin by antistreptolysin O antibodies in serum.	**Increased in:** Recent infection with group A β-hemolytic streptococci: scarlet fever, erysipelas, streptococcal pharyngitis/tonsillitis (40–50%), rheumatic fever (80–85%), poststreptococcal glomerulonephritis. Some collagen-vascular diseases. Certain serum lipoproteins, bacterial growth products, or oxidized streptolysin O may result in inhibition of hemolysis and thus cause false-positive results.	Standardization of (Todd) units may vary significantly from laboratory to laboratory. ASO titers are not useful in management of acute streptococcal pharyngitis. In patients with rheumatic fever, test may be a more reliable indicator of recent streptococcal infection than throat culture. An increasing titer is more suggestive of acute streptococcal infection than a single elevated level. Even with severe infection, ASO titers rise in only 70–80% of patients. Normal range increases with age. Am Fam Physician 2005;71:1949. [PMID: 15926411]

	Antithrombin III			α₁-Antitrypsin		
Antithrombin III (AT III), plasma 84–123% (enzymatic activity, qualitative) 80–130% (antigen, quantitative) Blue $$ Transport to lab on ice. Plasma must be separated and frozen in a polypropylene tube within 2 hours.	Antithrombin III is a serine protease inhibitor that protects against thrombus formation by inhibiting thrombin and factors IXa, Xa, XIa, XIIa, plasmin, and kallikrein. It accounts for 70–90% of the anticoagulant activity of human plasma. Its activity is enhanced 100-fold by heparin. There are two types of assay: functional/enzymatic (qualitative) and immunologic (quantitative). Since the immunologic assay cannot rule out functional AT III deficiency, a functional assay should be ordered first. Functional assays test AT III activity in inhibiting thrombin or factor Xa. Given an abnormal functional assay, the quantitative immunologic test indicates whether there is decreased synthesis of AT III (type I deficiency) or intact synthesis of a dysfunctional protein (type II deficiency).		**Increased by:** Oral anticoagulants. **Decreased in:** Congenital and acquired AT III deficiency (nephrotic syndrome, chronic liver disease), oral contraceptive use, chronic disseminated intravascular coagulation (DIC), acute venous thrombosis (consumption), L-asparaginase treatment and heparin therapy.	Congenital or acquired AT III deficiency results in a hypercoagulable state, venous thromboembolism, and heparin resistance. Congenital AT III deficiency is present in 1:2000–1:5000 people and is autosomal codominant. Heterozygotes have AT III levels 20–60% of normal. Evaluation of AT III should be considered in patients with venous thrombosis, especially for thrombosis in unusual sites or associated with heparin resistance. Testing should be performed at least 2 months after the thrombotic event, at a time when the patient is not receiving anticoagulants. Int J Biochem Cell Biol 2004;36:386. [PMID: 14687916] J Thromb Haemost 2005;3:459. [PMID: 15748234] Haematologica 2006;91:695. [PMID: 16670075]		
α₁-Antitrypsin (α₁-Antiprotease) serum 110–270 mg/dL [1.1–2.7 g/L] SST $$				α₁-Antiprotease is an α₁-globulin glycoprotein serine protease inhibitor (Pi) whose deficiency leads to excessive protease activity and panacinar emphysema in adults or liver disease in children (seen as ZZ and SZ phenotypes). Cirrhosis of the liver and liver cancer in adults are also associated with the Pi Z phenotype.	**Increased in:** Inflammation, infection, rheumatic disease, malignancy, and pregnancy as an acute-phase reactant. **Decreased in:** Congenital α₁-antitrypsin deficiency, nephrotic syndrome.	Smoking is a much more common cause of chronic obstructive pulmonary disease in adults than is α₁-antitrypsin deficiency. Clin Chim Acta 2005;352:1 [PMID: 15653097] Semin Respir Crit Care Med 2005;26:154. [PMID: 16088434] Lancet 2005;365:2225. [PMID: 15978931] Curr Opin Gastroenterol 2006;22:215. [PMID: 16550035]

	Arterial blood gases	Aspartate aminotransferase

Test/Range/Collection	Physiologic Basis	Interpretation	Comments
Arterial blood gases (ABG), whole blood Heparinized syringe $$$ Collect arterial blood in a heparinized syringe, and send to laboratory immediately.	Blood gas determination provides information about cardiopulmonary and metabolic status. When integrated with the history and physical examination, the rapidly available arterial blood gas (ABG) analysis is useful in the resuscitation of the acutely ill or injured patient.	See carbon dioxide, oxygen, and pH.	Emerg Med Clin North Am 1986;4:235. [PMID: 3084205]
Aspartate aminotransferase, serum (AST, SGOT, GOT) 0–35 IU/L [0–0.58 mckat/L] (laboratory-specific) SST $	Intracellular enzyme involved in amino acid metabolism. Present in large concentrations in liver, skeletal muscle, brain, red cells, and heart. Released into the bloodstream when tissue is damaged, especially in liver injury.	**Increased in:** Acute viral hepatitis (ALT > AST), biliary tract obstruction (cholangitis, choledocholithiasis), alcoholic hepatitis and cirrhosis (AST > ALT), liver abscess, metastatic or primary liver cancer; right heart failure, ischemia or hypoxia, injury to liver ("shock liver"), extensive trauma. Drugs that cause cholestasis or hepatotoxicity. **Decreased in:** Pyridoxine (vitamin B_6) deficiency.	Test is not indicated for diagnosis of myocardial infarction. AST/ALT ratio >1 suggests cirrhosis in patients with hepatitis C. See Liver function tests (Tables 8–12 & 8–13) Clin Gastroenterol Hepatol 2005;3:852. [PMID: 16234021] CMAJ 2005;172:367. [PMID: 15684121]

B cell immunoglobulin heavy chain gene rearrangement

B cell immunoglobulin heavy chain (IgH) gene rearrangement		Positive in:	
Whole blood, bone marrow, frozen or paraffin-embedded tissue Lavender $$$$	In general, the percentage of B lymphocytes with identical immunoglobulin heavy chain gene rearrangements is very low; in malignancies, however, the clonal expansion of one population leads to a large number of cells with identical B cell immunoglobulin heavy chain gene rearrangements. B-cell clonality can be assessed by restriction fragment Southern blot hybridization and polymerase chain reaction (PCR).	**Positive in:** B-cell neoplasms such as lymphoma (monoclonal B-cell proliferation).	The diagnostic sensitivity and specificity are heterogeneous and laboratory- and method-specific. The Southern blot analysis is considered the diagnostic gold standard. Results of the test must always be interpreted in the context of morphologic and other relevant data (eg, flow cytometry), and should not be used alone for a diagnosis of malignancy. The test is not intended to detect minimal residual disease. J Mol Diagn 2002;4:81. [PMID: 11986398] N Engl J Med 2003;348:1777. [PMID: 12724484]

bcr/abl, t(9;22) translocation by RT-PCR

Test/Range/Collection	Physiologic Basis	Interpretation	Comments
bcr/abl, t(9;22) **translocation by RT-PCR**, qualitative Blood Lavender $$$$	Approximately 95% of cases of CML have the characteristic t(9;22)(q34;q11) that results in a bcr/abl gene fusion on the derived chromosome 22 called the Philadelphia (Ph) chromosome. The remaining cases either have a cryptic translocation between 9q34 and 22q11 that cannot be identified by routine cytogenetic analysis, or have variant translocations involving a third or even a fourth chromosome besides 9 and 22. The bcr/abl fusion transcript is found in all cases of chronic myelogenous leukemia (CML), including those with a cryptic or variant translocation. A subset of acute lymphoblastic leukemia (ALL) and occasionally acute myelogenous leukemia (AML, mostly CML blast crisis) also have the Ph chromosome, and therefore are positive for bcr/abl, t(9;22) translocation.	**Positive in:** All chronic myelogenous leukemia (CML), a subset of acute lymphoblastic leukemia (ALL), and rare acute myeloid leukemia (eg, CML blast crisis).	This assay can also be used to distinguish between the major and minor transcripts. The major transcript, characterized by the p210 fusion gene product, is typically detected in CML. The minor transcript, characterized by the p190 fusion gene product, is typically detected in ALL. Small amounts of p190 transcript can be detected in the majority of patients with CML, due to alternative splicing of the bcr gene. When monitoring a patient for genetic recurrence and minimal residual disease, the bcr/abl, t(9;22) translocation quantitative RT-PCR assay should be used. The quantitative assay may not distinguish between the major and minor bcr/abl products. Clin Cancer Res 2003;9:160. [PMID: 12538464] Cancer Genet Cytogenet 2006;166:89. [PMID: 16616117] Ann Int Med 2006;145:913. [PMID: 17179059]

bcr/abl mutation analysis (Bcr/Abl genotyping) Blood Lavender $$$$	The Bcr/Abl tyrosine kinase inhibitor imatinib (STI571 or Gleevec) is effective in Philadelphia chromosome–positive (Ph-positive) leukemias (eg, chronic myeloid leukemia, CML), but relapse occurs, mainly as a result of the outgrowth of leukemic subclones with bcr/abl mutations that interfere with imatinib binding. The bcr/abl mutation analysis can assist physicians in evaluating resistance to imatinib therapy and facilitate appropriate adjustments to treatment (eg, increase in imatinib dosage or switch to dasatinib).	**Positive in:** Imatinib-resistant chronic myeloid leukemia; imatinib-resistant Ph-positive precursor B lymphoblastic leukemia.	The analysis involves direct DNA sequencing of the PCR-amplified bcr/abl products. The sequence is then compared with an Abl kinase domain reference sequence to identify single or multiple mutations. Mutations at 17 different amino acid positions within the Bcr-Abl kinase domain have been associated with clinical resistance to imatinib. Patients with T315I mutation are resistant to both imatinib and dasatinib. Science 2004;305:399. [PMID: 15256671] N Engl J Med 2006;354:2531. [PMID: 16775234]

Table header (spanning): bcr/abl mutation analysis

	Bilirubin	
Test/Range/Collection	**Physiologic Basis**	**Interpretation**	**Comments**

Test/Range/Collection	Physiologic Basis	Interpretation	Comments
Bilirubin, serum 0.1–1.2 mg/dL [2–21 mcmol/L] Direct (conjugated to gluc- uronide) bilirubin: 0.1–0.4 mg/dL [<7 mcmol/L]; Indirect (unconjugated) bilirubin: 0.2–0.7 mg/dL [<12 mcmol/L] SST $$	Bilirubin, a product of hemoglobin metabolism, is conjugated in the liver to mono- and diglucuronides and excreted in bile. Some conjugated bilirubin is bound to serum albumin, so-called D (delta) bilirubin. Elevated serum bilirubin occurs in liver disease, biliary obstruction, or hemolysis.	**Increased in:** Acute or chronic hepatitis, cirrhosis, biliary tract obstruction, toxic hepatitis, neonatal jaundice, congenital liver enzyme abnormalities (Dubin-Johnson, Rotor, Gilbert, Crigler-Najjar syndromes), fasting, hemolytic disorders. Hepato-toxic drugs.	Assay of total bilirubin includes conjugated (direct) and unconjugated (indirect) bilirubin plus delta bilirubin (conjugated bilirubin bound to albumin). It is usually clinically unnecessary to fractionate total bilirubin. The fractionation is unreliable by the diazo reaction and may underestimate unconjugated bilirubin. Only conjugated bilirubin appears in the urine, and it is indicative of liver disease; hemolysis is associated with increased unconjugated bilirubin. Persistence of delta bilirubin in serum in resolving liver disease means that total bilirubin does not effectively indicate the time course of resolution. Am Fam Physician 2004;69:299. [PMID: 14765767] CMAJ 2005;172:367. [PMID: 15684121]

Blood urea nitrogen

| **Blood urea nitrogen,** serum (BUN)

8–20 mg/dL
[2.9–7.1 mmol/L]

SST
$ | Urea, an end product of protein metabolism, is excreted by the kidney. BUN is directly related to protein intake and nitrogen metabolism and inversely related to the rate of excretion of urea.

Urea concentration in glomerular filtrate is the same as in plasma, but its tubular reabsorption is inversely related to the rate of urine formation. Thus, the BUN is a less useful measure of glomerular filtration rate than the serum creatinine (Cr). | **Increased in:** Renal failure (acute or chronic), urinary tract obstruction, dehydration, shock, burns, CHF, GI bleeding. Nephrotoxic drugs (eg, gentamicin).
Decreased in: Hepatic failure, nephrotic syndrome, cachexia (low-protein and high-carbohydrate diets). | Urease assay method commonly used. BUN/Cr ratio (normally 12:1–20:1) is decreased in acute tubular necrosis, advanced liver disease, low protein intake, and following hemodialysis. BUN/Cr ratio is increased in dehydration, GI bleeding, and increased catabolism.
Cleve Clin J Med 2002;69:569. [PMID: 12109642]
Semin Dial 2006;19:165. [PMID: 16551296] |

	B-type Natriuretic peptide		
Test/Range/Collection	Physiologic Basis	Interpretation	Comments
B-type Natriuretic peptide (BNP), plasma Lavender 0–100 pg/mL [0–347 pmol/L] $$ Point-of-care immunoassays also available.	BNP has biologic effects similar to those of atrial natriuretic peptide (ANP) and is stored mainly in the myocardium of the cardiac ventricles. Blood BNP levels are elevated in hypervolemic states such as congestive heart failure (CHF). BNP is useful for guiding and monitoring heart failure treatment and for prognosis prediction. Clinical applications in the setting of CHF include: to determine the cause of diagnostic symptoms (eg, dyspnea); to estimate the degree of severity of heart failure; to estimate the risk of disease progression; and to screen for less symptomatic disease in high-risk populations.	**Increased in:** CHF (cut-off concentration: >100 pg/mL; sensitivity 90%, specificity 73%. BNP <100 pg/mL has a negative predictive value of 90%). BNP is also increased in a variety of other cardiac and noncardiac diseases including coronary artery disease, acute coronary syndrome, left ventricular dysfunction, valvular aortic stenosis, and pulmonary embolism.	BNP testing is not a substitute for careful cardiopulmonary evaluation and should not be the sole criterion for admission/discharge of a patient. Although normal levels indicate a low probability of CHF, they do not exclude it or other serious cardiopulmonary disorders. Increased levels are not specific for CHF and can occur with a variety of cardiac and noncardiac diseases. BNP is not recommended for screening for left ventricular dysfunction or hypertrophy in the general population. It is also unnecessary to test BNP in patients with obvious CHF (eg, NYHA class IV). Treatment of CHF has been reported to decrease BNP levels in parallel with improving clinical symptoms. Tests for N-terminal fragment of pro-BNP (NT-pro-BNP) are also available, and its diagnostic performance is comparable to that of BNP. Congest Heart Fail 2004;10(Suppl:1). [PMID: 14872150] Clin Chem 2005;51:486. [PMID: 15738513] JAMA 2005;294:2866. [PMID: 16352794] Heart 2006;92:843. [PMID: 16698841]

	Brucella antibody	C-peptide
Brucella antibody, serum <1:80 titer SST $	Patients with acute brucellosis generally develop an agglutinating antibody titer of >1:160 within 3 weeks. The titer may rise during the acute infection, with relapses, brucellergin skin testing, or use of certain vaccines (see Interpretation). The agglutinin titer usually declines after 3 months or after successful therapy. Low titers may persist for years. Indirect ELISA measuring IgM, IgG, and IgA antibodies have higher sensitivity and specificity than the agglutinating antibody test. Future routine use of PCR testing needs further clinical evaluation.	This test detects antibodies against all of the *Brucella* species except *B canis*. A fourfold or greater rise in titer in separate specimens drawn 1–4 weeks apart is indicative of recent exposure. Since titers can remain high for a prolonged period, they are not suitable for patient follow-up. Final diagnosis depends on isolation of organism by culture. Expert Rev Mol Diagn 2004;4:115. [PMID: 14711354] N Engl J Med 2005;352:2325. [PMID: 15930423] **Increased in:** *Brucella* infection (except *B canis*) (97% within 3 weeks of illness); recent brucellergin skin test; infections with *Francisella tularensis, Yersinia enterocolitica,* salmonella, Rocky Mountain spotted fever; vaccinations for cholera and tularemia. **Normal in:** *B canis* infection.
C-peptide, serum 0.8–4.0 ng/mL [mcg/L] (0.26–1.3 nmol/L) SST $$$ Fasting sample preferred.	C-peptide is an inactive by-product of the cleavage of proinsulin to active insulin. Its presence indicates endogenous release of insulin. C-peptide is largely excreted by the kidney.	Test is most useful to detect factitious insulin injection (increased insulin, decreased C-peptide) or to detect endogenous insulin production in diabetic patients receiving insulin (C-peptide present). A random C peptide level has reasonable discriminatory power for determining type 1 vs. type 2 diabetes. A molar ratio of insulin to C-peptide in peripheral venous blood >1.0 in a hypoglycemic patient is consistent with surreptitious or inadvertent insulin administration but not insulinoma. C-peptide levels of 2 nmol/L or greater suggest insulinoma. Ann Endocrinol (Paris) 2004;65:88. Surg Clin North Am 2004;84:775. [PMID: 15145234] **Increased in:** Renal failure, ingestion of oral hypoglycemic drugs, insulinomas, B cell transplants. **Decreased in:** Factitious hypoglycemia due to insulin administration, pancreatectomy, type I diabetes mellitus (decreased or undetectable).

C-reactive protein, high sensitivity			
Test/Range/Collection	**Physiologic Basis**	**Interpretation**	**Comments**
C-reactive protein, high sensitivity (hs-CRP), serum <1.0 mg/dL (lower 95th percentile) SST $	CRP is an acute-phase reactant protein. Hepatic secretion is stimulated in response to inflammatory cytokines. Unlike other acute phase proteins, CRP is not affected by hormones. CRP activates the complement system, binds to Fc receptors, and serves as an opsonin for some microorganisms. Rapid, marked increases in CRP occur with inflammation, infection, trauma and tissue necrosis, malignancies, and autoimmune disorders. CRP levels are not only valuable in the clinical assessment of chronic inflammatory disorders, but also in assessing vascular inflammation and cardiovascular risk stratification. CRP level has been shown to be an independent risk factor for atherosclerotic disease. Elevated CRP levels are associated with increased cardiovascular morbidity and mortality in patients with coronary artery disease.	**Increased in:** Inflammatory states, including arteriosclerotic disorders.	CRP is a very sensitive but nonspecific marker of inflammation. A variety of conditions other than arteriosclerosis may cause dramatic increases in CRP levels. CRP levels increase within 2 hours of acute insult (eg, surgery, infection) and should peak and begin decreasing within 48 hours if no other inflammatory event occurs. In patients with rheumatoid arthritis, persistently elevated CRP concentrations are present when the disease is active and usually fall to normal during periods of complete remission. Patients with high hs-CRP concentrations are more likely to develop stroke, myocardial infarction, and severe peripheral vascular disease. hs-CRP results are used to assign risk as follows: <1.0 mg/L lowest tertile, lowest risk; 1.0–3.0 mg/L middle tertile, average risk; >3.0 mg/L highest tertile, highest risk. Noncardiovascular cause should be considered if CRP values are >10 mg/dL with repeat measurements. Circulation 2003;107:499 [PMID: 12551878] Curr Opin Rheumatol 2004;16:18. [PMID: 1473384] Autoimmun Rev 2006;5:331. [PMID: 16782558]

C1 esterase inhibitor

| C1 esterase inhibitor (C1 INH), serum

Method-dependent

SST
$$ | C1 esterase inhibitor (C1 INH) is an α-globulin, which controls the first stage of the classic complement pathway and inhibits thrombin, plasmin, and kallikrein. Deficiency results in spontaneous activation of C1, leading to consumption of C2 and C4. The functional assay involves the measurement of C1 INH as it inhibits the hydrolysis of a substrate ester by C1 esterase. Immunoassay of C1 INH is also available. | **Decreased in:** Hereditary angio-edema (HAE) (85%) (15% of patients with HAE will have normal levels by immunoassay, but the protein is non-functional and levels determined by the functional assay will be low). | C1 esterase inhibitor deficiency is an uncommon cause of angioedema. There are two subtypes of HAE. In one, the protein is absent; in the other, it is nonfunctional. Acquired angioedema has been attributed to massive consumption of C1 INH (presumably by tumor or lymphoma-related immune complexes) or to anti-C1 INH autoantibody. When clinical suspicion exists, a serum C4 level screens for HAE. Low levels of C4 are present in all cases during an attack. C1 esterase inhibitor levels are not indicated unless either the C4 level is low or there is a very high clinical suspicion of HAE in a patient with normal C4 during an asymptomatic phase between attacks. In acquired C1 INH deficiency, the C1 level is also significantly decreased (often 10% of normal), whereas in HAE the C1 level is normal or only slightly decreased. Clin Exp Dermatol 2005;30:460. [PMID: 15953110] Immunol Allergy Clin North Am 2006;26:653. [PMID: 17085283] |

	Calcitonin

Test/Range/Collection	Physiologic Basis	Interpretation	Comments
Calcitonin, plasma Male: <90 pg/mL [ng/L] Female: <70 pg/mL [ng/L] Green $$$ Fasting sample required. Place on ice.	Calcitonin is a 32-amino-acid poly-peptide hormone secreted by the parafollicular C cells of the thyroid. It decreases osteoclastic bone resorption and lowers serum calcium levels.	**Increased in:** Medullary thyroid carcinoma (>500 pg/mL on two occasions), Zollinger-Ellison syndrome, pernicious anemia, pregnancy (at term), newborns, carcinoma (breast, lung, pancreas), chronic renal failure.	Test is useful to diagnose and monitor medullary thyroid carcinoma, although stimulation tests may be necessary (eg, pentagastrin test). Genetic testing is now available for the diagnosis of multiple endocrine neoplasia type II. (MEN II is the most common familial form of medullary thyroid carcinoma.) J Clin Endocrinol Metab 2004;89:163. [PMID: 14715844] Ann R Coll Surg Engl 2006;88:433. [PMID: 17002842] Curr Opin Oncol 2007;19:18. [PMID: 17133107]

Calcium, serum

| Calcium, serum (Ca²⁺) 8.5–10.5 mg/dL [2.1–2.6 mmol/L] **Panic:** <6.5 or >13.5 mg/dL SST $ Prolonged venous stasis during collection causes false increase in serum calcium. | Serum calcium is the sum of ionized calcium plus complexed calcium and calcium bound to proteins (mostly albumin). Level of ionized calcium is regulated by parathyroid hormone and vitamin D. | **Increased in:** Hyperparathyroidism, malignancies secreting parathyroid hormone–related protein (PTHrP) (especially squamous cell carcinoma of lung and renal cell carcinoma), vitamin D excess, milk-alkali syndrome, multiple myeloma, Paget disease of bone with immobilization, sarcoidosis, other granulomatous disorders, familial hypocalciuria, vitamin A intoxication, thyrotoxicosis, Addison disease. Drugs: antacids (some), calcium salts, chronic diuretic use (eg, thiazides), lithium, others. **Decreased in:** Hypoparathyroidism, vitamin D deficiency, renal insufficiency, pseudohypoparathyroidism, magnesium deficiency, hyperphosphatemia, massive transfusion, hypoalbuminemia. | Need to know serum albumin to interpret calcium level. For every decrease in albumin by 1 mg/dL, calcium should be corrected upward by 0.8 mg/dL. In 10% of patients with malignancies, hypercalcemia is attributable to coexistent hyperparathyroidism, suggesting that serum PTH levels should be measured at initial presentation of all hypercalcemic patients (see Figure 8–12). Am Fam Physician 2003;67:1959. [PMID: 12751658] J Clin Endocrinol Metab 2005;90:6316. [PMID: 16131579] |

	Calcium, ionized		

Test/Range/Collection	Physiologic Basis	Interpretation	Comments
Calcium, ionized, serum 4.4–5.4 mg/dL (at pH 7.4) [1.1–1.3 mmol/L] Whole blood specimen must be collected anaerobically and anticoagulated with standardized amounts of heparin. Tourniquet application must be brief. Specimen should be analyzed promptly. SST $$	Calcium circulates in three forms: as free Ca²⁺ (47%), protein-bound to albumin and globulins (43%), and as calcium–ligand complexes (10%) (with citrate, bicarbonate, lactate, phosphate, and sulfate). Protein binding is highly pH-dependent, and acidosis results in an increased free calcium fraction. Ionized Ca²⁺ is the form that is physiologically active. Ionized calcium is a more accurate reflection of physiologic status than total calcium in patients with altered serum proteins (renal failure, nephrotic syndrome, multiple myeloma, etc), altered concentrations of calcium-binding ligands, and acid–base disturbances. Measurement of ionized calcium is by ion-selective electrodes.	**Increased in:** ↓ Blood pH. **Decreased in:** ↑ Blood pH, citrate, heparin, EDTA.	Ionized calcium measurements are not needed except in special circumstances, eg, massive blood transfusion, liver transplantation, neonatal hypocalcemia, cardiac surgery, and possibly monitoring of patients with secondary hyperparathyroidism from renal failure. Validity of test depends on sample integrity. See diagnostic algorithms for hypercalcemia and hypocalcemia (Figures 8–12 & 8–13). Nephrol Dial Transplant 2005;20:2126. [PMID: 16030044]

Calcium, urine

| **Calcium, urine** (U_{Ca})

100–300 mg/24 h
[2.5–7.5 mmol/24 h or
2.3–3.3 mmol/12 h]

Urine bottle containing
hydrochloric acid
$$$
Collect 24-hour urine or
12-hour overnight urine. | Ordinarily there is moderate urinary calcium excretion, the amount depending on dietary calcium, parathyroid hormone (PTH) level, and protein intake.

Renal calculi occur much more often in hyperparathyroidism than in other hypercalcemic states. | **Increased in:** Hyperparathyroidism, osteolytic bone metastases, myeloma, osteoporosis, vitamin D intoxication, distal RTA, idiopathic hypercalciuria, thyrotoxicosis, Paget disease, Fanconi syndrome, hepatolenticular degeneration, schistosomiasis, sarcoidosis, malignancy (breast, bladder), osteitis deformans, immobilization. Drugs: acetazolamide, calcium salts, cholestyramine, corticosteroids, dihydrotachysterol, initial diuretic use (eg, furosemide), others. **Decreased in:** Hypoparathyroidism, pseudohypoparathyroidism, rickets, osteomalacia, nephrotic syndrome, acute glomerulonephritis, osteoblastic bone metastases, hypothyroidism, celiac disease, steatorrhea, hypocalciuric hypercalcemia, other causes of hypocalcemia. Drugs: aspirin, bicarbonate, chronic diuretic use (eg, thiazides, chlorthalidone), estrogens, indomethacin, lithium, neomycin, oral contraceptives. | Approximately one-third of patients with hyperparathyroidism have normal urine calcium excretion.
The extent of calcium excretion can be expressed as a urine calcium (U_{Ca})/ urine creatinine (U_{Cr}) ratio.
Normally,

$$\frac{U_{Ca}\,(mg/dL)}{U_{Cr}\,(mg/dL)} < 0.14$$

and

$$\frac{U_{Ca}\,(mmol/L)}{U_{Cr}\,(mmol/L)} < 0.40$$

Hypercalciuria is defined as a ratio of >0.20 or >0.57, respectively.
Test is useful in the evaluation of renal stones but is not usually needed for the diagnosis of hyperparathyroidism, which can be made using serum calcium (see above) and PTH measurements (see Figure 9–8). It may be useful in hypercalcemic patients to rule out familial hypocalciuric hypercalcemia.
In the diagnosis of hypercalciuria, U_{Ca}/U_{Cr} ratios in random single-voided urine specimens correlate well with 24-hour calcium excretions.
J Clin Pathol 2005;58:134. [PMID: 15677531]
Am Fam Physician 2006;74:86. [PMID: 16848382] |

Test/Range/Collection	Physiologic Basis	Interpretation	Comments
Carbon dioxide, partial pressure (Pco₂), whole blood Arterial: 32–48 mm Hg (4.26–6.38 kPa) Heparinized syringe $$$ Specimen must be collected in heparinized syringe and immediately transported on ice to lab without exposure to air.	The partial pressure of carbon dioxide in arterial blood (Pco₂) provides important information with regard to adequacy of ventilation, and acid–base balance.	**Increased in:** Respiratory acidosis: decreased alveolar ventilation (eg, COPD, respiratory depressants), neuromuscular diseases (eg, myasthenia gravis). **Decreased in:** Respiratory alkalosis: hyperventilation (eg, anxiety), sepsis, liver disease, fever, early salicylate poisoning, and excessive artificial ventilation.	See laboratory characteristics of acid–base disturbances (Figure 8–1, Table 8–1). Br J Nurs 2004;13:522. [PMID: 15215728] Dis Mon 2004;50:122. [PMID: 15069420] J Nephrol 2006;19(Suppl 9):S86. [PMID: 16736446]

Carbon dioxide, partial pressure

Carbon dioxide, (total bicarbonate) serum		Carboxyhemoglobin	
Carbon dioxide, (total bicarbonate) serum 22–28 meq/L [mmol/L] *Panic:* <15 or >40 meq/L [mmol/L] SST $	Bicarbonate-carbonic acid buffer is one of the most important buffer systems in maintaining normal body fluid pH. Total CO_2 is measured as the sum of bicarbonate concentration plus carbonic acid concentration plus dissolved CO_2. Because bicarbonate makes up 90–95% of the total CO_2 content, total CO_2 is a useful surrogate for bicarbonate concentration.	**Increased in:** Primary metabolic alkalosis, compensated respiratory acidosis, volume contraction, mineralocorticoid excess, congenital chloridorrhea. Drugs: diuretics (eg, thiazide, furosemide). **Decreased in:** Metabolic acidosis, compensated respiratory alkalosis. Fanconi syndrome, volume overload. Drugs: acetazolamide, outdated tetracycline.	Total CO_2 determination is indicated for all seriously ill patients on admission. If arterial blood gas studies are done, total CO_2 test is redundant. Simultaneous measurement of pH and Pco_2 is required to fully characterize a patient's acid–base status. See Acid–base disturbance (Table 8–1; Figure 8–1). Respir Care 2001;46:366. [PMID: 11262556] Respir Care 2001;46:342. [PMID: 11262554]
Carboxyhemoglobin, whole blood (COHb) <9% [<0.09] Blood gas syringe or Green $$ Specimen should be collected before treatment with oxygen is started. Do not remove stopper or cap.	Carbon monoxide (CO) is an odorless and nonirritating gas formed by hydrocarbon combustion. CO binds to hemoglobin with much greater affinity (~240 times) than oxygen, forming carboxyhemoglobin (COHb) and resulting in impaired oxygen transport/delivery and utilization. CO can also precipitate an inflammatory cascade that results in CNS lipid peroxidation and delayed neurologic sequelae.	**Increased in:** Carbon monoxide poisoning. Exposure to automobile exhaust, smoke from fires, coal gas, and defective furnaces. Cigarette smokers can have up to 9% carboxyhemoglobin, while nonsmokers have <2%.	Laboratory CO-oximetry is widely available for rapid evaluation of CO poisoning. Toxic effects (headache, dizziness, nausea, confusion, and/or unconsciousness) occur if the COHb level is higher than 10–15%. Levels above 40% may be fatal if not treated immediately with oxygen. Po_2 is usually normal in CO poisoning. J Emerg Med 2006;31:13. [PMID: 16798147] JAMA 2006;295:398. [PMID: 16434630]

Test/Range/Collection	Physiologic Basis	Interpretation	Comments
Carcinoembryonic antigen, serum (CEA) 0–2.5 ng/mL [mcg/L] Marbled $$	CEA is an oncofetal antigen, a glycoprotein associated with certain malignancies, particularly epithelial, tumors.	**Increased in:** Colon cancer (72%), lung cancer (76%), pancreatic cancer (91%), stomach cancer (61%), cigarette smokers, benign liver disease (acute 50% and chronic 90%), benign GI disease (peptic ulcer, pancreatitis, colitis). Elevations >20 ng/mL are generally associated with malignancy. For breast cancer recurrence (using 5 ng/mL cutoff), sensitivity 44.4% and specificity 95.5%.	**Screening:** Test is not sensitive or specific enough to be useful in cancer screening. **Monitoring after surgery:** Test is used to follow progression of colon cancer after surgery (elevated CEA levels suggest recurrence 3–6 months before other clinical indicators), although such monitoring has not yet been shown to improve survival rates. If monitoring is done, the same assay method must be used consistently in order to eliminate any method-dependent variability. Ann Clin Biochem 2004;41:370. [PMID: 15333188] Cancer Invest 2005;23:338. [PMID: 16100946]

CD4 cell count		
CD4 cell count, absolute, whole blood CD4: 359–1725 cells/mcL (29–61%) Lavender $$$ For an absolute CD4 count, order T-cell subsets and a CBC with differential.	Lymphocyte identification depends on specific cell surface CD (clusters of differentiation) antigens, which can be detected by flow cytometry analysis using monoclonal antibodies. The CD4 cells (helper T cells) express both CD3 (a pan–T-cell marker) and CD4. The CD8 cells (suppressor T cells) express both CD3 and CD8. CD4 cell levels are a criterion for categorizing HIV-related clinical conditions by CDC's classification system for HIV infection. The measurement of CD4 cell levels has been used to establish decision points for initiating prophylaxis and antiviral therapy and to monitor the efficacy of treatment. It has been recommended that CD4 cell levels be monitored every 3–6 months in all HIV-infected persons.	**Increased in:** Rheumatoid arthritis, type I diabetes mellitus, SLE without renal disease, primary biliary cirrhosis, atopic dermatitis, Sézary syndrome, psoriasis, chronic autoimmune hepatitis. **Decreased in:** AIDS/HIV infection, SLE with renal disease, acute cytomegalovirus (CMV) infection, burns, graft-versus-host disease, sunburn, myelodysplastic syndromes, acute lymphoblastic leukemia in remission, recovery from bone marrow transplantation, herpes infection, infectious mononucleosis, measles, ataxia-telangiectasia, vigorous exercise.	During HIV infection, antiviral therapy is often initiated when the absolute CD4 count drops below 500 cells/μL. When the absolute CD4 count drops below 200 cells/μL, therapeutic prophylaxis against phencyclidine (PCP) and other opportunistic infections may be initiated. When the absolute CD4 count drops below 100 cells/μL, prophylaxis against *Mycobacterium avium* complex is recommended. For longitudinal studies involving serial monitoring, specimen collections should be performed at the same time of day. JAMA 2006;296:827. [PMID: 16905788] JAMA 2006;296:1498. [PMID: 17003398] N Engl J Med 2006;355:1141. [PMID: 16971720]

Test/Range/Collection	Physiologic Basis	Interpretation	Comments
Centromere antibody, serum (ACA) Negative SST $$	Centromere antibodies are antibodies to nuclear proteins of the kinetochore plate.	**Positive in:** CREST (70–90%), scleroderma (10–15%), Raynaud disease (10–30%).	In patients with connective tissue disease, the predictive value of a positive test is >95% for scleroderma or related disease (CREST, Raynaud disease). Diagnosis of CREST is made clinically (calcinosis, Raynaud disease, esophageal dysmotility, sclerodactyly, and telangiectasia). In the absence of clinical findings, the test has low predictive value. (See also Autoantibodies, Table 8–6) Arthritis Res Ther 2003;5:80. [PMID: 12718748] Rheumatology (Oxford) 2005;44:1212. [PMID: 15870151]
Ceruloplasmin, serum 20–35 mg/dL [200–350 mg/L] SST $$	Ceruloplasmin, a 120,000–160,000 MW α_2-glycoprotein synthesized by the liver, is the main (95%) copper-carrying protein in human serum.	**Increased in:** Acute and chronic inflammation, pregnancy. Drugs: oral contraceptives, phenytoin. **Decreased in:** Wilson disease (hepatolenticular degeneration) (95%), CNS disease other than Wilson (15%), liver disease other than Wilson (23%), malabsorption, malnutrition, primary biliary cirrhosis, nephrotic syndrome, severe copper deficiency, Menkes disease (X-linked inherited copper deficiency).	Serum ceruloplasmin level and slit-lamp examination for Kayser-Fleischer rings are initial recommended tests for diagnosis of Wilson disease. Slit-lamp exam is only 50–60% sensitive in patients without neurological symptoms. Equivocal cases may need 24-hour urinary copper measurement. Serum copper level is rarely indicated. Over 5% of patients with Wilson disease have low–normal levels of ceruloplasmin. Aliment Pharmacol Ther 2004;19:157. [PMID: 14723607] Lancet 2007;369:397. [PMID: 17276780]

Chloride		
Chloride, serum (Cl⁻) 98–107 meq/L [mmol/L] SST $	Chloride, the principal inorganic anion of extracellular fluid, is important in maintaining normal acid–base balance and normal osmolality. If chloride is lost (as HCl or NH_4Cl), alkalosis ensues; if chloride is ingested or retained, acidosis ensues.	**Increased in:** Renal failure, nephrotic syndrome, renal tubular acidosis, dehydration, overtreatment with saline, hyperparathyroidism, diabetes insipidus, metabolic acidosis from diarrhea (loss of HCO_3^-), respiratory alkalosis, hyperadrenocorticism. Drugs: acetazolamide (hyperchloremic acidosis), androgens, hydrochlorothiazide, salicylates (intoxication). **Decreased in:** Vomiting, diarrhea, gastrointestinal suction, renal failure combined with salt deprivation, over-treatment with diuretics, chronic respiratory acidosis, diabetic ketoacidosis, excessive sweating, SIADH, salt-losing nephropathy, acute intermittent porphyria, water intoxication, expansion of extracellular fluid volume, adrenal insufficiency, hyperaldosteronism, metabolic alkalosis. Drugs: chronic laxative or bicarbonate ingestion, corticosteroids, diuretics.	Test is helpful in assessing normal and increased anion gap metabolic acidosis. It is somewhat helpful in distinguishing hypercalcemia due to primary hyperparathyroidism (high serum chloride) from that due to malignancy (normal serum chloride). Clin Chim Acta 2005;353:1. [PMID: 15698586]

	Cholesterol

Test/Range/Collection	Physiologic Basis	Interpretation	Comments
Cholesterol, Total, serum Desirable: <200 mg/dL [<5.2 mmol/L] Borderline: 200–239 mg/dL [5.2–6.1 mmol/L] High risk: >240 mg/dL [>6.2 mmol/L] SST $ Fasting specimen is required for LDL-C determination. HDL-C but total cholesterol can be measured with nonfasting specimen.	Cholesterol level is determined by lipid metabolism, which is in turn influenced by heredity, diet, and liver, kidney, thyroid, and other endocrine organ functions. Screening for total cholesterol (TC) may be done with nonfasting specimens, but a complete lipoprotein profile or LDL cholesterol (LDL-C) determination must be performed on fasting specimens. TC, triglyceride (TG), and high-density lipoprotein cholesterol (HDL-C) are directly measured. Although methods have been developed for direct LDL-C measurement, in practice, LDL-C is often indirectly determined by use of the Friedewald equation: $[LDL-C] = [TC] - [HDL-C] - [TG] / 5.$ Note that this calculation is not valid for specimens having TG >400 mg/dL [>4.52 mmol/L], for patients with type III hyperlipoproteinemia or chylomicronemia, or nonfasting specimens.	**Increased in:** Primary disorders: polygenic hypercholesterolemia, familial hypercholesterolemia (deficiency of LDL receptors), familial combined hyperlipidemia, familial dysbetalipoproteinemia. Secondary disorders: hypothyroidism, uncontrolled diabetes mellitus, nephrotic syndrome, biliary obstruction, anorexia nervosa, hepatocellular carcinoma, Cushing syndrome, acute intermittent porphyria. Drugs: corticosteroids. **Decreased in:** Severe liver disease (acute hepatitis, cirrhosis, malignancy), hyperthyroidism, severe acute or chronic illness, malnutrition, malabsorption (eg, HIV), extensive burns, familial (Gaucher disease, Tangier disease), abetalipoproteinemia, intestinal lymphangiectasia.	National Cholesterol Education Program (NCEP) expert panel has published clinical recommendations for cholesterol assessment and management. According to NCEP guidelines, HDL-C <40 mg/dL is a risk factor for coronary heart disease (CHD), and HDL-C ≥60 mg/dL is a "negative" risk factor. In addition, there is a direct relation between LDL-C and the incidence of CHD. Treatment decisions and therapeutic goals are primarily based on LDL-C concentrations. The recommended LDL-C intervention goals are <100 mg/dL for high-risk patients (eg, patients with CHD), <130 mg/dL for moderate-risk patients (≥2 risk factors), and <160 mg/dL for low-risk patients (no or 1 risk factor). See Table 8–10 for risk factor assessment for CHD. Am J Prevent Med 2001;20(3 Suppl):77. JAMA 2001;285:2486. Mayo Clinic Proc 2006;81:1225. [PMID: 16970219] Med Gen Med 2006;8:54. [PMID: 16915184]

Chorionic gonadotropin, β-subunit, quantitative		
Chorionic gonadotropin, β-subunit, quantitative, serum (β-hCG) Males and nonpregnant females: undetectable or <2 mIU/mL [IU/L] SST $$	Human chorionic gonadotropin is a glycoprotein made up of two subunits (α and β). Human glycoproteins such as LH, FSH, and TSH share the α-subunit of hCG, but the β-subunit is specific for hCG, and its detection in serum or urine is the basis for pregnancy testing. Serum hCG can be detected as early as 24 hours after implantation at a concentration of 5 mIU/mL. During normal pregnancy, serum levels double every 2–3 days and are 50–100 mIU/mL at the time of the first missed menstrual period. Peak levels are reached 60–80 days after the last menstrual period (LMP) (30,000–100,000 mIU/mL), and levels then decrease to a plateau of 5,000–10,000 mIU/mL at about 120 days after LMP and persist until delivery.	**Increased in:** Pregnancy (including ectopic pregnancy), hyperemesis gravidarum, trophoblastic tumors (hydatidiform mole, choriocarcinoma of uterus), some germ cell tumors (teratomas of ovary or testicle, seminoma), ectopic hCG production by other malignancies (stomach, pancreas, lung, colon, liver). Failure of elevated serum levels to decrease after surgical resection of trophoblastic tumor indicates metastatic tumor; levels rising from normal indicate tumor recurrence. **Decreasing over time:** Threatened abortion.	Routine pregnancy testing is done by *qualitative* serum or urine hCG test. Test is positive (>50 mIU/mL) in most pregnant women at the time of or shortly after the first missed menstrual period. *Quantitative* hCG testing is indicated for: (1) the evaluation of suspected ectopic pregnancy (where levels are lower than in normal pregnancy at the same gestational age) if the routine pregnancy test is negative and (2) the evaluation of threatened abortion. In both situations, hCG levels fail to demonstrate the normal early pregnancy increase. Viable pregnancies exhibit an hCG increase of at least 50% over 2 days. Test is also indicated for following the course of trophoblastic and germ cell tumors. Clin Obstet Gynecol 2003;46:523. [PMID: 12972735] CMAJ 2005;173:905. [PMID: 16217116]

Test/Range/Collection	Physiologic Basis	Interpretation	Comments
Clostridium difficile enterotoxin, stool Negative (≤1:10 titer) Urine or stool container $$$ Must be tested within 12 hours of collection as toxin (B) is labile.	_Clostridium difficile_, a motile, gram-positive rod, is the major recognized agent of antibiotic-associated diarrhea, which is toxigenic in origin (see Antibiotic-associated colitis). There are two toxins (A and B) produced by _C difficile_. Cell culture is used to detect the cytopathic effect of the toxins, whose identity is confirmed by neutralization with specific antitoxins. Toxin A (more weakly cytopathic in cell culture) is enterotoxic and produces enteric disease. Toxin B (more easily detected in standard cell culture assays) fails to produce intestinal disease.	**Positive in:** Antibiotic-associated diarrhea (15–25%), antibiotic-associated colitis (50–75%), and pseudomembranous colitis (90–100%). About 3% of healthy adults and 10–20% of hospitalized patients have _C difficile_ in their colonic flora. There is also a high carrier rate of _C difficile_ and its toxin in healthy neonates.	Definitive diagnosis of disease caused by _C difficile_ toxin is by endoscopic detection of pseudomembranous colitis. Direct examination of stool for leukocytes, gram-positive rods, or blood is not helpful. Culture of _C difficile_ is not routinely performed, because it would isolate numerous nontoxigenic _C difficile_ strains. CMAJ 2004;171:51. [PMID: 15238498] Am Fam Physician 2005;71:921. [PMID: 15768622] Cleve Clin J Med 2006;73:187. [PMID: 16478043]

Coccidioides antibodies		
Coccidioides antibodies, serum or CSF Negative SST $$	Screens for presence of antibodies to *Coccidioides immitis.* Some centers use the mycelial-phase antigen, coccidioidin, to detect antibody. IgM antibodies appear early in disease in 75% of patients, begin to decrease after week 3, and are rarely seen after 5 months. They may persist in disseminated cases, usually in the immunocompromised. IgG antibodies appear later in the course of the disease. Meningeal disease may have negative serum IgG and require CSF IgG antibody titers.	**Positive in:** Infection by coccidioides (90%). **Negative in:** Coccidioidin skin testing, many patients with chronic cavitary coccidioides; 5% of meningeal coccidioides is negative by CSF complement fixation (CF) test.	Diagnosis is based on culture and serologic testing. Precipitin and CF tests detect 90% of primary symptomatic cases. Precipitin test is most effective in detecting early primary infection or an exacerbation of existing disease. Test is diagnostic but not prognostic. CF test becomes positive later than precipitin test, and titers can be used to assess severity of infection. Titers rise as the disease progresses and decline as the patient improves. Enzyme immunoassay now available; data suggest good test performance characteristics. Clin Infect Dis 2005;41:1217. [PMID: 16206093] Clin Infect Dis 2006;42:103. [PMID: 16323099]

	Cold agglutinins		
Test/Range/Collection	Physiologic Basis	Interpretation	Comments
Cold agglutinins, serum or plasma <1:32 titer Red, lavender $$ Specimen should be kept in warm water (37°C) before separation from cells.	Cold agglutinins are autoantibodies that are capable of agglutinating red blood cells (RBCs) at temperature below 35°C (strongly at 4°C, weakly at 24°C, and weakly or not at all at 37°C). Cold agglutinins can be monoclonal or polyclonal, and have been associated with various diseases, particularly infections, neoplasms, and collagen vascular diseases. Cold agglutinins are not necessarily pathologic, and may be detected in asymptomatic individuals during routine blood typing and cross-matching. If the agglutination is not reversible after incubation at 37°C, then the reaction is not due to cold agglutinins.	**Increased in:** Chronic cold agglutinin disease, lymphoproliferative disorders (eg, Waldenström macroglobulinemia, chronic lymphocytic leukemia), autoimmune hemolytic anemia, myeloma, collagen-vascular diseases, *Mycoplasma pneumoniae* pneumonia, infectious mononucleosis, mumps orchitis, cytomegalovirus, listeriosis, tropical diseases (eg, trypanosomiasis, malaria).	Patients with cold agglutinins develop anti-i or anti-I antibodies which are usually of the IgM class and react with adult human RBCs at temperature below 35°C, resulting in agglutination. In *Mycoplasma* pneumonia, titers of anti-I rise late in the first week or during the second week, are maximal at 3–4 weeks after onset, and then disappear rapidly. A rise in cold agglutinin antibody titer is suggestive of recent mycoplasma infection. Haematologica 2006;91:439. [PMID: 16585009] Transfusion 2006;46:324. [PMID: 16533272]

	Complement C3	Complement C4
Complement C3, serum 64–166 mg/dL [640–1660 mg/L] SST $$	The classic and alternative complement pathways converge at the C3 step in the complement cascade. Low levels indicate activation by one or both pathways. Most diseases with immune complexes show decreased C3 levels. Test is usually performed as an immunoassay (by radial immunodiffusion or nephelometry).	**Increased in:** Many inflammatory conditions as an acute-phase reactant, active phase of rheumatic diseases (eg, rheumatoid arthritis, SLE), acute viral hepatitis, myocardial infarction, cancer, diabetes mellitus, pregnancy, sarcoidosis, amyloidosis, thyroiditis. **Decreased by:** Decreased synthesis (protein malnutrition, congenital deficiency, severe liver disease), increased catabolism (immune complex disease, membranoproliferative glomerulonephritis [75%], SLE, Sjögren syndrome, rheumatoid arthritis, DIC, paroxysmal nocturnal hemoglobinuria, autoimmune hemolytic anemia, gram-negative bacteremia), increased loss (burns, gastroenteropathies).	Complement C3 levels may be useful in following the activity of immune complex diseases. The best test to detect inherited deficiencies is CH50. N Engl J Med 1987;316:1525. [PMID: 3295544] Intern Med 2001;40:1254. [PMID: 11813855] Curr Rheumatol Rep 2004;6:375. [PMID: 15355750]
Complement C4, serum 15–45 mg/dL [150–450 mg/L] SST $$	C4 is a component of the classic complement pathway. Depressed levels usually indicate classic pathway activation. Test is usually performed as an immunoassay and not a functional assay.	**Increased in:** Various malignancies (not clinically useful). **Decreased by:** Decreased synthesis (congenital deficiency), increased catabolism (SLE, rheumatoid arthritis, proliferative glomerulonephritis, HAE), and increased loss (burns, protein-losing enteropathies).	Low C4 accompanies acute attacks of HAE, and C4 is used as a first-line test for the disease. C1 esterase inhibitor levels are not indicated for the evaluation of hereditary HAE unless C4 is low. Congenital C4 deficiency occurs with an SLE-like syndrome. N Engl J Med 1987;316:1525. [PMID: 3295544] Am J Med 1990;88:656. [PMID: 2189311]

Complement CH50

Test/Range/Collection	Physiologic Basis	Interpretation	Comments
Complement CH50, plasma or serum (CH50) 22–40 U/mL (laboratory-specific) SST $$$	The quantitative assay of hemolytic complement activity depends on the ability of the classic complement pathway to induce hemolysis of red cells sensitized with optimal amounts of anti–red cell antibodies. For precise titrations of hemolytic complement, the dilution of serum that lyse 50% of the indicator red cells is determined as the CH50. This arbitrary unit depends on the conditions of the assay and is therefore laboratory-specific.	**Decreased with:** >50–80% deficiency of classic pathway complement components (congenital or acquired deficiencies). **Normal in:** Deficiencies of the alternative pathway complement components.	This is a functional assay of biologic activity. Sensitivity to decreased levels of complement components depends on exactly how the test is performed. It is used to detect congenital and acquired severe deficiency disorders of the classic complement pathway. N Engl J Med 1987;316:1525. [PMID: 3295544] Pediatr Clin North Am 2000;47:1339. [PMID: 11130999]

Complete blood cell count		
Complete blood cell count (CBC), blood Refer to individual test for reference range Lavender $	The CBC consists of a panel of tests that examines different parts of the whole blood and includes the following: total white blood cell count (WBC, $\times 10^3$/mcL) and white blood cell differential (%), red blood cell count (RBC, $\times 10^6$/mcL), hemoglobin concentration (Hb, g/L), hematocrit (Hct, %), platelet count (Plt, $\times 10^3$/mcL), red cell indices including mean corpuscular volume (MCV, fL), mean corpuscular hemoglobin (MCH, pg), mean corpuscular hemoglobin concentration (MCHC, g/L), and red cell distribution width (RDW, %). Automated laboratory hematology analyzers are widely available. The basic principles used for the cell counting and white cell differential are instrument-dependent.	Refer to individual test for detailed information. Also see Table 8–29 for white cell count and differential.	The CBC test provides important information about the types and numbers of cells in the blood, especially red cells, white cells, and platelets. It helps in evaluating symptoms (eg, weakness, fatigue, fever or bruising), diagnosing conditions/diseases (eg, anemia, infection, leukemia, and many other disorders), and determining the stages of a particular disease. Hct, MCH, and MCHC are typically calculated from RBC, Hb and MCV. If significantly abnormal CBC values are obtained, a peripheral blood smear should be prepared and examined (eg, red cell morphology, WBC differential, platelet count estimation, identification of immature and malignant cells). (see Figure 2–2). Lab Hematol 2005;11:285. [PMID: 16475476] Mayo Clin Proc 2005;80:923. [PMID: 16007898] Arch Pathol Lab Med 2006;130:596. [PMID: 16683868] Lab Hematol 2006;12:15. [PMID: 16513543]

Test/Range/Collection	Physiologic Basis	Interpretation	Comments
Cortisol, plasma or serum 8:00 AM: 5–20 mcg/dL [140–550 nmol/L] SST, lavender, or green $$	Release of corticotropin-releasing factor (CRF) from the hypothalamus stimulates release of ACTH from the pituitary, which in turn stimulates release of cortisol from the adrenal. Cortisol provides negative feedback to this system. Test measures both free cortisol and cortisol bound to cortisol-binding globulin (CBG). Morning levels are higher than evening levels.	**Increased in:** Cushing syndrome, acute illness, surgery, trauma, septic shock, depression, anxiety, alcoholism, starvation, chronic renal failure, increased CBG (congenital, pregnancy, estrogen therapy). **Decreased in:** Addison disease; decreased CBG (congenital, liver disease, nephrotic syndrome).	Cortisol levels are useful only in the context of standardized suppression or stimulation tests. See Cosyntropin stimulation test and Dexamethasone suppression tests for details. Circadian fluctuations in cortisol levels limit usefulness of single measurements. Analysis of diurnal variation of cortisol is not useful diagnostically. J Endocrinol Invest 2003;26(7 Suppl):74. [PMID: 14604069] J Clin Endocrinol Metab 2006;91:3746. [PMID: 16866050]
Cortisol (urinary free), urine 10–110 mcg/24 h [30–300 nmol/d] Urine bottle containing boric acid. $$$ Collect 24-hour urine.	Urinary free cortisol measurement is useful in the initial evaluation of suspected Cushing syndrome (see Cushing syndrome algorithm, Figure 8–8).	**Increased in:** Cushing syndrome, acute illness, stress. **Not increased in:** Obesity.	Urinary free cortisol is the initial diagnostic test of choice for Cushing syndrome. Not useful for the diagnosis of adrenal insufficiency. A shorter (12-hour) overnight collection and measurement of the ratio of urine-free cortisol to urine creatinine appears to perform nearly as well as a 24-hour collection for urine-free cortisol. Ann Intern Med 2003;138:980. [PMID: 12809455] Am J Med 2005;118:1340. [PMID: 16378774]

	Cosyntropin stimulation test	Creatine kinase
Cosyntropin stimulation test, serum or plasma Marbled, green, or lavender $$$ First draw a cortisol level. Then administer cosyntropin (1 mcg or 250 mcg IV). Draw another cortisol level in 30 minutes.	Cosyntropin (synthetic ACTH preparation) stimulates the adrenal to release cortisol. A normal response is a doubling of basal levels or an increment of 7 mcg/dL (200 nmol/L) to a level above 18 mcg/dL (>504 nmol/L). A poor cortisol response to cosyntropin indicates adrenal insufficiency (see Adrenocortical insufficiency algorithm, Figure 8–3).	**Decreased in:** Adrenal insufficiency, pituitary insufficiency, AIDS.	Test does not distinguish primary from secondary (pituitary) adrenal insufficiency, because in secondary adrenal insufficiency the atrophic adrenal may be unresponsive to cosyntropin. Test may not reliably detect pituitary insufficiency. Metyrapone test may be useful to assess the pituitary-adrenal axis. AIDS patients with adrenal insufficiency may have normal ACTH stimulation tests. Ann Intern Med 2003;139:194. [PMID: 12809455] J Clin Endocrinol Metab 2005;90:4973. [PMID: 16087959]
Creatine kinase, serum (CK) 32–267 IU/L [0.53–4.45 mckat/L] (method-dependent) SST $	Creatine kinase splits creatine phosphate in the presence of ADP to yield creatine and ATP. Skeletal muscle, myocardium, and brain are rich in the enzyme. CK is released by tissue damage.	**Increased in:** Myocardial infarction (MI), myocarditis, muscle trauma, rhabdomyolysis, muscular dystrophy, polymyositis, severe muscular exertion, malignant hyperthermia, hypothyroidism, cerebral infarction, surgery, Reye syndrome, tetanus, generalized convulsions, alcoholism, IM injections, DC countershock. Drugs: clofibrate, HMG-CoA reductase inhibitors.	CK is as sensitive a test as aldolase for muscle damage, so aldolase is not needed. During an MI, serum CK level rises rapidly (within 3–5 hours); elevation persists for 2–3 days post-MI. Total CK is not specific enough for use in diagnosis of MI, but a normal total CK has a high negative predictive value. A more specific test is needed for diagnosis of MI or acute coronary syndrome (eg, CK-MB, now largely replaced by cardiac troponin I). Prog Cardiovasc Dis 2004;46:404. [PMID: 15179629] Crit Care 2005;9:158. [PMID: 15774072] Curr Rheumatol Rep 2006;8:178. [PMID: 16901075]

Creatine kinase MB

Test/Range/Collection	Physiologic Basis	Interpretation	Comments
Creatine kinase MB, serum enzyme activity (CK-MB) <16 IU/L [<0.27 mckat/L] or <4% of total CK or <7 mcg/L mass units (laboratory-specific) SST $$	CK consists of three isoenzymes, made up of 2 subunits, M and B. The fraction with the greatest electrophoretic mobility is CK1 (BB), CK2 (MB) is intermediate, and CK3 (MM) moves slowest toward the anode. Skeletal muscle is characterized by isoenzyme MM and brain by isoenzyme BB. Myocardium has approximately 40% MB isoenzyme. Assay techniques include isoenzyme separation by electrophoresis (isoenzyme activity units) or immunoassay using antibody specific for MB fraction (mass units).	**Increased in:** Myocardial infarction, cardiac trauma, certain muscular dystrophies, and polymyositis. Slight persistent elevation reported in a few patients on hemodialysis.	CK-MB is a relatively specific test for MI. It appears in serum approximately 4 hours after infarction, peaks at 12–24 hours, and declines over 48–72 hours. CK-MB mass concentration is a more sensitive marker of MI than CK-MB isoenzymes or total CK within 4–12 hours after infarction. Cardiac troponin I levels are useful in the late (after 48 hours) diagnosis of MI because, unlike CK-MB levels, they remain elevated for 5–7 days. Within 48 hours, sensitivity and specificity of troponin I are similar to CK-MB. Specificity of troponin I is higher than CK-MB in patients with skeletal muscle injury or renal failure, or postoperatively. Cardiac troponin I is therefore the preferred test. Estimation of CK-MM and CK-BB is not clinically useful. Use total CK. Prog Cardiovasc Dis 2004;46:404. [PMID: 15179629]

Creatinine		
Creatinine, serum (Cr) 0.6–1.2 mg/dL [50–100 mcmol/L] SST $	Endogenous creatinine is excreted by filtration through the glomerulus and by tubular secretion. Creatinine clearance is an acceptable clinical measure of glomerular filtration rate (GFR), although it sometimes overestimates GFR (eg, in cirrhosis). For each 50% reduction in GFR, serum creatinine approximately doubles.	**Increased in:** Acute or chronic renal failure, urinary tract obstruction, nephrotoxic drugs, hypothyroidism. **Decreased in:** Reduced muscle mass.	In the alkaline picrate method, substances other than Cr (eg, acetoacetate, acetone, β-hydroxybutyrate, α-ketoglutarate, pyruvate, glucose) may give falsely high results. Therefore, patients with diabetic ketoacidosis may have spuriously elevated Cr. Cephalosporins may spuriously increase or decrease Cr measurement. Increased bilirubin may spuriously decrease Cr. Chronic renal insufficiency may be underrecognized. Age, male gender, and black race are predictors of kidney disease. Serum creatinine levels frequently do not reflect decreased renal function because creatinine production rate is decreased with reduced lean body mass. Increased intravascular volume and increased volume of distribution associated with anasarca may also mask decreased renal function by reducing serum creatinine levels. See glomerular filtration rate, estimated (eGFR). Am Fam Physician 2004;70:1091. [PMID: 15456118] Am Fam Physician 2005;72:1723. [PMID: 16300034]

Test/Range/Collection	Physiologic Basis	Interpretation	Comments
Creatinine clearance (Cl_{Cr}) Adults: 90–130 mL/ min/1.73 m^2 BSA $$ Collect carefully timed 24-hour urine and simultaneous serum/plasma creatinine sample. Record patient's weight and height.	Widely used test of glomerular filtration rate. Theoretically reliable, but often compromised by incomplete urine collection. Creatinine clearance is calculated from measurement of urine creatinine (U_{Cr} [mg/dL]), plasma/serum creatinine (P_{Cr} [mg/dL]), and urine flow rate (V [mL/min]) according to the formula: $$Cl_{Cr}(mL/min) = \frac{U_{Cr} \times V}{P_{Cr}}$$ where $$V(mL/min) = \frac{24\text{-hour urine volume (mL)}}{1440(min/24h)}$$ Creatinine clearance is often "corrected" for body surface area (BSA [m^2]) according to the formula: $$Cl_{Cr} \atop (corrected) = \frac{Cl_{Cr}}{(corrected)} \times \frac{1.73}{BSA}$$	**Increased in:** High cardiac output, exercise, acromegaly, diabetes mellitus (early stage), infections, hypothyroidism. **Decreased in:** Acute or chronic renal failure, decreased renal blood flow (shock, hemorrhage, dehydration, CHF). Drugs: nephrotoxic drugs.	Serum Cr may, in practice, be a more reliable indicator of renal function than 24-hour Cl_{Cr} unless urine collection is carefully monitored. An 8-hour collection provides results similar to those obtained with a 24-hour collection. Cl_{Cr} will overestimate glomerular filtration rate to the extent that Cr is secreted by the renal tubules (eg, in cirrhosis). Cl_{Cr} can be estimated from the serum creatinine using the following formula: $$Cl_{Cr} \atop (mL/min) = \frac{(140 - Age) \times Wt(kg)}{72 \times P_{Cr}}$$ Serial decline in Cl_{Cr} is the most reliable indicator of progressive renal dysfunction. Also see GFR, estimated (eGFR). Clin Chem 2006;52:5. [PMID: 16332993]

		Cryoglobulins	Cryptococcal antigen
Cryoglobulins, serum Negative SST $ Patients should be fasting and blood sample must be immediately transported to lab in warm water (37°C)	Cryoglobulins are immunoglobulins (IgG, IgM, IgA, or light chains) which precipitate on exposure to cold. The sample is stored at 4°C and examined daily for the presence or absence of cryoglobulins over a period of 3–5 days. Type I cryoglobulins (25%) are monoclonal immunoglobulins, most commonly IgM, occasionally IgG, and rarely IgA or Bence Jones protein. Type II (25%) are mixed cryoglobulins with a monoclonal component (usually IgM but occasionally IgG or IgA) that complexes with polyclonal normal IgG in the cryoprecipitate. Type III (50%) are mixed polyclonal cryoglobulins (IgM and IgG).	**Positive in:** Immunoproliferative disorders (multiple myeloma, Waldenström macroglobulinemia, chronic lymphocytic leukemia, lymphoma), collagen-vascular disease (SLE, polyarteritis nodosa, rheumatoid arthritis, Sjögren syndrome), hemolytic anemia, infections (eg, HCV, HIV), glomerulonephritis, chronic liver disease. The term "essential mixed cryoglobulinemia" (a vasculitic syndrome) is used to refer to patients with no primary disease other than Sjögren syndrome; other cases are classified as secondary mixed cryoglobulinemia.	All types of cryoglobulins may cause cold-induced symptoms, including Raynaud phenomenon, vascular purpura, and urticaria. Patients with type I cryoglobulinemia usually suffer from underlying disease (eg, multiple myeloma). Patients with type II and III cryoglobulinemia often have immune complex disease, with vascular purpura, bleeding tendencies, arthritis, and nephritis. Typing of cryoglobulins by electrophoresis is not necessary for diagnosis or clinical management. About 50% of essential mixed cryoglobulinemia patients have evidence of hepatitis C infection. Ann Clin Lab Sci 2006;36:395. [PMID: 17127726] Curr Opin Rheumatol 2006;18:54. [PMID: 16344620]
Cryptococcal antigen, serum or CSF Negative SST (serum) or glass or plastic tube (CSF) $$	The capsular polysaccharide of *Cryptococcus neoformans* potentiates opportunistic infections by the yeast. The cryptococcal antigen test used is often a latex agglutination test.	**Increased in:** Cryptococcal infection.	False-positive and false-negative results have been reported. False-positives due to rheumatoid factor can be reduced by pretreatment of serum using pronase before testing. Sensitivity and specificity of serum cryptococcal antigen titer for cryptococcal meningitis are 91% and 83%, respectively. Ninety-six percent of cryptococcal infections occur in AIDS patients. Infect Dis Clin North Am 2001;15:567. [PMID: 11447710] Murray PR et al (editors): *Manual of Clinical Microbiology*, 8th ed. ASM Press, 2003.

Cytomegalovirus antibody			
Test/Range/Collection	Physiologic Basis	Interpretation	Comments
Cytomegalovirus antibody, serum (CMV) Negative SST $$$	Detects the presence of antibody to CMV, either IgG or IgM. CMV infection is usually acquired during childhood or early adulthood. By age 20–40 years, 40–90% of the population has CMV antibodies.	**Increased in:** Previous or active CMV infection. False-positive CMV IgM tests occur when rheumatoid factor or infectious mononucleosis is present.	Serial specimens exhibiting a greater than fourfold titer rise suggest a recent infection. Active CMV infection must be documented by viral isolation. Useful for screening of potential organ donors and recipients. Universal prophylaxis reduces infection in transplant recipients. Detection of CMV IgM antibody in the serum of a newborn usually indicates congenital infection. Detection of CMV IgG antibody is not diagnostic, because maternal CMV IgG antibody passed via the placenta can persist in newborn's serum for 6 months. CMV seronegative blood components are more efficacious than leukocyte-reduced blood components in preventing transfusion-acquired CMV infection. Ann Intern Med 2005;143:870. [PMID: 16365468] Transfus Med Rev 2005;19:181. [PMID: 16010649]

	D-dimer	Dexamethasone suppression test (low dose)
D-dimer, plasma Negative Blue $$	D-dimer is one of the fibrin degradation products. The presence of D-dimers indicates that a fibrin clot was formed and subsequently degraded by plasmin. Essentially, a D-dimer is present whenever the coagulation system has been activated, followed by fibrinolysis. **Increased in:** Deep vein thrombosis (DVT), disseminated intravascular coagulation (DIC), pulmonary embolism (PE), arterial thromboembolism, pregnancy (especially postpartum period), malignancy, surgery, thrombolytic therapy.	D-dimer assay is a very sensitive test for DIC, DVT and PE. The D-dimer can be measured by a variety of methods: semiquantitative vs quantitative, manual vs automated, latex agglutination vs ELISA. The newly developed highly sensitive automated D-dimer tests reportedly may be used to exclude PE and DVT: a negative test essentially rules out thrombosis, and further testing (eg, ultrasound) is recommended. See Figure 8–20 and Table 8–18 for its use in pulmonary embolism evaluation. N Engl J Med 2003;349:1227. [PMID: 14507948] Ann Intern Med 2004;140:589. [PMID: 15096330] Intern Emerg Med 2006;1:59. [PMID: 16941816]
Dexamethasone suppression test (single low dose, overnight), serum 8:00 AM serum cortisol level: <5 mcg/dL [<140 nmol/L] $$ Give 1 mg dexamethasone at 11:00 PM. At 8:00 AM, draw serum cortisol level.	In normal patients, dexamethasone suppresses the 8:00 AM serum cortisol level below 5 mcg/dL. Patients with Cushing syndrome have 8:00 AM levels >10 mcg/dL (>276 nmol/L). **Positive in:** Cushing syndrome (sensitivity is high in severe cases but less so in mild ones; specificity is 70–90% in patients with chronic illness or hospitalized patients.).	Good screening test for Cushing syndrome. If this test is abnormal, use high-dose dexamethasone suppression test (see below) to determine etiology. (See also Cushing syndrome algorithm, Figure 8–8.) Patients taking phenytoin may fail to suppress because of enhanced dexamethasone metabolism. Depressed patients may also fail to suppress morning cortisol level. N Engl J Med 2007;356:601. [PMID: 17287480]

Test/Range/Collection	Physiologic Basis	Interpretation	Comments
Dexamethasone suppression test (high-dose, overnight), serum 8:00 AM serum cortisol level: <5 mcg/dL [<140 nmol/L] $$ Give 8 mg dexamethasone dose at 11:00 PM. At 8:00 AM, draw cortisol level.	Suppression of plasma cortisol levels to <50% of baseline with dexamethasone indicates Cushing disease (pituitary-dependent ACTH hypersecretion) and differentiates this from adrenal and ectopic Cushing syndrome (see Cushing syndrome algorithm, Figure 8–8).	**Positive in:** Cushing disease (88–92% sensitivity; specificity 57–100%).	Test indicated only after a positive low-dose dexamethasone suppression test (see above). Sensitivity and specificity depend on sampling time and diagnostic criteria. Measurement of urinary 17-hydroxycorticosteroids has been replaced in this test by measurement of serum cortisol. Bilateral sampling of the inferior petrosal sinuses for ACTH after administration of corticotrophin-releasing hormone has been used to identify the site of adenoma before surgery. Eur J Endocrinol 2006;155 (Suppl 1):S93. [PMID: 17075004]
Double-stranded-DNA antibody (ds-DNA Ab), serum <1:10 titer SST $$	IgG or IgM antibodies directed against host double-stranded DNA.	**Increased in:** Systemic lupus erythematosus (60–70% sensitivity, 95% specificity) based on >1:10 titer. **Not increased in:** Drug-induced lupus.	High titers are seen only in SLE. Titers of ds-DNA antibody correlate moderately well with disease activity and with occurrence of glomerulonephritis. (See also Autoantibodies, Table 8–6.) Curr Opin Rheumatol 2000;12:364. [PMID: 10990170] Clin Chem 2004;50:2169. [PMID: 15502090] Lupus 2006;15:397. [PMID: 16898172]

	Drug abuse screen, urine	Epstein-Barr virus antibodies
Drug abuse screen, urine Negative $	Testing for drugs of abuse usually involves testing a single urine specimen for a number of drugs, such as cocaine, opiates, barbiturates, amphetamines, benzodiazepines, cannabinoids, methadone, oxycodone, phencyclidine (PCP), tricyclic antidepressants. Screening tests are often immunoassays, which may not be specific for the tested drug. A positive test may warrant further confirmatory test by gas chromatography-mass spectrometry (GC/MS), the most widely accepted method for drug confirmation.	**Positive in:** Chronic and casual drug users. (sensitivity and specificity are assay-dependent).	It is important to know which drugs are included in the drug abuse screen and to understand that the test is qualitative and not quantitative. A single urine drug test detects only fairly recent drug use, and does not differentiate casual use from chronic drug use. The latter requires sequential drug testing and clinical evaluation. Urine drug testing does not determine the degree of impairment, the dose of drug taken, or the exact time of drug use. *Handbook of Workplace Drug Testing,* Washington, DC, AACC Press, 1995. Clin Chem 2003;49:357. [PMID: 12600948]
Epstein-Barr virus antibodies, serum (EBV Ab) Negative Marbled $$	Antiviral capsid antibodies (anti-VCA) (IgM) often reach their peak at clinical presentation and last up to 3 months; anti-VCA IgG antibodies last for life. Early antigen antibodies (anti-EA) are next to develop, are most often positive at 1 month after presentation, typically last for 2–3 months, and may last up to 6 months in low titers. Anti-EA may also be found in some patients with Hodgkin disease, chronic lymphocytic leukemia, and some other malignancies. Anti-EB nuclear antigen (anti-EBNA) antibody begins to appear in a minority of patients in the third or fourth week but is uniformly present by 6 months.	**Increased in:** EB virus infection, infectious mononucleosis. Antibodies to the diffuse (D) form of antigen (detected in the cytoplasm and nucleus of infected cells) are greatly elevated in nasopharyngeal carcinoma. Antibodies to the restricted (R) form of antigen (detected only in the cytoplasm of infected cells) are greatly elevated in Burkitt lymphoma.	Most useful in diagnosing infectious mononucleosis in patients who have the clinical and hematologic criteria for the disease but who fail to develop the heterophile agglutinins (10%) (see Heterophile antibody). EBV antibodies cannot be used to diagnose "chronic" mononucleosis. Chronic fatigue syndrome is not caused by EBV. The best indicator of primary infection is a positive anti-VCA IgM (check for false-positives caused by rheumatoid factor). Rose NR et al (eds.): *Manual of Clinical Laboratory Immunology,* 6th ed. American Society for Microbiology, 2002. Am Fam Physician 2004;70:1279. [PMID: 15508538]

	Erythrocyte sedimentation rate		
Test/Range/Collection	**Physiologic Basis**	**Interpretation**	**Comments**
Erythrocyte sedimentation rate, whole blood (ESR) Male: <10 Female: <15 mm/h (laboratory-specific) Lavender $ Test must be run within 2 hours after sample collection.	In plasma, erythrocytes (red blood cells [RBCs]) usually settle slowly. However, if they aggregate for any reason (usually because of plasma proteins called acute-phase reactants, eg, fibrinogen), they settle rapidly. Sedimentation of RBCs occurs because their density is greater than plasma. ESR measures the distance in millimeters that erythrocytes fall during 1 hour.	**Increased in:** Infections (osteomyelitis, pelvic inflammatory disease [75%]), inflammatory disease (temporal arteritis, polymyalgia rheumatica, rheumatic fever), malignant neoplasms, paraproteinemias, anemia, pregnancy, chronic renal failure, GI disease (ulcerative colitis, regional ileitis). For endocarditis, sensitivity is approximately 93%. **Decreased in:** Polycythemia, sickle cell anemia, spherocytosis, anisocytosis, poikilocytosis, hypofibrinogenemia, hypogammaglobulinemia, congestive heart failure, microcytosis, certain drugs (eg, high-dose corticosteroids).	There is a good correlation between ESR and C-reactive protein, but ESR is less expensive. Test is useful and indicated only for diagnosis and monitoring of temporal arteritis, and polymyalgia rheumatica. The test is not sensitive or specific for other conditions. ESR is higher in women, blacks, and older persons. Low value is of no diagnostic significance. ESR should not be used to screen asymptomatic persons for disease due to its low sensitivity and specificity. Ann Intern Med 1986;104:515. [PMID: 3954279] JAMA 2002;287:92. [PMID: 11754714] Am J Clin Pathol 2004;122:802. [PMID: 15491977] Am Fam Physician 2006;74:1547. [PMID: 17111894]

	Erythropoietin	Ethanol
Erythropoietin, serum or non-EDTA plasma (EPO) 5–30 mIU/mL [5–30 IU/L] SST $$$	Erythropoietin (EPO) is a glycoprotein hormone produced in the kidney that induces RBC production by stimulating proliferation, differentiation, and maturation of erythroid precursors. Hypoxia is the usual stimulus for production of EPO. EPO has also been shown to have an important cytoprotective function in the neuronal and cardiovascular systems.	**Increased in:** Anemias associated with bone marrow hyporesponsiveness (aplastic anemia, iron deficiency anemia), hemolytic anemia, secondary polycythemia (high-altitude hypoxia, COPD, pulmonary fibrosis), EPO producing tumors (cerebellar hemangioblastomas, pheochromocytomas, renal tumors), kidney transplant rejection, pregnancy, polycystic kidney disease, treatment with recombinant human EPO (eg, Epogen). **Decreased in:** Anemia of chronic disease, renal failure, inflammatory states, primary polycythemia (polycythemia vera) (39%), HIV infection with AZT treatment.	EPO levels are useful in differentiating primary from secondary polycythemia and in detecting recurrence of EPO-producing tumors. See diagnostic evaluation of polycythemia (Figure 8–18). Because virtually all patients with severe anemia due to chronic renal failure respond to EPO therapy, pre-therapy EPO levels are not necessary. Patients receiving recombinant human EPO as chronic therapy should have iron studies performed routinely. JAMA 2005;293:90. [PMID: 15632341] N Engl J Med 2005;352:1011. [PMID: 15758012] Mayo Clin Proc 2006;81:1188. [PMID: 16970215]
Ethanol, serum (EtOH) 0 mg/dL [mmol/L] SST $$ Do not use alcohol swab. Do not remove stopper.	Measures serum level of ethyl alcohol (ethanol).	**Present in:** Ethanol ingestion.	Whole blood alcohol concentrations are about 15% lower than serum concentrations. Each 0.1 mg/dL of ethanol contributes about 22 mosm/kg to serum osmolality (see Table 8–14). Legal intoxication in many states is defined as >80 mg/dL (>17 mmol/L). N Engl J Med 1976;294:757. [PMID: 3733] Accid Anal Prev 2005;37:149. [PMID: 15607286]

Test/Range/Collection	Physiologic Basis	Interpretation	Comments
		Factor assays	**Factor II (prothrombin) mutation**
Factor assays (coagulation factors II, V, VII, VIII, IX, X, XI, and XII) Blood Blue 50–150% $$$ Deliver immediately to laboratory on ice. Stable for 2 hours. Freeze if assay is delayed >2 hours.	The partial thromboplastin time (PTT) and prothrombin time (PT) are the bases for factor assays. Factors VIII, IX, XI, and XII are PTT-based. Factors II, V, VII, and X are PT-based. The factor assay is based on the ability of specific factor-deficient plasma. Quantitative results are obtained from comparing the ability of patient plasma to correct the PTT or PT of a standard curve made from dilutions of normal reference plasma.	**Decreased in:** Hereditary factor deficiency (eg, Factor VIII in hemophilia A, B); acquired factor deficiency secondary to acquired factor-specific inhibitor (eg, factor VIII inhibitor), liver disease (except factor VIII) and DIC (consumptive coagulopathy); vitamin K deficiency or warfarin (II, VII, IX, and X), etc. Severe factor II deficiency may occur in rare patients with lupus anticoagulant. Acquired factor X deficiency may occur in patients with amyloidosis. Patients with von Willebrand disease may have low factor VIII levels.	Although factor assays are typically PTT- or PT-based, chromogenic and immunogenic factor assays are also available for some factors including factor VIII. Heparin, hirudin, and argatroban can act as inhibitors and interfere with specific factor assays. Lab Hematol 2005;11:118. [PMID: 16024335] Semin Thromb Hemost 2005;31:17. [PMID: 15706471] Hamostaseologie 2006;26:38. [PMID: 16444320]
Factor II (prothrombin) G20210A mutation Blood Lavender $$$$	The factor II (prothrombin) 20210A mutation is a common genetic risk factor for thrombosis and is associated with elevated prothrombin levels. Higher concentrations of prothrombin lead to increased rates of thrombin generation, resulting in excessive growth of fibrin clots. It is an autosomal dominant disorder, with heterozygotes being at a 3- to 11-fold greater risk for thrombosis. Although homozygosity is rare, inheritance of two G20210A mutations would further increase the risk for developing thrombosis. The estimated frequency of factor II G20210A in white populations is between 1% and 6%.	**Positive in:** Hypercoagulability secondary to factor II (prothrombin) G20210A mutation (sensitivity and specificity approach 100%).	If a patient is heterozygous for both the pro-thrombin G20210A and the factor V Leiden mutation, the combined heterozygosity leads to an earlier onset of thrombosis and tends to be more severe than single-gene heterozygotsity. Polymerase chain reaction (PCR) is the most commonly used method for the detection of factor II G20210A mutation. Mol Genet Metab 2005;86:91. [PMID: 16185908] Arch Intern Med 2006;166:729. [PMID: 16606808]

	Factor V (Leiden) mutation	Factor VIII assay
	The factor V Leiden mutation is the most common genetic risk factor for thrombosis and accounts for greater than 90% of cases with APC resistance. The presence of the mutation is only a risk factor for thrombosis, not an absolute marker for disease. Homozygotes have a 50- to 100-fold increase in risk of thrombosis (relative to the general population), and heterozygotes have a 7-fold increase in risk. Polymerase chain reaction (PCR) is the most commonly used method for the detection of the Leiden mutation of factor V. Mol Genet Metab 2005;86:91. [PMID: 16185908] Arch Intern Med 2006;166:729. [PMID: 16606808]	Normal hemostasis requires at least 25% of factor VIII activity. Symptomatic hemophiliacs usually have levels ≤5%. Disease levels are defined as severe (<1%), moderate (1–5%), and mild (>5%). Factor VIII assays are used to guide replacement therapy in patients with hemophilia. Factor deficiency can be distinguished from factor inhibitor by an inhibitor screen. Hemophilia 2002;8:644. [PMID: 12199673] Lab Hematol 2005;11:118. [PMID: 16024335]
	Positive in: Hypercoagulability secondary to factor V$_{Leiden}$ mutation (sensitivity and specificity approach 100%).	**Increased in:** Inflammatory states (acute-phase reactant, last trimester of pregnancy, oral contraceptives. **Decreased in:** Hemophilia A, von Willebrand disease, DIC, acquired factor VIII inhibitor.
Factor V (Leiden) mutation Blood Lavender $$$$	The Leiden mutation is a single nucleotide base mutation (G1691A) in the factor V gene, leading to an amino acid substitution (Arg506Glu) at one of the sites where coagulation factor V is cleaved by activated protein C (APC). This mutation results in a substantially reduced anticoagulant response to APC, because factor Va$_{Leiden}$ is inactivated about 10 times more slowly than normal factor Va. The frequency of factor V$_{Leiden}$ in white populations is between 2–15%. Factor V mutations may be present in up to half of the cases of unexplained venous thrombosis and are seen in more than 90% of patients with APC resistance.	
Factor VIII assay, plasma 50–150% of normal (varies with age) Blue $$$ Deliver immediately to laboratory on ice. Stable for 2 hours. Freeze if the assay is delayed >2 hours. $$$	Measures activity of factor VIII (antihemophilic factor), a key factor of the intrinsic clotting cascade.	

	Fecal fat

Test/Range/Collection	Physiologic Basis	Interpretation	Comments
Fecal fat, stool Random: <60 droplets of fat/high power field 72 hour: <7 g/d $$$ Qualitative: random stool sample is adequate. Quantitative: dietary fat should be at least 50–150 g/d for 2 days before collection. Then all stools should be collected for 72 hours and refrigerated.	In healthy people, most dietary fat is completely absorbed in the small intestine. Normal small intestinal lining, bile acids, and pancreatic enzymes are required for normal fat absorption.	**Increased in:** Malabsorption from small bowel disease (regional enteritis, celiac disease, tropical sprue), pancreatic insufficiency, diarrhea with or without malabsorption.	A random, qualitative fecal fat (so-called Sudan stain) is only useful if positive. Furthermore, it does not correlate well with quantitative measurements. Sudan stain appears to detect triglycerides and lipolytic by-products, whereas 72-hour fecal fat measures fatty acids from a variety of sources, including phospholipids, cholesteryl esters, and triglycerides. The quantitative method can be used to measure the degree of fat malabsorption initially and then after a therapeutic intervention. A normal quantitative stool fat reliably rules out pancreatic insufficiency and most forms of generalized small intestine disease. Am J Gastroenterol 2001;96:3237. [PMID: 11774931]

Fecal occult blood		
Fecal occult blood, stool Negative $ Dietary (meat, fish, turnips, horseradish) and medication (aspirin, nonsteroidal anti-inflammatory drugs) restrictions are often recommended to reduce false positive results, but available evidence does not suggest large effect on positivity rates in non-rehydrated testing. To avoid false-negatives, patients should avoid taking vitamin C. Patient collects two specimens from three consecutive bowel movements.	Measures blood in the stool using gum guaiac as an indicator reagent. In the Hemoccult test, gum guaiac is impregnated in a test paper that is smeared with stool using an applicator. Hydrogen peroxide is used as a developer solution. The resultant phenolic oxidation of guaiac in the presence of blood in the stool yields a blue color.	**Positive in:** Upper GI disease (peptic ulcer, gastritis, variceal bleeding, esophageal and gastric cancer), lower GI disease (diverticulosis, colonic polyps, colon carcinoma, inflammatory bowel disease, vascular ectasias, hemorrhoids).	Although fecal occult blood testing is an accepted screening test for colon carcinoma, the sensitivity and specificity of an individual test are low. The usefulness of fecal occult blood testing after digital rectal examination is low. Three randomized controlled trials have shown reductions in colon cancer mortality with yearly (33% reduction) or biennial (15–21% reduction) testing. About 1000 fifty-year-olds must be screened for 10 years to save one life. Colonoscopy is the procedure of choice for colon cancer screening. Ann Intern Med 2005;142:81. [PMID: 15657155]

			Ferritin
Test/Range/Collection	**Physiologic Basis**	**Interpretation**	**Comments**
Ferritin, serum Males 16–300 ng/mL [mcg/L] Females 4–161 ng/mL [mcg/L] SST $$	Ferritin is the body's major iron stor-age protein. The serum ferritin level correlates with total body iron stores. The test is used to detect iron defi-ciency, to monitor response to iron therapy, and, in iron overload states, to monitor iron removal therapy. It is also used to predict homozygosity for hemochromatosis in relatives of affected patients. In the absence of liver disease, it is a more sensitive test for iron deficiency than serum iron and iron-binding capacity (transferrin saturation).	**Increased in:** Iron overload (hemo-chromatosis [sensitivity 85%, speci-ficity 95%], hemosiderosis), acute or chronic liver disease, alcoholism, various malignancies (eg, leukemia, Hodgkin disease), chronic inflamma-tory disorders (eg, rheumatoid arthri-tis, adult Still disease), thalassemia minor, hyperthyroidism, HIV infec-tion, non–insulin-dependent diabetes mellitus, and postpartum state. **Decreased in:** Iron deficiency (60–75%).	Serum ferritin is clinically useful in distinguishing between iron deficiency anemia (serum ferritin levels diminished) and anemia of chronic disease or thalassemia (levels usually normal or elevated). Test of choice for diagnosis of iron deficiency anemia. **Ferritin (ng/mL)** **Likelihood Ratio (LR) for Iron Deficiency** >100 — 0.08 45–100 — 0.54 35–45 — 1.83 25–35 — 2.54 15–25 — 8.83 ≤15 — 52.00 Liver disease increases serum ferritin levels and may mask the diagnosis of iron deficiency. Serum ferritin <1000 ng/mL may predict absence of cirrhosis in hemochromatosis. Eur J Gastroenterol Hepatol 2002;14:217. [PMID: 11953684] Ann Intern Med 2005;143:522. [PMID: 16204165]

α-Fetoprotein		
α-Fetoprotein, serum (AFP) 0–15 ng/mL [mcg/L] SST $$ Avoid hemolysis.	α-Fetoprotein is a glycoprotein produced both early in fetal life and by some tumors.	**Increased in:** Hepatocellular carcinoma (72%), massive hepatic necrosis (74%), viral hepatitis (34%), chronic active hepatitis (29%), cirrhosis (11%), regional enteritis (5%), benign gynecologic diseases (22%), testicular carcinoma (embryonal) (70%), teratocarcinoma (64%), teratoma (37%), ovarian carcinoma (57%), endometrial cancer (50%), cervical cancer (53%), pancreatic cancer (23%), gastric cancer (18%), and colon cancer (5%). **Negative in:** Seminoma.	The test is not sensitive or specific enough to be used as a general screening test for hepatocellular carcinoma. However, screening may be justified in populations at very high risk for hepatocellular cancer. In hepatocellular cancer or germ cell tumors associated with elevated AFP, the test may be helpful in detecting recurrence after therapy. AFP is also used to screen pregnant women at 15–20 weeks gestation for possible fetal neural tube defects. AFP level in maternal serum or amniotic fluid is compared with levels expected at a given gestational age. Ann Intern Med 2003;139:46. [PMID: 12834318] Ann Oncol 2003;14:1463. [PMID: 14504044] Gastroenterology 2004;127(5 Suppl 1):S113. [PMID: 15508074] J Fam Pract 2006;55:155. [PMID: 16451784]

Test/Range/Collection	Physiologic Basis	Interpretation	Comments
Fibrinogen (functional), plasma 150–400 mg/dL [1.5–4.0 g/L] ***Panic:*** <75 mg/dL Blue $$	Fibrinogen is synthesized in the liver and has a half-life of about 4 days. Thrombin cleaves fibrinogen to form insoluble fibrin monomers, which polymerize to form a clot.	**Increased in:** Inflammatory states (acute-phase reactant), use of oral contraceptives, pregnancy, postmenopausal women, smoking, and exercise. **Decreased in:** Acquired deficiency: liver disease, consumptive coagulopathies such as DIC, and thrombolytic therapy; hereditary deficiency, resulting in an abnormal (dysfibrinogenemia), reduced (hypofibrinogenemia), or absent fibrinogen (afibrinogenemia).	Fibrinogen assay is typically performed in the investigation of unexplained bleeding, prolonged PT or PTT, or as part of a DIC panel. An elevated fibrinogen level has also been used as a predictor of arterial thrombotic events. Fibrinogen is generally measured by a clotting-based functional (activity) assay. The Clauss assay, based on a high concentration of thrombin added to diluted patient plasma, is the most commonly used method. Diagnosis of dysfibrinogenemia depends upon the discrepancy between antigen (eg, ELISA) and activity levels. Arch Pathol Lab Med 2002;126:499. [PMID: 11900586] Br J Haematol 2003;121:396. [PMID: 12716361]

	Fluorescent treponemal antibody-absorbed	Folic acid (RBC)
Test / Specimen	**Fluorescent treponemal antibody-absorbed,** serum (FTA-ABS) Nonreactive SST $$	**Folic acid (RBC),** whole blood 165–760 ng/mL [370–1720 nmol/L] Lavender $$$
Description	Detects specific antibodies against *Treponema pallidum*. Patient's serum is first diluted with nonpathogenic treponemal antigens (to bind nonspecific antibodies). The absorbed serum is placed on a slide that contains fixed *T pallidum*. Fluorescein-labeled antihuman gamma globulin is then added to bind to and visualize (under a fluorescence microscope) the patient's antibody on treponemes.	Folate is a vitamin necessary for methyl group transfer in thymidine formation, and hence DNA synthesis. Deficiency can result in megaloblastic anemia. The naturally occurring folate polyglutamates are hydrolyzed to monoglutamate forms before absorption by the small intestine. In the liver, folate monoglutamates are converted to N^5-methyltetrahydrofolate (MeTHF), which is excreted in bile. This methylated form of folate is reabsorbed from the gut but not taken up by the liver and therefore becomes the major circulating form of folate.
Interpretation	**Reactive in:** Syphilis: primary (95%), secondary (96%), late (96%), latent (100%); also rarely positive in collagen–vascular diseases in the presence of antinuclear antibody.	**Decreased in:** Tissue folate deficiency (from dietary folate deficiency), vitamin B_{12} deficiency (50–60%, since cellular uptake of folate depends on vitamin B_{12}).
Comments	Used to confirm a reactive nontreponemal screening serologic test for syphilis such as RPR or VDRL. Once positive, the FTA-ABS may remain positive for life. However, one study found that at 36 months after treatment, 24% of patients had nonreactive FTA-ABS tests. Ann Intern Med 1991;114:1005. [PMID: 2029095] Murray PR et al (editors): *Manual of Clinical Microbiology*, 8th ed. ASM Press, 2003.	Red cell folate level correlates better than serum folate level with tissue folate deficiency. A low red cell folate level may indicate either folate or vitamin B_{12} deficiency. A therapeutic trial of folate (and not red cell or serum folate testing) is indicated when the clinical and dietary history is strongly suggestive of folate deficiency and the peripheral smear shows hypersegmented polymorphonuclear leukocytes. However, the possibility of vitamin B_{12} deficiency must always be considered in the setting of megaloblastic anemia, since folate therapy treats the hematologic, but not the neurologic, sequelae of vitamin B_{12} deficiency. Am J Clin Nutr 2005;82:1346. [PMID: 16332669] Blood Rev 2006;20:299. [PMID: 16716475]

Test/Range/Collection	Physiologic Basis	Interpretation	Comments
	Follicle-stimulating hormone		
Follicle-stimulating hormone, serum (FSH) Male: 1–10 mIU/mL Female: (mIU/mL) Follicular 4–13 Luteal 2–13 Midcycle 5–22 Postmenopausal 20–138 (laboratory-specific) SST $$	FSH is stimulated by the hypothalamic hormone GnRH and is then secreted from the anterior pituitary in a pulsatile fashion. Levels rise during the preovulatory phase of the menstrual cycle and then decline. FSH is necessary for normal pubertal development and fertility in males and females.	**Increased in:** Primary (ovarian) gonadal failure, ovarian or testicular agenesis, castration, postmenopause, Klinefelter syndrome, drugs. **Decreased in:** Hypothalamic disorders, pituitary disorders, pregnancy, anorexia nervosa. Drugs: corticosteroids, oral contraceptives.	Test indicated in the work-up of amenorrhea in women (see Amenorrhea algorithm, Figure 8–4), delayed puberty, impotence, and infertility in men. Impotence work-up should begin with serum testosterone measurement. Basal FSH levels in premenopausal women depend on age, smoking history, and menstrual cycle length and regularity. Because of its variability, FSH is an unreliable guide to menopausal status during the transition into menopause. JAMA 2003;289:895. [PMID: 12588275] Am J Med 2005;118 (Suppl 12B):8. [PMID: 16414322] BJOG 2006;113:1472. [PMID: 17176280]
	Free erythrocyte protoporphyrin		
Free erythrocyte protoporphyrin, whole blood (FEP) <35 mcg/dL (method-dependent) Lavender $$$	Protoporphyrin is produced in the next to last step of heme synthesis. In the last step, iron is incorporated into protoporphyrin to produce heme. Enzyme deficiencies, lack of iron, or presence of interfering substances (lead) can disrupt this process and cause elevated FEP.	**Increased in:** Decreased iron incorporation into heme (iron deficiency, infection, and lead poisoning), erythropoietic protoporphyria.	FEP can be used to screen for lead poisoning in children provided that iron deficiency has been ruled out. Test does not discriminate between uroporphyrin, coproporphyrin, and protoporphyrin, but protoporphyrin is the predominant porphyrin measured. Best Pract Res Clin Haematol 2005;18:347. [PMID: 15737895]

	Fructosamine	Gamma-glutamyl transpeptidase	Gastrin
Test	**Fructosamine,** serum 1.6–2.6 mmol/L SST $	**Gamma-glutamyl trans-peptidase,** serum (GGT) 9–85 U/L [0.15–1.42 mckat/L] (laboratory-specific) SST $	**Gastrin,** serum <100 pg/mL [ng/L] SST $$ Overnight fasting required.
Description	Glycation of albumin produces fructosamine, a less expensive marker of glycemic control than HbA$_{1c}$.	GGT is an enzyme present in liver, kidney, and pancreas. It is induced by alcohol intake and is an extremely sensitive indicator of liver disease, particularly alcoholic liver disease.	Gastrin is secreted from G cells in the stomach antrum and stimulates acid secretion from the gastric parietal cells. Values fluctuate throughout the day but are lowest in the early morning.
Interpretation	**Increased in:** Diabetes mellitus.	**Increased in:** Liver disease: acute viral or toxic hepatitis, chronic or subacute hepatitis, alcoholic hepatitis, cirrhosis, biliary tract obstruction (intrahepatic or extrahepatic), primary or metastatic liver neoplasm, and mononucleosis. Drugs (by enzyme induction): phenytoin, carbamazepine, barbiturates, alcohol.	**Increased in:** Gastrinoma (Zollinger-Ellison syndrome) (80–93% sensitivity), antral G cell hyperplasia, hypochlorhydria, achlorhydria, chronic atrophic gastritis, pernicious anemia. Drugs: antacids, cimetidine, and other H$_2$ blockers; omeprazole and other proton pump inhibitors. **Decreased in:** Antrectomy with vagotomy.
Comments	Fructosamine correlates well with fasting plasma glucose ($r = .74$) but cannot be used to predict precisely the HbA$_{1c}$. Br J Nutr 2004;92:367. [PMID: 15469640]	GGT is useful in follow-up of alcoholics undergoing treatment because the test is sensitive to modest alcohol intake. GGT is elevated in 90% of patients with liver disease. GGT is used to confirm hepatic origin of elevated serum alkaline phosphatase. Ann Clin Biochem 2002;39:22. [PMID: 11853185] Addict Behav 2004;29:1427. [PMID: 15345274] Clin Cornerstone 2001;3:1. [PMID: 11501190]	Gastrin is the first-line test for determining whether a patient with active ulcer disease has a gastrinoma. Gastric acid analysis is not indicated. Before interpreting an elevated level, be sure that the patient is not taking antacids, H$_2$ blockers, or proton pump inhibitors. Both fasting and post-secretin infusion levels may be required for diagnosis. Minerva Med 2005;96:187. [PMID: 16175161]

Test/Range/Collection	Physiologic Basis	Interpretation	Comments
Glomerular filtration rate, estimated (eGFR) (see Creatinine, serum) >60 mL/min/1.73 m² 	The National Kidney Disease Education Program (NKDEP) recommends the use of the estimation of GFR from serum creatinine in adults (>18 years) with chronic kidney disease (CKD) and those at risk for CKD (diabetes, hypertension, and family history of kidney failure). The recommended equation (http://www.nkdep.nih.gov) involves the serum creatinine, urea nitrogen, and albumin concentrations, and the age, gender, and race of the patient.	**Decreased in:** CKD, kidney failure.	CKD is defined as either kidney damage or GFR <60 mL/min/1.73 m² for at least 3 months. Kidney damage is defined as pathologic abnormalities or markers of damage, including abnormalities in blood or urine tests (eg, albuminuria) or imaging studies. Kidney failure is defined as GFR <15 mL/min. Clinical laboratories are not routinely using the recommended equation and its calculation may be too complex for direct clinical use. Kidney Int 2005;67:2089. [PMID: 15882252] Ann Intern Med 2006;145:247. [PMID: 16908915] N Engl J Med 2006;354:2473. [PMID: 16760447]
Glucose, serum 60–110 mg/dL [3.3–6.1 mmol/L] **Panic:** <40 or >500 mg/dL SST $ Overnight fasting usually required.	Normally, the glucose concentration in extracellular fluid is closely regulated so that a source of energy is readily available to tissues and so that no glucose is excreted in the urine.	**Increased in:** Diabetes mellitus, Cushing syndrome (10–15%), chronic pancreatitis (30%). Drugs: corticosteroids, phenytoin, estrogen, thiazides. **Decreased in:** Pancreatic islet cell disease with increased insulin, insulinoma, adrenocortical insufficiency, hypopituitarism, diffuse liver disease, malignancy (adrenocortical, stomach, fibrosarcoma), infant of a diabetic mother, enzyme deficiency diseases (eg, galactosemia). Drugs: insulin, ethanol, propranolol; sulfonylureas, tolbutamide, and other oral hypoglycemic agents.	Diagnosis of diabetes mellitus requires a fasting plasma glucose of >126 mg/dL on more than one occasion or a casual plasma glucose level ≥200 mg/dL (11.1mmol/L) along with symptoms of diabetes. Hypoglycemia is defined as a glucose of <50 mg/dL in men and <40 mg/dL in women. While random serum glucose levels correlate with home glucose monitoring results (weekly mean capillary glucose values), there is wide fluctuation within individuals. Thus, glycosylated hemoglobin levels are favored to monitor glycemic control. The American Diabetes Association recommends that adults age 45 years or older should be evaluated for diabetes by measuring fasting glucose levels. Long-term outcome studies are needed to provide evidence for this recommendation. Diabetes Care 2006;29:S43. [PMID: 16373932]

The table header spanning columns reads: **Glomerular filtration rate, estimated** and **Glucose**

Glucose tolerance test

| Glucose tolerance test, serum | The test determines the ability of a patient to respond appropriately to a glucose load. | **Increased glucose rise (decreased glucose tolerance) in:** Diabetes mellitus, impaired glucose tolerance, gestational diabetes, severe liver disease, hyperthyroidism, stress (infection), increased absorption of glucose from GI tract (hyperthyroidism, gastrectomy, gastroenterostomy, vagotomy, excess glucose intake), Cushing syndrome, pheochromocytoma. Drugs: diuretics, oral contraceptives, glucocorticoids, nicotinic acid, phenytoin. **Decreased glucose rise (flat glucose curve) in:** Intestinal disease (celiac sprue, Whipple disease), adrenal insufficiency (Addison disease, hypopituitarism), pancreatic islet cell tumors, or hyperplasia. | Test is not generally required for diagnosis of diabetes mellitus. In screening for gestational diabetes, the glucose tolerance test is performed between 24 and 28 weeks of gestation. After a 50-g oral glucose load, a 2-hr postprandial blood glucose is measured as a screen. If the result is >140 mg/dL, then the full test with 100 g glucose load is done using the following reference ranges:

Fasting: <105
1-hour: <190
2-hour: <165
3-hour: <145 mg/dL

Clin Chem Lab Med 2003;41:1239. [PMID: 14598876]
Diabetes Care 2005;28:2626. [PMID: 16249530]
Clin Chem Lab Med 2006;44:99. [PMID: 16375594] |

Fasting: <100
1-hour: <200
2-hour: <140 mg/dL
[Fasting: <5.6
1-hour: <11.0
2-hour: <7.7 mmol/L]

SST
$$

Subjects should receive a 150- to 200-g/d carbohydrate diet for at least 3 days before the test. A 75-g glucose dose is dissolved in 300 mL of water for adults (1.75 g/kg for children) and given after an overnight fast. Serial determinations of plasma or serum venous blood glucoses are obtained at baseline, 1 hour, and 2 hours.

Test/Range/Collection	Physiologic Basis	Interpretation	Comments
			G6PD screen
Glucose-6-phosphate dehydrogenase screen, whole blood (G6PD) 5–14 units/g Hb [0.1–0.28 mckat/L] Green or blue $$	G6PD is an enzyme in the hexose monophosphate shunt that is essential in generating reduced glutathione and NADPH, which protect hemoglobin from oxidative denaturation. Numerous G6PD isoenzymes have been identified. Most African Americans have G6PD-A(+) isoenzyme. 10–15% have G6PD-A(−), which has only 15% of normal enzyme activity. It is transmitted in an X-linked recessive manner. Some Mediterranean people have the B− variant that has extremely low enzyme activity (1% of normal).	**Increased in:** Young erythrocytes (reticulocytosis). **Decreased in:** G6PD deficiency.	In deficient patients, hemolytic anemia can be triggered by oxidant agents: antimalarial drugs (eg, chloroquine), nalidixic acid, nitrofurantoin, dapsone, phenacetin, vitamin C, and some sulfonamides. Any African American about to be given an oxidant drug should be screened for G6PD deficiency. (Also screen people from certain Mediterranean areas: Greece, Italy, etc.) Hemolytic episodes can also occur in deficient patients who eat fava beans, in patients with diabetic acidosis, and in infections. G6PD deficiency may be the cause of hemolytic disease of newborns in Asians and Mediterraneans. G6PD activity levels may be measured as normal during an acute episode, because only nonhemolyzed young red cells are assessed. If deficiency is still suspected, assay should be repeated in 2–3 months when cells of all ages are present. Am Fam Physician 2004;69:2599. [PMID: 15202694] Am Fam Physician 2005;72:1277. [PMID: 16225031]
			Glutamine
Glutamine, CSF Glass or plastic tube 6–15 mg/dL **Panic:** >40 mg/dL $$$	Glutamine is synthesized in the brain from ammonia and glutamic acid. Elevated CSF glutamine is associated with hepatic encephalopathy.	**Increased in:** Hepatic encephalopathy.	Test is not indicated if albumin, ALT, bilirubin, and alkaline phosphatase are normal or if there is no clinical evidence of liver disease. Hepatic encephalopathy is essentially ruled out if the CSF glutamine is normal. Arch Intern Med 1971;127:1033. [PMID: 5578559]

	Glycohemoglobin	
Glycohemoglobin; glycated (glycosylated) hemoglobin, (HbA$_{1c}$) 3.9–6.9% (method-dependent) Lavender $$	During the life span of each RBC, glucose combines with hemoglobin to produce stable glycated hemoglobin. The level of glycated hemoglobin is related to the mean plasma glucose level during the prior 1–3 months. There are three glycated A hemoglobins: HbA$_{1a}$, HbA$_{1b}$, and HbA$_{1c}$. Some assays quantitate HbA$_{1c}$, some quantitate total HbA$_1$, and some quantitate all glycated hemoglobins, not just A. Hemoglobin variants may interfere with HbA$_{1c}$ determinations.	**Increased in:** Diabetes mellitus, splenectomy. Falsely high results can occur depending on the method used and may be due to presence of hemoglobin F or uremia. **Decreased in:** Any condition that shortens red cell life span (hemolytic anemias, congenital spherocytosis, acute or chronic blood loss, sickle cell disease, hemoglobinopathies).	HbA$_{1c}$ is useful for quantifying the risk of diabetic complications and for monitoring glycemic control. It is not recommended for the initial diagnosis of diabetes. There is a clear relationship between glycemic control as reflected by HbA$_{1c}$ and the progression of microvascular complications in both type I and type II diabetes. Intervention to lower blood glucose in the two landmark clinical trials, the UK Prospective Diabetes Study (UKPDS) and the Diabetes Control and Complications Trial (DCCT), led to a reduction in the microvascular complications of diabetes. The UKPDS indicated that each 1% decrease in HbA$_{1c}$ reduced the risk for mortality associated with diabetes by 21% and the risk for myocardial infarction by 14%. Target HbA$_{1c}$ is <7%, but encouraging patients to aim slightly lower (eg, by 0.5%) can result in significant reduction in complication risk. Clin Chem Lab Med 2003;41:1182. [PMID: 14598868] Angiology 2005;56:571. [PMID: 16193196] Aust Fam Physician 2005;34:663. [PMID: 16113704] Endocr Pract 2006;12 (Suppl 1):63. [PMID: 16627384]

Test/Range/Collection	Physiologic Basis	Interpretation	Comments
Growth hormone, serum (GH) 0–5 ng/mL [mcg/L] SST $$$	GH is a single-chain polypeptide of 191 amino acids that induces the generation of somatomedins, which directly stimulate collagen and protein synthesis. GH levels are subject to wide fluctuations during the day.	**Increased in:** Acromegaly (90% have GH levels >10 ng/mL), Laron dwarfism (defective GH receptor), starvation. Drugs: dopamine, levodopa. **Decreased in:** Pituitary dwarfism, hypopituitarism.	Nonsuppressibility of GH levels to <2 ng/mL after 100 g oral glucose and elevation of IGF-1 levels are the two most sensitive tests for acromegaly. Random determinations of GH are rarely useful in the diagnosis of acromegaly. For the diagnosis of hypopituitarism or GH deficiency in children, an insulin hypoglycemia test has been used. Failure to increase GH levels to >5 ng/mL after insulin (0.1 unit/kg) is consistent with GH deficiency. Pituitary dysfunction may occur after traumatic brain injury or post-partum hypotension (apoplexy). N Engl J Med 2006;355:2558. [PMID: 17167139] Eur J Endocrinol 2006;155:663. [PMID: 17062881]
Haptoglobin, serum 46–316 mg/dL [0.5–3.2 g/L] SST $$	Haptoglobin is a glycoprotein synthesized in the liver that binds free hemoglobin.	**Increased in:** Acute and chronic infection (acute-phase reactant), malignancy, biliary obstruction, ulcerative colitis, myocardial infarction, and diabetes mellitus. **Decreased in:** Newborns and children, posttransfusion intravascular hemolysis, autoimmune hemolytic anemia, liver disease (10%). May be decreased following uneventful transfusion (10%) for unknown reasons.	Low haptoglobin is considered an indicator of hemolysis, but it is of uncertain clinical predictive value because of the greater prevalence of other conditions associated with low levels and because of occasional normal individuals who have very low levels. It thus has low specificity. High normal levels probably rule out significant intravascular hemolysis. Low haptoglobin levels aid in early recognition of the HELLP syndrome (**h**emolytic anemia, **e**levated liver enzymes, and **l**ow **p**latelet count). J Perinat Med 2000;28:249. [PMID: 11031696] Am J Clin Pathol 2004;121:S97. [PMID: 15298155]

Helicobacter pylori antibody		
***Helicobacter pylori* antibody,** serum Negative SST $$	*Helicobacter pylori* is a gram-negative spiral bacterium that is found on gastric mucosa. It induces acute and chronic inflammation in the gastric mucosa and a positive serologic antibody response. Serologic testing for *H pylori* antibody (IgG) is by ELISA.	**Increased (positive) in:** Histologic (chronic or chronic active) gastritis due to *H pylori* infection (with or without peptic ulcer disease). Sensitivity 98%, specificity 48%. Asymptomatic adults: 15–50%.	95% of patients with duodenal ulcers and >70% of patients with gastric ulcers have chronic infection with *H pylori* along with associated histologic gastritis. All patients with peptic ulcer disease and positive *H pylori* serology should be treated to eradicate *H pylori* infection. The prevalence of *H pylori*-positive serologic tests in asymptomatic adults is approximately 35% overall but is >50% in patients over age 60. Fewer than one in six adults with *H pylori* antibody develop peptic ulcer disease. Treatment of asymptomatic adults is not currently recommended. The role of *H pylori* in patients with chronic dyspepsia is controversial. There is currently no role for treatment of such patients except in clinical trials. After successful eradication, serologic titers fall over a 3- to 6-month period but remain positive in up to 50% of patients at 1 year. J Pediatr 2005;146:S21. [PMID: 15758899] Gastroenterol Clin North Am 2006;35:229. [PMID: 16880064]

Test/Range/Collection	Physiologic Basis	Interpretation	Comments
Hematocrit, whole blood (Hct) Male: 39–49% Female: 35–45% (age-dependent) Lavender $	The Hct represents the percentage of whole blood volume composed of erythrocytes. Laboratory instruments calculate the Hct from the erythrocyte count (RBC) and the mean corpuscular volume (MCV) by the formula: $Hct = RBC \times MCV$	**Increased in:** Hemoconcentration (as in dehydration, burns, vomiting), polycythemia, extreme physical exercise. **Decreased in:** Macrocytic anemia (liver disease, hypothyroidism, vitamin B_{12} deficiency, folate deficiency), normocytic anemia (early iron deficiency, anemia of chronic disease, hemolytic anemia, acute hemorrhage), and microcytic anemia (iron deficiency, thalassemia).	Conversion from hemoglobin (Hb) to hematocrit is roughly $Hb \times 3 = Hct$. The Hct reported by clinical laboratories is not a spun Hct. The spun Hct may be spuriously high if the centrifuge is not calibrated, if the specimen is not spun to constant volume, or if there is "trapped plasma." In determining transfusion need, the clinical picture must be considered in addition to the Hct. Point-of-care instruments may not measure Hct accurately in all patients. In hemodialysis patients, maintaining an Hct in the range of 33–36% provides best outcomes in studies of hospitalizations and mortality. Clin Nephrol 2002;58:S58. [PMID: 12227728] Crit Care Med 2006;34:S102. [PMID: 16617252]
Hemoglobin A_2, whole blood (HbA_2) 1.5–3.5% of total hemoglobin (Hb) Lavender $$	HbA_2 is a minor component of normal adult hemoglobin (<3.5% of total Hb).	**Increased in:** β-Thalassemia minor (HbA_2 levels 4–9% of total Hb, HbF 1–5%), β-thalassemia major (HbA_2 levels normal or increased, HbF 80–100%). **Decreased in:** Untreated iron deficiency, hemoglobin H disease. Patients with the combination of iron deficiency and β-thalassemia may have a normal HbA_2 level.	Test is useful in the diagnosis of β-thalassemia minor (in absence of iron deficiency, which decreases HbA_2 and can mask the diagnosis). Quantitated by column chromatographic or automated HPLC techniques. Normal HbA_2 levels are seen in δβ-thalassemia or very mild β-thalassemias. See thalassemia syndromes (Table 8–23). Clin Chem 2004;50:1736. [PMID: 15388656] Am J Clin Pathol 2005;123:657. [PMID: 15981805] Hemoglobin 2005;29:293. [PMID: 16370492]

Hemoglobin electrophoresis		
Hemoglobin (Hb) elec-trophoresis, whole blood HbA: >95% HbA₂: 1.5–3.5% HbF: <2% (age-dependent) Lavender, blue, or green $$	Hemoglobin electrophoresis is used as a screening test to detect and differentiate variant and abnormal hemoglobins. Alkaline and/or citrate agar electrophoresis is the commonly used method. Separation of hemoglobins is based on different rates of migration of charged hemoglobin molecules in an electric field.	Presence of HbS with HbA > HbS: sickle cell trait (HbAS) or sickle α-thalassemia; HbS and F, no HbA: sickle cell anemia (HbSS), sickle β⁰-thalassemia (hereditary persistence of fetal hemolyglubinuria), or sickle-HPFH; HbS > HbA and F: sickle β⁺-thalassemia. Presence of HbC: HbA > HbC: HbC trait (HbAC); HbC and F, no HbA: HbC disease (HbCC); HbC-β⁰-thalassemia, or HbC-HPFH; HbC > HbA: HbC β⁺-thalassemia. Presence of HbS and HbC: HbSC disease. Presence of HbH: HbH disease. Increased HbA₂: β-thalassemia minor. Increased HbF: Hereditary persistence of fetal hemoglobin, sickle cell anemia, β-thalassemia, HbC disease, HbE disease.	Evaluation of a suspected hemoglobinopathy should include electrophoresis of a hemolysate to detect abnormal hemoglobins, quantitation of hemoglobins A₂ and F by column chromatography, and solubility test if HbS is detected. Interpretation of Hb electrophoresis results should be put in the clinical context, including the family history, serum iron studies, red cell morphology, hemoglobin, hematocrit, and red cell indices (eg, MCV). Automated HPLC instruments are proving to be useful alternative methods for hemoglobinopathy screening. Molecular testing aids in genetic counseling of patients with thalassemia and combined hemo-globinopathies. Clin Chem 2004;50:1736. [PMID: 15386656] Clin Lab Haematol 2005;27:111. [PMID: 15784126]

Hemoglobin, fetal

Test/Range/Collection	Physiologic Basis	Interpretation	Comments
Hemoglobin, fetal, whole blood (HbF) Adult: <2% (varies with age) Lavender, blue, or green $$	Fetal hemoglobin constitutes about 75% of total hemoglobin at birth and declines to 50% at 6 weeks, 5% at 6 months, and <1.5% by 1 year. During the first year, adult hemoglobin (HbA) becomes the predominant hemoglobin.	**Increased in:** Hereditary disorders: eg, β-thalassemia major (20–100% of total Hb is HbF), β-thalassemia minor (2–5% HbF), HbE β-thalassemia (10–80% HbF), sickle cell anemia (1–20% HbF), hereditary persistence of fetal hemoglobin (10–40% HbF). Acquired disorders (<10% HbF): aplastic anemia, megaloblastic anemia, paroxysmal nocturnal hemoglobinuria (PNH), leukemia (eg, juvenile myelomonocytic leukemia). **Decreased in:** Hemolytic anemia of the newborn.	Semiquantitative acid elution test provides an estimate of fetal hemoglobin only and varies widely between laboratories. It is useful in distinguishing hereditary persistence of fetal hemoglobin (all RBCs show an increase in fetal hemoglobin) from β-thalassemia minor (only a portion of RBCs are affected). Enzyme-linked antiglobulin test and flow cytometry are used to detect fetal red cells in the Rh(–) maternal circulation in suspected cases of Rh sensitization and to determine the amount of RhoGAM to administer (1 vial/15 mL fetal RBC). Prenatal diagnosis of hemoglobinopathies may be made from quantitative hemoglobin levels using HPLC or molecular diagnostic techniques. Clin Lab Haematol 2003;25:405. [PMID: 14641146] Cytometry B Clin Cytom 2005;67:27. [PMID: 16059876]7

Hemoglobin, total	Hemosiderin
Hemoglobin, total, whole blood (Hb) Male: 13.6–17.5 Female: 12.0–15.5 g/dL (age-dependent) [Male: 136–175 Female: 120–155 g/L] ***Panic:*** ≤7 g/dL Lavender $	Hemosiderin, urine Negative Urine container $$ Fresh, random sample.
Hemoglobin is the major protein of erythrocytes that transports oxygen from the lungs to peripheral tissues. It is measured by spectrophotometry on automated instruments after hemolysis of red cells and conversion of all hemoglobin to cyanmethemoglobin.	Hemosiderin is a protein produced by the digestion of hemoglobin. Its presence in the urine indicates acute or chronic release of free hemoglobin into the circulation with accompanying depletion of the scavenging proteins, hemopexin, and haptoglobin. Presence of hemosiderin usually indicates intravascular hemolysis or recent transfusion.
Increased in: Hemoconcentration (as in dehydration, burns, vomiting), polycythemia, extreme physical exercise. **Decreased in:** Macrocytic anemia (liver disease, hypothyroidism, vitamin B_{12} deficiency, folate deficiency), normocytic anemia (early iron deficiency, anemia of chronic disease, hemolytic anemia, acute hemorrhage), and microcytic anemia (iron deficiency, thalassemia).	**Increased in:** Intravascular hemolysis: hemolytic transfusion reactions, paroxysmal nocturnal hemoglobinuria (PNH), cold hemagglutinin disease, microangiopathic hemolytic anemia, mechanical destruction of erythrocytes (heart valve hemolysis), sickle cell anemia, thalassemia major, oxidant drugs with G6PD deficiency (eg, dapsone), clostridial exotoxemia; hemochromatosis.
The cyanmethemoglobin technique is the method of choice selected by the International Committee for Standardization in Hematology. The method measures all hemoglobin derivatives except sulfhemoglobin by hemolyzing the specimen and adding a reducing agent. As such, this method does not distinguish between intracellular versus extracellular hemoglobin (hemolysis). Hypertriglyceridemia and very high white blood cell counts can cause false elevations of Hb. Clin Nephrol 2002;58:S58. [PMID: 12227728] Crit Care Med 2006;34:S102. [PMID: 16617252]	Hemosiderin can be qualitatively detected in urinary sediment using Prussian blue stain. Hemosiderin is not detected in alkaline urine. J Vasc Surg 2003;37:132. [PMID: 12514590] Br J Radiol 2004;77:953. [PMID: 15507422]

	Heparin anti-Xa assay		
Test/Range/Collection	**Physiologic Basis**	**Interpretation**	**Comments**
Heparin anti-Xa assay, plasma Undetectable (<0.05 U/mL) Blue $$	The anti-Xa assay is a chromogenic assay that measures heparin level indirectly. Antithrombin and factor Xa are used as assay reagents. Heparin in patient's plasma binds with the added excess antithrombin and inhibits excess Xa. The quantity of residual Xa is then measured using a chromogenic substrate, and the released colored compound is measured spectrophotometrically. The quantity of residual Xa is inversely proportional to the amount of heparin present in plasma.	**Therapeutic ranges:** Unfractionated heparin: 0.35–0.70 U/mL. Low molecular weight heparin (LMWH): 0.50–1.10 U/mL. Note that the therapeutic ranges are laboratory- and method-specific.	The test can precisely determine the level of heparin in patient's plasma, and is used to monitor heparin therapy. PTT is the most commonly used test for monitoring unfractionated heparin therapy. But for patients with documented lupus anticoagulant, PTT is unreliable and therefore heparin level by anti-Xa assay should be used. Low molecular weight heparin (LMWH; eg, enoxaparin) generally does not prolong the PTT. Therefore the anti-Xa assay is used if monitoring of LMWH is required (eg, obesity with >100 kg body weight, renal insufficiency, and pregnancy). Blood sample is typically collected 4 hours after subcutaneous injection. Blood Coagul Fibrinolysis 2005;16:173. [PMID: 15795534] Am J Clin Pathol 2006;126:416. [PMID: 16880140] Br J Haematol 2006;133:19. [PMID: 16512825]

Heparin-associated antibody detection		
Heparin-associated antibody detection (heparin-induced thrombocytopenia), serum Negative SST $$	Heparin-induced thrombocytopenia (HIT) is a life-threatening disorder follows exposure to unfractionated or (less commonly) low-molecular-weight heparin. The HIT antibodies are directed at heparin and platelet factor 4 (PF4) and may appear on exposure to heparin. The formed immune complexes propagate platelet activation, leading to release of more PF4 and thrombosis. However, only a minority of patients who form HIT antibodies actually develop thrombocytopenia and/or thrombosis. An enzyme-linked immunosorbent assay (ELISA) method is typically used for the detection of HIT antibodies.	**Positive in:** Heparin-induced thrombocytopenia.	There are two types of HIT. Type I HIT is generally considered a benign condition and is not antibody-mediated. In Type II HIT, thrombocytopenia is usually more severe and is antibody-mediated. Patients with Type II HIT are at risk for developing arterial or venous thrombosis if heparin therapy is continued. The ELISA-based antigenic assay is very sensitive and is designed to detect antibody binding to PF4/heparin (usually IgG). However, the test may also detect nonpathogenic IgA and IgM antibodies. Functional assays (serotonin release assay, heparin-induced platelet aggregation study, and flow cytometry analysis) are more specific, but are technically demanding and usually done in reference laboratories. Arch Pathol Lab Med 2002;126:1415. [PMID: 12421151] N Engl J Med 2006;355:809. [PMID: 16928996]

Test/Range/Collection	Physiologic Basis	Interpretation	Comments
		Hepatitis A antibody	**Hepatitis B surface antigen**
Hepatitis A antibody, serum (Anti-HAV) Negative SST $$	Hepatitis A is caused by a nonenveloped 27-nm RNA virus of the enterovirus-picornavirus group and is usually acquired by the fecal–oral route. IgM antibody is detectable within 1 week after symptoms develop and persists for 6 months. IgG antibody appears 4 weeks later than IgM and persists for years (see Figure 9–5 for time course of serologic changes).	**Positive in:** Acute hepatitis A (IgM), convalescence from hepatitis A (IgG).	The most commonly used test for hepatitis A antibody is an immunoassay that detects total IgG and IgM antibodies. This test can be used to establish immune status. Specific IgM testing is necessary to diagnose acute hepatitis A. IgG antibody positivity is found in 40–50% of adults in the United States and Europe (higher rates in developing nations). Testing for anti-HAV (IgG) may reduce cost of HAV vaccination programs. Ann Intern Med 2005;142:67. [PMID: 15630110] Am J Med 2005;118 (Suppl 10A):28S. [PMID: 16271538] J Viral Hepat 2005;12:101. [PMID: 15655056]
Hepatitis B surface antigen, serum (HBsAg) Negative SST $$	In hepatitis B virus infection, surface antigen is detectable 2–5 weeks before onset of symptoms, rises in titer, and peaks at about the time of onset of clinical illness. Generally it persists for 1–5 months, declining in titer and disappearing with resolution of clinical symptoms (see Figure 9–6 for time course of serologic changes).	**Increased in:** Acute hepatitis B, chronic hepatitis B (persistence of HBsAg for >6 months, positive HBcAb [total]), HBsAg-positive carriers. May be undetectable in acute hepatitis B infection. If clinical suspicion is high, HBcAb (IgM) test is then indicated.	First-line test for the diagnosis of acute or chronic hepatitis B. If positive, no other test is needed. HBeAg is a marker of extensive viral replication found only in HBsAg-positive sera. Persistently HBeAg-positive patients are more infectious than HBeAg-negative patients and more likely to develop chronic liver disease. Hosp Med 2002;63:16. [PMID: 11828810] Am J Gastroenterol 2006;101(Suppl):S1. [PMID: 16448446]

Test / Specimen	Interpretation	Comments
Hepatitis B surface antibody, serum (HBsAb, anti-HBs) Negative SST $$ Test detects antibodies to hepatitis B virus (HBV), which are thought to confer immunity to hepatitis B. Because several subtypes of hepatitis B exist, there is a possibility of subsequent infection with a second subtype.	**Increased in:** Hepatitis B immunity due to HBV infection or hepatitis B vaccination. **Absent in:** Hepatitis B carrier state, nonexposure.	Test indicates immune status. It is not useful for the evaluation of acute or chronic hepatitis. (See Figure 9–6 for time course of serologic changes.) Am J Med 2005;118 (Suppl 10A):26S. [PMID: 16271538]
Hepatitis B core antibody, total, serum (HBcAb, anti-HBc) Negative SST $$ HbcAb (IgG and IgM) will be positive (as IgM) about 2 months after exposure to hepatitis B. Its persistent positivity may reflect chronic hepatitis (IgM) or recovery (IgG). (See Figure 9–6 for time course of serologic changes.)	**Positive in:** Hepatitis B (acute and chronic), hepatitis B carriers (high levels), prior hepatitis B (immune) when IgG present in low titer with or without HBsAb. **Negative:** After hepatitis B vaccination.	HBcAb (total) is useful in evaluation of acute or chronic hepatitis only if HBsAg is negative. An HBcAb (IgM) test is then indicated only if the HBcAb (total) is positive. HBcAb (IgM) may be the only serologic indication of acute HBV infection. Clin Liver Dis 2004;8:267. [PMID: 15481340]
Hepatitis B e antigen/antibody (HBeAg/Ab), serum Negative SST $$ HBeAg is a soluble protein secreted by HBV, related to HBcAg, indicating viral replication and infectivity. Two distinct serologic types of hepatitis B have been described, one with a positive HBeAg and the other with a negative HBeAg and a positive anti-HBe antibody.	**Increased (positive) in:** HBV (acute, chronic) hepatitis.	The assumption has been that loss of HBeAg and accumulation of HBeAb are associated with decreased infectivity. Testing has proved unreliable, and tests are not routinely needed as indicators of infectivity. All patients positive for HBsAg must be considered infectious. Anti-HBeAb is used to select patients for clinical trials of interferon therapy or liver transplantation. Cochrane Database Syst Rev 2002;2:CD000345. [PMID: 12076393]

	Hepatitis B virus DNA, quantitative		
Test/Range/Collection	**Physiologic Basis**	**Interpretation**	**Comments**
Hepatitis B virus DNA, quantitative (HBV-DNA), serum negative (detection limit: 40 HBV DNA IU/mL, assay-specific) SST or lavender $$$$	The presence of HBV-DNA in serum or plasma confirms active hepatitis B infection and implies infectivity of serum. Current use of the assay is primarily for assessing responses of hepatitis B to therapy, such as interferon-α, lamivudine, or adefovir. HBV-DNA is also used before and after liver transplantation, and for low-level viral replication by mutant strains of HBV that do not make normal surface antigen. HBV-DNA can be detected using very sensitive techniques (eg, real-time PCR) even in patients thought to have recovered from HBV infection who are positive for anti-HBs and anti-HBc.	**Positive in:** Acute hepatitis B, chronic hepatitis B, silent HBV carriers.	Viral load fluctuates over time in most patients and may vary by as much as 10^2–10^4 in serial measurements. The World Health Organization has recognized an international standard, a genotype A subtype adw2 isolate, for HBV-DNA quantification. Assays are commonly reported in International Units (IU) based on comparison with the standard. One IU/mL of HBV DNA is approximately 5 copies/mL. However, correlation between copies/mL and IU is variable. Hepatology 2003;37:1309. [PMID: 12774009] J Med Virol 2004;73:522. [PMID: 15221895]

Hepatitis C antibody

| Hepatitis C antibody, serum (HCAb)\n\nNegative\n\nSST\n$$ | Detects antibody to hepatitis C virus, which is a single-stranded RNA virus of the *Flaviviridae* family.\n\nCurrent screening test (ELISA) detects antibodies to proteins expressed by putative structural (HC34) and non-structural (HC31, C100-3) regions of the HCV genome. The presence of these antibodies indicates that the patient has been infected with HCV, may harbor infectious HCV, and may be capable of transmitting HCV.\n\nA recombinant immunoblot assay (RIBA), equivalent to Western blot, is available as a confirmatory test.\n\nSee Figure 9–7 for hepatitis C serologic changes. | **Increased in:** Acute hepatitis C (only 20–50%; seroconversion may take 6 months or more), posttransfusion chronic non-A, non-B hepatitis (70–90%), sporadic chronic non-A, non-B hepatitis (30–80%), blood donors (0.5–1%), non-blood-donating general public (2–3%), hemophiliacs (75%), intravenous drug abusers (40–80%), hemodialysis patients (1–30%), male homosexuals (4%). | Sensitivity of current assays is 86%, specificity 99.5%.\n\nSeropositivity for hepatitis C documents previous exposure, not necessarily acute infection.\n\nSamples that are weakly positive (signal to cutoff value ratio <3.9 for ELISA assay) are usually negative on RIBA, and CDC guidelines recommend confirmation with RIBA before reporting these as positive. HCV-RNA can also be obtained if there is high clinical suspicion of HCV despite a negative anti-HCV, especially in immunocompromised individuals or in the setting of acute hepatitis.\n\nAnti-HCV and the RIBA often do not become positive during an acute infection; thus repeat testing several months later is required if clinically indicated.\n\nClin Chem 2003;49:479. [PMID: 12600961]\nClin Chem 2003;49:940. [PMID: 12765991] |

Test/Range/Collection	Physiologic Basis	Interpretation	Comments
Hepatitis C RNA (HCV-RNA), quantitative Negative (detection limit: 50 IU/mL, assay-specific) SST or lavender. $$$$ Separate serum or plasma and freeze at –20°C within 2 hours. Analysis should be done within 2 hours.	Detection of HCV-RNA is used to confirm current infection and to monitor treatment with interferon-α (with or without ribavirin). Widely used methods include reverse-transcriptase PCR (RT-PCR) and branched DNA (b-DNA) transcription-mediated amplification (TMA). Cross-contamination with RNA from other specimens causing false-positive results is possible, particularly with b-DNA TMA method.	**Positive in:** Hepatitis C.	RNA is very susceptible to degradation; thus, improper specimen handling can cause false-negative results. Assays are generally reported in IU/mL, with standardization using WHO reference material. A negative result does not rule out the presence of PCR inhibitors in the patient specimen or hepatitis C virus RNA concentrations below the level of detection by the assay. A less than 2 log decrease in viral load after 12 weeks of treatment indicates lack of response to therapy. Hepatology 2002;36:S1. [PMID: 12407571] Hepatology 2004;39:1147. [PMID: 15057920]
Hepatitis C virus genotyping SST or lavender $$$$ Separate serum or plasma from cells within 2 hours of collection.	Patient RNA is assayed using reverse transcription polymerase chain reaction (RT-PCR) to amplify a specific portion of the 5′ untranslated region (5′ UTR) of the hepatitis C virus. The amplified nucleic acid is sequenced bidirectionally. Results are based on comparison with databases derived from GenBank sequences and published information. The test may be unsuccessful if the HCV RNA viral load is less than 1,000 HCV RNA copies per mL of plasma.	**Positive in:** Hepatitis C. Isolates of hepatitis C virus are grouped into six major genotypes. These genotypes are subtyped according to sequence characteristics and are designated as 1a, 1b, 2a, 2b, 3a, 3b, 4, 5a, and 6a.	Genotyping to identify the HCV subtype is performed to determine potential responses to therapy. Reports suggest that patient prognosis and disease course may be genotype dependent. For example, hepatitis C virus type 1 and type 4 infections may be associated with more severe disease and decreased responsiveness to therapy. In contrast, types 2 and 3 may be treated with shorter durations of therapy. Arch Pathol Lab Med 2002;126:285. [PMID: 11603001] J Clin Microbiol 2002;40:4407. [PMID: 12454127] Lancet 2003;362:2095. [PMID: 14697814] J Clin Virol 2005;34:108. [PMID: 16157261]

Test		Interpretation
Hepatitis D antibody, serum (anti-HDV) Negative Marbled $$	This antibody is a marker for acute or persisting infection with the delta agent, a defective RNA virus that can only infect HBsAg-positive patients. HBV plus hepatitis D virus (HDV) infection may be more severe than HBV infection alone. Antibody to HDV ordinarily persists for about 6 months following acute infection. Further persistence indicates carrier status. **Positive in:** Hepatitis D.	Test only indicated in HBsAg-positive patients. Chronic HDV hepatitis occurs in 80–90% of HBsAg carriers who are superinfected with delta, but in less than 5% of those who are coinfected with both viruses simultaneously. Hepatology 2006;44:536, 713, 728. [PMID: 16941704, 16941685, 16941695]
Heterophile antibody, serum (Monospot, Paul-Bunnell test) Negative SST $	Infectious mononucleosis (IM) is an acute saliva-transmitted infectious disease due to the Epstein-Barr virus (EBV). The virus preferentially infects B cells, and causes immune responses including the activation of T cells. Heterophile (Paul-Bunnell) antibodies (IgM) appear in 60% of mononucleosis patients within 1–2 weeks and in 80–90% within the first month. They are not specific for EBV but are found only rarely in other disorders. Titers are substantially diminished by 3 months after primary infection and are not detectable by 6 months. **Positive in:** Infectious mononucleosis (IM) (90–95%). **Negative in:** Heterophile-negative mononucleosis: CMV, heterophile-negative EBV, toxoplasmosis, hepatitis viruses, HIV-1 seroconversion, listeriosis, tularemia, brucellosis, cat scratch disease, Lyme disease, syphilis, rickettsial infections, medications (phenytoin, sulfasalazine, dapsone), collagen-vascular diseases (especially systemic lupus erythematosus), subacute infective endocarditis.	The test is used as an aid in the diagnosis of IM. The three classic laboratory features of IM are lymphocytosis, a "significant number" (>10–20%) of atypical lymphocytes (altered T cells) on Wright-stained peripheral blood smear, and positive heterophile test. If heterophile test is negative in the setting of hematologic and clinical evidence of a mononucleosis-like illness, a repeat test in 1–2 weeks may be positive. EBV serology (anti-VCA, anti-EBNA, anti-EA) may also be indicated, especially in children and teenage patients who may have negative heterophile tests. Am J Fam Physician 2004;70:1279. [PMID: 15508538] Am J Hematol 2004;76:315. [PMID: 15282662] J Infect Dis 2005;192:1505. [PMID: 16206064]

Histoplasma capsulatum antigen

Test/Range/Collection	Physiologic Basis	Interpretation	Comments
***Histoplasma capsulatum* antigen,** urine, serum, CSF (HPA) Negative SST $$ Deliver urine, CSF in a clean plastic or glass container tube. Urine is the best specimen for the test.	Histoplasmosis is the most common systemic fungal infection and typically starts as a pulmonary infection with influenza-like symptoms. This may heal, progress, or lie dormant with reinfection occurring at a later time. Heat-stable *H capsulatum* polysaccharide is detected by enzyme immunoassay antigen (EIA) using alkaline phosphatase or horseradish peroxidase-conjugated antibodies. EIA has replaced the previously used RIA as the mainstream method.	**Increased in:** Disseminated histoplasmosis (90–97% in urine, 50–78% in blood, and approximately 42% in CSF), localized disease (16% in urine), blastomycosis (urine and serum), coccidioidomycosis (CSF).	Histoplasmosis is usually seen in the Mississippi and Ohio River valleys but may appear elsewhere. Detection of *Histoplasma* antigenemia or antigenuria is recommended for the diagnosis of disseminated histoplasmosis and may be useful in the early acute stage of pulmonary histoplasmosis before the appearance of antibodies. The test can also used to monitor therapy or to follow relapse in immunocompromised patients. EIA for *H capsulatum var capsulatum* polysaccharide antigen in urine is a useful test in diagnosis of disseminated histoplasmosis and in assessing efficacy of treatment or in detecting relapse, especially in AIDS patients and when serologic tests for antibodies may be negative. It is not useful for ruling out localized pulmonary histoplasmosis. In bronchoalveolar lavage fluid, HPA has 70% sensitivity for the diagnosis of pulmonary histoplasmosis. The antigenuria tests high sensitivity and specificity have dispelled the confusion in interpreting antibody test results. Clin Microbiol Rev 2002;15:465. [PMID: 12097252] J Antimicrob Chemother 2002;49(Suppl 1):11. [PMID: 11801576] Semin Respir Infect 2002;17:158. [PMID: 12070835] Diagn Microbiol Infect Dis 2006;54:283. [PMID: 16466889]

	Histoplasma capsulatum precipitins		*Histoplasma capsulatum* CF antibody
***Histoplasma capsulatum* precipitins,** serum Negative SST (acute and convalescent samples, collected 2–3 weeks apart) $$	This test screens for presence of Histoplasma antibody by detecting precipitin "H" and "M" bands by immunodiffusion. Positive H band indicates active infection, but is rarely found alone; M band indicates acute or chronic infection or prior skin testing. Presence of both is highly suggestive of active histoplasmosis.	**Positive in:** Previous, chronic, or acute histoplasma infection, recent histoplasmin skin testing. Cross-reactions at low levels in patients with blastomycosis and coccidioidomycosis.	Test is useful as a screening test or as an adjunct to complement fixation test (see below) in diagnosis of systemic histoplasmosis. Rose NR et al (editors): *Manual of Clinical Laboratory Immunology,* 6th ed. ASM Press, 2002. Murray PR et al (editors): *Manual of Clinical Microbiology,* 8th ed. ASM Press, 2003.
***Histoplasma capsulatum* complement fixation (CF) antibody,** serum; CSF <1:4 titer SST $$ Submit paired sera, one specimen collected within 1 week after onset of illness and another 2 weeks later.	The standard method for the diagnosis of histoplasmosis remains culture isolation and identification of the organism. However, culture often requires 2–4 weeks. Antibody detection offers a more rapid alternative and is valuable in the diagnosis of acute, chronic, disseminated, and meningeal histoplasmosis. Antibodies in primary pulmonary infections are generally found within 4 weeks after exposure and frequently are present at the time symptoms appear. Two types of CF test are available based on mycelial antigen and yeast phase antigen. The yeast phase test is considerably more sensitive. Latex agglutination (LA) and ELISA tests are also available but are less reliable.	**Increased in:** Previous, chronic, or acute histoplasma infection (75–80%), recent histoplasmin skin testing (20%), other fungal disease, leishmaniasis. Cross-reactions in patients with blastomycosis and coccidioidomycosis.	Elevated CF titers of >1:16 are suggestive of infection. Titers of >1:32 or rising titers are usually indicative of active infection. Histoplasmin skin test is not recommended for diagnosis because it interferes with subsequent serologic tests. The CF test is usually positive in CSF from patients with chronic meningitis. About 3.5–12% of clinically normal persons have positive titers, usually less than 1:16. Rose NR et al (editors): *Manual of Clinical Laboratory Immunology,* 6th ed. American Society for Microbiology, 2002. Murray PR et al (editors): *Manual of Clinical Microbiology,* 8th ed. ASM Press, 2003.

Test/Range/Collection	Physiologic Basis	Interpretation	Comments
HIV antibody, serum Negative SST $$	This test detects antibody against the human immunodeficiency virus-1 (HIV-1), the etiologic agent of the vast majority of all HIV infections in the US. Antibodies become detectable approximately 22–27 days after acute infection. Early detection is crucial for the institution of highly active antiretroviral therapy (HAART). HIV antibody test is considered positive only when a repeatedly reactive enzyme immunoassay (EIA) is confirmed by a Western blot (WB) analysis. Immunofluorescent antibody test (IFA) is also performed in some laboratories for screening and/or as a substitute for WB. Rapid HIV antibody tests are available and provide timely detection of antibody to HIV in cases of needle stick injury or exposure to potentially HIV-contaminated materials.	**Positive in:** HIV infection: EIA sensitivity >99% after first 2–4 months of infection, specificity 99%. When combined with confirmatory test, specificity is 99.995%.	Although Western blot test is currently the most sensitive and specific assay for HIV serodiagnosis, it is highly dependent on the proficiency of the laboratory performing the test and on the standardization of the procedure. The CDC recommends that all pregnant women be offered HIV testing. There are at least three rapid HIV tests approved by the US FDA and available in the US: OraQuick Rapid HIV-1 Antibody Test, Reveal Rapid HIV-1 Antibody Test, and Uni-Gold Recombigen HIV Test. JAMA 1991;266:2861. Murray PR et al (editors): *Manual of Clinical Microbiology*, 8th ed. ASM Press, 2003. MLO Med Lab Obs 2004;36:12. [PMID: 15318787]

HIV antibody

HIV RNA, quantitative		
HIV RNA, quantitative (viral load), plasma <75 [copies per mL] (assay-specific) Lavender $$$$	Monitoring HIV-1 RNA level (viral load) in sera of infected patients is used to assess disease progression and patient response to antiviral therapy. Currently, there are three FDA-approved commercially developed assays to monitor HIV viral load. Two assays are based on target amplification (Roche Amplicor HIV Monitor and bioMerieux NucliSens HIV-1 RNA QT), and one is based on signal amplification (Bayer Versant HIV-1 RNA 3.0 bDNA). The HIV viral load assays are intended for use in conjunction with clinical presentation and other laboratory markers of disease progression.	The Amplicor and bDNA assays are generally more sensitive than the NucliSens assay. The analytic measurement/quantification range of the Amplicor and bDNA assays are 400–750,000 copies per mL (Amplicor with standard specimen processing procedure), 50–75,000 copies per mL (Amplicor with ultrasensitive specimen processing procedure), and 75–500,000 copies per mL (bDNA), respectively. Refer to test report for details.	The clinical significance of changes in HIV-1 viral load has not been fully established; however, a threefold change (0.5 log) in copies/mL may be significant. Caution should be taken in the interpretation of any single viral load determination. Lennette EH, Smith TF (editors): *Laboratory Diagnosis of Viral Infections*, 3rd ed. Marcel Dekker, 1999. Murray PR et al (editors): *Manual of Clinical Microbiology*, 8th ed. ASM Press, 2003.

	HIV resistance testing	
Test/Range/Collection	**Physiologic Basis**	**Interpretation**	**Comments**
HIV resistance testing, serum Lavender $$$$	Testing for resistance to antiretroviral agents is considered to be standard of care and is widely used in the management of HIV-infected persons. It is an important tool in optimizing the efficacy of the combination therapy to treat HIV infection. The identification of resistance mutations allows the care providers to select antiviral agents with maximum therapeutic benefit and minimum toxic side effects. Both phenotypic and genotypic resistance tests are available.	Positive in: HIV-1 infection with drug resistance (per report).	Phenotypic resistance tests (eg, PhenoSense from ViroLogic, Inc) rely on PCR amplification of viral protease and reverse transcriptase (RT) gene sequence in lieu of viral isolation. The ViroLogic test involves cloning and expression of the amplified viral RNA in an HIV-1 vector that lacks these regions and contains luciferase reporter gene in place of the viral envelope gene. The replication of the recombinant virus in the presence of various antiviral agents is monitored by the amount of expressed luciferase. Genotypic resistance assays (eg, LiPA assay) detect specific mutations in the viral genome that are associated with resistance to various antiretroviral agents. The initial step of the assay is PCR amplification of viral protease and a 250–400 codon segment of HIV RT gene. This is followed by either direct sequencing or by hybridization-based detection of the amplified products to assess the presence of mutations associated with resistance to antiretroviral agents. Ann Clin Lab Sci 2002;32:406. [PMID: 12458895] J Infect Dis 2006;194 (Suppl 1):S59. [PMID: 16921474]

HLA typing		
HLA typing, serum and blood (HLA) SST (2 mL) and Yellow (40 mL) $$$$ Specimens must be <24 hours old. Refrigerate serum, but not blood in yellow tubes.	The human leukocyte antigen (HLA) system consists of four closely linked loci (HLA-A, -B, -C, and -DR) located on the short arm of chromosome 6. The previous 'gold standard' technique for HLA typing was the complement-dependent cytotoxicity test. This is a complement-mediated serologic assay in which antiserum containing specific anti-HLA antibodies is added to peripheral blood lymphocytes. Cell death indicates that the lymphocytes carried the specific targeted antigen. The three HLA-A, -B, and -C are determined in this manner. The HLA-D locus (DR or D-related) is determined by mixed lymphocyte culture. DNA-based methods for HLA genotyping have now replaced traditional HLA testing based on serologic assays.	**Useful in:** Evaluation of transplant candidates and potential donors and for paternity and forensic testing.	HLA typing is usually performed for transplantation candidates matching, in blood product matching (eg, platelets), and in paternity testing. Although diseases associated with particular HLA antigens have been identified, HLA typing for the diagnosis of these diseases is not generally indicated. JAMA 1995;273:586. [PMID: 7837393] Arch Pathol Lab Med 2002;126:281. [PMID: 11860300]

HLA-B27 typing

Test/Range/Collection	Physiologic Basis	Interpretation	Comments
HLA-B27 typing, whole blood Negative $$$ Specimens must be <24 hours old.	The HLA-B27 allele is found in approximately 8% of the US white population. It occurs less frequently in the African American population. PCR-based HLA-B27 testing is available.	There is an increased incidence of spondyloarthritis among patients who are HLA-B27–positive. HLA-B27 is present in 88% of patients with ankylosing spondylitis. It is also associated with the development of Reiter syndrome (80%) following infection with enteric organisms, such as *Yersinia, Shigella,* or *Salmonella.*	The best diagnostic test for ankylosing spondylitis is a lumbar spine film and not HLA-B27 typing. HLA-B27 testing is not usually clinically indicated. Ann Intern Med 2002;136:896. [PMID: 12069564] Rheumatology (Oxford) 2002;41:857. [PMID: 12154202]

Homocystein

Homocysteine, plasma Male: 4–12 mcmol/L Female: 4–10 mcmol/L (method- and age-dependent) Lavender (green and SST also acceptable) (Fasting specimen is required; plasma or serum must be separated from cells within 1 hour of collection) $$	Homocysteine is a naturally occurring, sulfur-containing amino acid produced during catabolism of methionine, an essential amino acid. It is metabolized by two major pathways: remethylation and transsulfuration. Several vitamins function as cofactors and substrates in these pathways: folic acid and vitamin B_{12} regulate the remethylation pathway catalyzed by methylenetetrahydrofolate reductase (MTHFR) and methionine synthase, respectively, whereas vitamin B_6 is a cofactor for cystathionine β-synthase, a key enzyme in the transsulfuration pathway. Deficiencies in one or more of these vitamins can lead to acquired hyperhomocysteinemia. Homocystinuria is a rare autosomal recessive disorder that usually results from defective activity of cystathionine β-synthase.	**Increased in:** Homocystinuria due to defects in cystathionine β-synthase, methionine synthase or intracellular cobalamin metabolism, MTHFR C677T mutation, deficiency in folic acid or B vitamins (eg, B_{12}, B_6), cigarette smoking, chronic alcohol ingestion, renal failure, systemic lupus erythematosus, hypothyroidism, diabetes mellitus, certain medications (eg, methotrexate, nicotinic acid, theophylline, L-dopa), and advanced age. **Decreased in:** Down syndrome, hyperthyroidism.	Hyperhomocysteinemia is typically defined as a total homocysteine level above the 95th percentile of a control population, which in most studies is approximately 15 mcmol/L. According to the 1999 Science Advisory from the American Heart Association, hyperhomocysteinemia may be classified as moderate (16–30 mcmol/L), intermediate (31–100 mcmol/L), and severe (>100 mcmol/L). Clinical and epidemiologic studies have demonstrated that hyperhomocysteinemia is an independent risk factor for atherosclerosis and coronary heart disease and for arterial and venous thromboembolism. Nevertheless, due to the lack of definitive evidence for clinical treatment outcome benefits from reducing homocysteine levels, routine screening for hyperhomocysteinemia is not recommended. It is reasonable to determine levels of fasting homocysteine in high-risk patients, especially those with strong family history of premature atherosclerosis or with arterial occlusive diseases, as well as their family members. For patients with elevated homocysteine concentration, it is important to check their vitamin status. Circulation 1999;99:178. [PMID: 9884399] J Am Acad Nurse Pract 2005;17:90. [PMID: 15748221] Clin Chem 2007;53:807. [PMID: 17468406] Semin Hematol 2007;44:62. [PMID: 17433897]

Test/Range/Collection	Physiologic Basis	Interpretation	Comments
	5-Hydroxyindoleacetic acid		**IgG index**
5-Hydroxyindoleacetic acid, urine (5-HIAA) 2–8 mg/24 h [10–40 mcmol/d] Urine bottle containing hydrochloric acid $$	Serotonin (5-hydroxytryptamine) is a neurotransmitter that is metabolized by monoamine oxidase (MAO) to 5-HIAA and then excreted into the urine. Serotonin is secreted by most carcinoid tumors, which arise from neuroendocrine cells in locations derived from the embryonic gut. Biochemical diagnosis of gastrointestinal carcinoids is established by demonstrating elevation of urinary 5-HIAA or plasma chromogranin A or serotonin.	**Increased in:** Metastatic carcinoid tumor (foregut, midgut, and bronchial). Nontropical sprue (slight increase). Diet: Bananas, walnuts, avocado, eggplant, pineapple, plums. Drugs: reserpine. **Negative in:** Rectal carcinoids (usually), renal insufficiency. Drugs: MAO inhibitors, phenothiazines. Test is often falsely positive because pretest probability is low. Using 5-HIAA/Cr ratio may improve performance.	Urinary 5-HIAA excretion is used as a biochemical tumor marker for clinical diagnosis, to monitor treatment effects, and as a prognostic predictor. A very high concentration of urinary 5-HIAA is an indicator that a gastrointestinal carcinoid tumor is malignant. Because most carcinoid tumors drain into the portal vein and serotonin is rapidly cleared by the liver, the carcinoid syndrome (flushing, bronchial constriction, diarrhea, hypotension, and cardiac valvular lesions) is a late manifestation of carcinoid tumors, appearing only after hepatic metastasis has occurred. Gastroenterology 2005;128:1717. [PMID: 15887161] J Surg Oncol 2005;89:151. [PMID: 15719376] J Surg Oncol 2005;89:161. [PMID: 15719373] J Clin Gastroenterol 2006;40:572. [PMID: 16917396]
IgG index, serum and CSF 0.29–0.59 ratio SST (for serum) and glass/plastic tube (for CSF) $$$ Collect serum and CSF simultaneously.	This test compares CSF IgG and albumin levels to serum levels. An increased ratio allegedly reflects synthesis of IgG within the central nervous system.	**Increased in:** Multiple sclerosis (80–90%), neurosyphilis, subacute sclerosing panencephalitis, other inflammatory and infectious CNS diseases.	Test is reasonably sensitive but not specific for multiple sclerosis. (Compare with Oligoclonal bands.) J Neuroimmunol 2002;125:149. [PMID: 11960651] J Neurol Sci 2003;216:61. [PMID: 14607304]

Immunofixation electrophoresis		
Immunofixation electro-phoresis (IFE), serum or urine Negative SST (serum) $$$	IFE is used to identify specific immunoglobulin (Ig) classes. Proteins are separated electrophoretically on several tracks on a gel. Antisera specific to individual classes of molecules are added to each track. If specific classes of heavy or light chain are present, insoluble complexes form with the antisera, which can then be stained and detected.	**Positive in:** Presence of identifiable monoclonal protein: plasma cell myeloma, Waldenström macroglobulinemia, heavy chain disease, primary amyloidosis, monoclonal gammopathy of undetermined significance, plasmacytoma, lymphoma, leukemia. The most common M-protein seen in myeloma is the IgG type.	IFE is indicated to define an overt or suspicious Ig spike seen on serum protein electrophoresis (SPEP) or urine protein electrophoresis (UPEP), to differentiate a polyclonal from a monoclonal increase (eg, M-protein in serum, Bence Jones protein in urine), and to identify the nature of a monoclonal increase. Immuno-subtraction capillary zone electrophoresis (CZE) is an alternative test to IFE, and is increasingly used in clinical laboratories. Clin Cancer Res 2005;11:8706. [PMID: 16361557] Clin Chem Lab Med 2006;44:609. [PMID: 16681432] N Engl J Med 2006;354:1362. [PMID: 16571879]

	Immunoglobulins		
Test/Range/Collection	Physiologic Basis	Interpretation	Comments
Immunoglobulins, serum (Ig) IgA: 0.78–3.67 g/L IgG: 5.83–17.6 g/L IgM: 0.52–3.35 g/L SST $$$	IgG makes up about 85% of total serum immunoglobulins and predominates late in immune responses. It is the only immunoglobulin to cross the placenta. IgM antibody predominates early in immune responses. Secretory IgA plays an important role in host defense mechanisms by blocking transport of microbes across mucosal surfaces.	↑ **IgG:** *Polyclonal:* Autoimmune diseases (eg, SLE, rheumatoid arthritis), sarcoidosis, chronic liver diseases, some parasitic diseases, chronic or recurrent infections. *Monoclonal:* Multiple myeloma (IgG type), lymphomas, or other malignancies. ↑ **IgM:** *Polyclonal:* Isolated infections such as viral hepatitis, infectious mononucleosis, early response to bacterial or parasitic infection. *Monoclonal:* Waldenström macroglobulinemia, lymphoma. ↑ **IgA:** *Polyclonal:* Chronic liver disease, chronic infections (especially of the GI and respiratory tracts). *Monoclonal:* Multiple myeloma (IgA). ↓ **IgG:** Immunosuppressive therapy, genetic (severe combined immunodeficiency disease [SCID], Wiskott-Aldrich syndrome, common variable immunodeficiency). ↓ **IgM:** Immunosuppressive therapy. ↓ **IgA:** Inherited IgA deficiency (ataxia-telangiectasia, combined immunodeficiency disorders).	Protein electrophoresis (PEP, serum and/or urine) followed by IFE will detect monoclonal immunoglobulin (paraprotein in serum, Bence Jones protein in urine). Quantitative immunoglobulin levels are indicated in the evaluation of immunodeficiency or the quantitation of a paraprotein. IgG deficiency is associated with recurrent and occasionally severe pyogenic infections. The most common form of multiple myeloma is the IgG type, followed by IgA type. Myeloma of IgM, IgD, or IgE type is rare. Clin Chem 2003;49:1909. [PMID: 14578323] Mayo Clin Proc 2006;81:693. [PMID: 16706268] N Engl J Med 2006;355:2765. [PMID: 17192542]

	Inhibitor screen (1:1 mix)	Insulin antibody
Inhibitor screen (1:1 mix), plasma — Negative — Blue — $$ — Fill tube completely.	Test is useful for evaluating a prolonged PTT, PT, or thrombin time. (Presence of heparin should first be excluded.) Patient's plasma is mixed with pooled normal plasma (1:1 mix) and a PTT is performed. If the patient has a factor deficiency, the post-mixing PTT will be normal (correction). If an inhibitor is present, the post-mixing PTT will still be prolonged (no correction) immediately and/or after incubation. **Positive in:** Presence of inhibitor: Antiphospholipid antibodies (lupus anticoagulant, LAC), factor-specific antibodies, or both. **Negative in:** Factor deficiencies. See evaluation of isolated prolongation of PTT (Figure 8–19).	LAC is a nonspecific inhibitor, which prolongs PTT on inhibitor screen (1:1 mix study) both immediately and after (1–2 hours) incubation. 1- to 2-hour incubation period is needed to detect factor-specific antibodies with low in vitro affinities (eg, post-mixing PTT is normal immediately, but is prolonged after incubation). N Engl J Med 2002;346:752. [PMID: 11882732] Semin Thromb Hemost 2005;31:17. [PMID: 15706471] Semin Thromb Hemost 2005;31:39. [PMID: 15706474]
Insulin antibody, serum — Negative — SST — $$$	Insulin antibodies develop in nearly all diabetics treated with insulin. Most antibodies are IgG and do not cause clinical problems. Occasionally, high-affinity antibodies can bind to exogenous insulin and cause insulin resistance. **Increased in:** Insulin therapy, type I diabetics before treatment (secondary to autoimmune pancreatic B-cell destruction).	Insulin antibodies interfere with most assays for insulin. Insulin antibody test is not sensitive or specific for the detection of surreptitious insulin use; use C-peptide level instead. Anti-insulin and islet cell antibodies are poor predictors of insulin-dependent diabetes and only roughly correlate with insulin requirements in patients with diabetes. Diabetes Metab Res Rev 2005;21:395. [PMID: 15895384]

Test/Range/Collection	Physiologic Basis	Interpretation	Comments
Insulin, immunoreactive, serum 6–35 mcU/mL [42–243 pmol/L] SST $$ Fasting sample required. Measure glucose concurrently.	Measures levels of insulin, either endogenous or exogenous.	**Increased in:** Insulin-resistant states (eg, obesity, type II diabetes mellitus, uremia, glucocorticoids, acromegaly), liver disease, surreptitious use of insulin or oral hypoglycemic agents, insulinoma (pancreatic islet cell tumor). **Decreased in:** Type I diabetes mellitus, hypopituitarism.	Measurement of serum insulin level has little clinical value except in the diagnosis of fasting hypoglycemia. An insulin-to-glucose ratio of >0.3 is presumptive evidence of insulinoma. C-peptide should be used as well as serum insulin to distinguish insulinoma from surreptitious insulin use, since C-peptide will be absent with exogenous insulin use. J Clin Endocrinol Metab 2000;85:3222. [PMID: 10999812]
Insulin-like growth factor-1, plasma (IGF-I, previously known as somatomedin C) 123–463 ng/mL (age- and sex-dependent) Lavender $$$$	Insulin-like growth factor-1 is a GH-dependent plasma peptide produced by the liver. It mediates the growth-promoting effect of GH. It has an anabolic, insulin-like action on fat and muscle and stimulates collagen and protein synthesis. Its level is relatively constant throughout the day. Its concentration is regulated by genetic factors, nutrient intake, GH and other hormones such as T4, cortisol, and sex steroids.	**Increased in:** Acromegaly (level correlates with disease activity better than GH level). **Decreased in:** Pituitary dwarfism, hypopituitarism, Laron dwarfism (end-organ resistance to GH), fasting for 5–6 days, poor nutrition, hypothyroidism, cirrhosis. Values may be normal in GH-deficient patients with hyperprolactinemia or craniopharyngioma.	IGF-1 is a sensitive test for acromegaly. Normal IGF-I levels rule out active acromegaly. In acromegaly, IGF-1 levels are useful for assessing the relative degree of GH excess, because changes in IGF-1 correlate with changes in symptoms and soft-tissue growth. IGF-1 is also very useful in monitoring the symptomatic response to therapy. IGF-I can be decreased in adult GH deficiency, but it is not a sensitive test. Minerva Endocrinol 2004;29:207. [PMID: 15765030] Nat Clin Pract Endocrinol Metab 2006;2:436. [PMID: 16932333] N Engl J Med 2006;355:2558. [PMID: 17167139] Nat Clin Pract Endocrinol Metab 2006;2:436. [PMID: 16932333]

	Iron	Iron-binding capacity
Iron, serum (Fe) 50–175 mcg/dL [9–31 mcmol/L] SST $ Hemolyzed sample unacceptable	Plasma iron concentration is determined by absorption from the intestine; storage in the liver, spleen, bone marrow; rate of breakdown or loss of hemoglobin; and rate of synthesis of new hemoglobin.	**Increased in:** Hemosiderosis (eg, multiple transfusions, excess iron administration), acute Fe poisoning (children), hemolytic anemia, pernicious anemia, aplastic or hypoplastic anemia, viral hepatitis, lead poisoning, thalassemia, hemochromatosis. Drugs: estrogens, ethanol, oral contraceptives. **Decreased in:** Iron deficiency, nephrotic syndrome, chronic renal failure, many infections, active hematopoiesis, remission of pernicious anemia, hypothyroidism, malignancy (carcinoma), postoperative state, kwashiorkor.	Absence of stainable iron on bone marrow aspirate differentiates iron deficiency from other causes of microcytic anemia (eg, thalassemia, sideroblastic anemia, some chronic disease anemias), but the procedure is invasive and expensive. Serum iron, iron-binding capacity, transferrin saturation, serum ferritin or soluble transferrin receptor may obviate the need for bone marrow examination. Serum iron, iron-binding capacity, and transferrin saturation are useful in screening family members for hereditary hemochromatosis. Recent transfusion confounds the test results. Am Fam Physician 2002;65:853. [PMID: 11898957] Eur J Gastroenterol Hepatol 2002;14:217. [PMID: 11953684] Hematology 2006;11:183. [PMID: 17325959] Can J Gastroenterol 2006;20:535. [PMID: 16955151]
Iron-binding capacity, total, serum (TIBC) 250–460 mcg/dL [45–82 mcmol/L] SST $$	Iron is transported in plasma complexed to transferrin, which is synthesized in the liver. Total iron-binding capacity is calculated from transferrin levels measured immunologically. Each molecule of transferrin has two iron-binding sites, so its iron-binding capacity is 1.47 mg/g. Normally, transferrin carries an amount of iron representing about 16–60% of its capacity to bind iron (eg, % saturation of iron-binding capacity is 16–60%).	**Increased in:** Iron deficiency anemia, late pregnancy, infancy, acute hepatitis. Drugs: oral contraceptives. **Decreased in:** Hypoproteinemic states (eg, nephrotic syndrome, starvation, malnutrition, cancer), hemochromatosis, thalassemia, hyperthyroidism, chronic infections, chronic inflammatory disorders, chronic liver disease, other chronic disease.	TIBC correlates with serum transferrin, but the relationship is not linear over a wide range of transferrin values and is disrupted in diseases affecting transferrin-binding capacity or other iron-binding proteins. Increased % transferrin saturation with iron is seen in iron overload (iron poisoning, hemolytic anemia, sideroblastic anemia, thalassemia, hemochromatosis, pyridoxine deficiency, aplastic anemia). Decreased % transferrin saturation with iron is seen in iron deficiency (usually saturation <16%). Transferrin levels can also be used to assess nutritional status. Recent transfusion confounds the test results. Curr Med Chem 2005;12:2683. [PMID: 16305465] Kidney Int Suppl 2006;101:S4. [PMID: 16830699]

	JAK2 (V617F) mutation	

Test/Range/Collection	Physiologic Basis	Interpretation	Comments
JAK2 (V617F) mutation Blood Lavender $$$$	*JAK2* stands for the Janus Kinase 2. Detection of the *JAK2* (V617F) mutation provides a qualitative diagnostic marker for the non-chronic myelogenous leukemia subgroup of myeloproliferative disorders, including polycythemia vera (PV), essential thrombocythemia (ET), and chronic idiopathic myelofibrosis (CIMF). The mutation, a valine-to-phenylalanine substitution at codon 617, leads to constitutive tyrosine phosphorylation activity which is believed to confer independence and/or hypersensitivity of myeloid progenitors to cytokines (eg, erythropoietin).	**Positive in:** (~80%), (50%), CIMF (40%).	A positive result identifies a *JAK2* (V617F) mutation and is strongly supportive of a diagnosis of PV, ET, or CIMF. It is particularly useful for establishing a diagnosis of PV in patients with marked erythrocytosis (eg, hemoglobin >18.5 g/dL in males or >16.5 g/dL in females). A negative result does not rule out the possibility of diagnosis of PV, ET, or CIMF. The test is polymerase chain reaction based. See diagnostic evaluation for polycythemia and thrombocytosis (Figures 8–18 and 8–23). Blood 2005;105:4187. [PMID: 15817681] Nature 2005;434:1144. [PMID: 15793561] Arch Pathol Lab Med 2006;130:1126. [PMID: 16879013]

Lactate dehydrogenase		
Lactate dehydrogenase, serum (LDH) 88–230 U/L [1.46–3.82 mckat/L] (laboratory-specific) SST $ Hemolyzed specimens are unacceptable.	LDH is an enzyme that catalyzes the interconversion of lactate and pyruvate in the presence of NAD/NADH. It is widely distributed in body cells and fluids. Because LDH is highly concentrated in RBCs, spuriously elevated serum levels occur if RBCs are hemolyzed during specimen collection.	**Increased in:** Tissue necrosis, especially in acute injury of cardiac muscle, RBCs, kidney, skeletal muscle, liver, lung, or skin. Commonly elevated in various carcinomas, in *Pneumocystis jiroveci* pneumonia (78–94%) and in chronic lymphocytic leukemia and other lymphomas. Marked elevations occur in hemolytic anemias, vitamin B$_{12}$ deficiency anemia, folate deficiency anemia, PV, thrombotic thrombocytopenic purpura (TTP), hepatitis, cirrhosis, obstructive jaundice, renal disease, musculoskeletal disease, and CHF. Drugs causing hepatotoxicity (eg, acetaminophen) or hemolysis. **Decreased in:** Drugs: clofibrate, fluoride (low dose).	In the Follicular Lymphoma International Prognostic Index, serum LDH is one of five prognostic factors (age, Ann Arbor stage, number of nodal sites, hemoglobin level, and serum LDH). Similarly, in chronic lymphocytic leukemia, the increase in serum LDH is used, along with lymphocyte count, bone marrow infiltration pattern and lymphocyte doubling time as a prognostic factor. Serum LDH is a useful prognostic biomarker in metastatic melanoma although serum S100B protein may be superior in predicting prognosis and response to treatment. LDH is not a useful liver function test, and it is not specific enough for the diagnosis of hemolytic or megaloblastic anemias. In diagnosis of myocardial infarction, serum LDH has been replaced by cardiac troponin I levels. LDH isoenzymes are not clinically useful. Clin Lymphoma 2005;6:21. [PMID: 15989702] Curr Opin Oncol 2005;17:167. [PMID: 15725923] Expert Rev Mol Diagn 2005;5:65. [PMID: 15723593] Haematologica 2005;90:391. [PMID: 15749671]

	Lactate

Test/Range/Collection	Physiologic Basis	Interpretation	Comments
Lactate, venous blood 0.5–2.0 meq/L [mmol/L] Gray $$ Collect on ice in gray-top tube containing fluoride to inhibit in vitro glycolysis and lactic acid production.	Severe tissue anoxia leads to anaerobic glucose metabolism with production of lactic acid (type A lactic acidosis). In other disorders, lactic acidosis (type B) occurs with no clinical evidence of inadequate tissue oxygen delivery.	**Increased in:** Lactic acidosis, ethanol ingestion, sepsis, shock, liver disease, diabetic ketoacidosis, muscular exercise, hypoxia; regional hypoperfusion (bowel ischemia); prolonged use of a tourniquet (spurious elevation); MELAS (mitochondrial myopathy, encephalopathy, lactic acidosis, and stroke-like episodes); type I glycogen storage disease, fructose 1,6-diphosphatase deficiency (rare), pyruvate dehydrogenase deficiency, non-Hodgkin and Burkitt lymphoma (rare). Drugs: phenformin, metformin (debated), isoniazid toxicity, nucleoside reverse-transcriptase inhibitors.	Lactic acidosis should be suspected when there is a markedly increased anion gap (>18 meq/L) in the absence of other causes (eg, renal failure, ketosis, ethanol, methanol, or salicylate). Lactic acidosis is characterized by lactate levels >5 mmol/L and serum pH <7.35. However, hypoalbuminemia may mask the anion gap and concomitant alkalosis may raise the pH. Blood lactate levels may indicate whether perfusion is being restored by therapy. J Intern Med 2004;255:179. [PMID: 14746555] J Intensive Care Med 2005;20:255. [PMID: 16145217]

	Lead	Lecithin/sphingomyelin ratio
Lead, whole blood (Pb) Child (<6 yrs): <10 mcg/dL Child (>6 yrs): <25 mcg/dL Adult: <40 mcg/dL [Child (<6 yrs): <0.48 mcmol/L Child (>6 yrs): <1.21 mcmol/L Adult: <1.93 mcmol/L] Industrial workers' limit: <50 mcg/dL Navy $$ Use trace metal-free navy blue top tube with heparin.	Lead salts are absorbed through ingestion, inhalation, or the skin. About 5–10% of ingested lead is found in blood, and 95% of this is in erythrocytes. 80–90% is taken up by bone, where it is relatively inactive. Lead poisons enzymes by binding to protein disulfide groups, leading to cell death. Lead levels fluctuate. Several specimens may be needed to rule out lead poisoning. There is substantial individual variability in vulnerability to lead.	**Increased in:** Lead poisoning, including abnormal ingestion (especially lead-containing paint, water from lead plumbing, moonshine whiskey), occupational exposures (metal smelters, miners, welders, storage battery workers, auto manufacturers, ship builders, paint manufacturers, printing workers, pottery workers, gasoline refinery workers, demolition and tank cleaning workers), retained bullets. Cognition may be impaired by modest elevations of blood lead concentrations. Neurologic impairment may be detectable in children with lead levels of 15 mcg/dL and in adults at 30 mcg/dL; full-blown symptoms appear at >60 mcg/dL. Most chronic lead poisoning leads to a moderate anemia with basophilic stippling of erythrocytes on peripheral blood smear. Acute poisoning is rare and associated with abdominal pain and constipation. Annu Rev Med 2004;55:209. [PMID: 14746518] Pediatrics 2004;113(4 Suppl):1016. [PMID: 15060194] Pediatrics 2005;116:1036. [PMID: 16199720] Clin Lab Med 2006;26:67. [PMID: 16567226]
Lecithin/sphingomyelin ratio, amniotic fluid (L/S ratio) >2.0 (method-dependent) $$$ Collect in a plastic tube.	This test is used to estimate lung maturity in fetuses at risk for hyaline membrane disease. As fetal pulmonary surfactant matures, there is a rapid rise in amniotic fluid lecithin content. To circumvent the dependency of lecithin concentrations on amniotic fluid volume and analytic recovery of lecithin, the assay examines the lecithin/sphingomyelin ratio.	**Increased in:** Contamination of amniotic fluid by blood, meconium, or vaginal secretions that contain lecithin (false-positives). **Decreased in:** Fetal lung immaturity; 95% of normal fetuses. Test identifies fetal lung maturity effectively only 60% of the time and has now been supplanted by amniotic fluid lamellar body counts. **Lamellar body counts** (using the platelet channel of automated hematology analyzers) can be used as a rapid screening test to predict lung maturation (<55,000/mcL suggests immaturity) with a negative predictive value of ~97%. Compared with the L/S ratio, lamellar body counting is faster, more objective, less labor intensive, less technique dependent, and less expensive than the L/S ratio. J Matern Fetal Neonatal Med 2003;14:373. [PMID: 15061315] Clin Biochem 2006;39:1. [PMID: 16303123] Pediatr Pulmonol 2007;42:3. [PMID: 17123320]

	Legionella antibody		
Test/Range/Collection	**Physiologic Basis**	**Interpretation**	**Comments**
Legionella antibody, serum <1:32 titer SST $$$ Submit paired sera, one collected within 2 weeks of illness and another 2–3 weeks later.	*Legionella pneumophila* is a weakly staining gram-negative bacillus that causes Pontiac fever (acute influenza-like illness) and Legionnaire disease (a pneumonia that may progress to a severe multisystem illness). It does not grow on routine bacteriologic culture media. There are at least six serogroups of *L pneumophila* and at least 22 species of *Legionella*. Indirect immunofluorescent assays for *L pneumophila* serogroup 1 (IgM and/or IgG) and serogroups 1–6 (IgM and/or IgG) are both available.	**Increased in:** Legionella infection (80% of patients with pneumonia have a fourfold rise in titer); cross-reactions with other infectious agents (*Yersinia pestis* [plague], *Francisella tularensis* [tularemia], *Bacteroides fragilis, Mycoplasma pneumoniae, Leptospira interrogans,* campylobacter serotypes).	The test provides only a retrospective lab diagnosis because it generally takes more than 3 weeks to mount a detectable antibody response. A greater than fourfold rise in titer to >1:128 in specimens gathered more than 3 weeks apart indicates recent infection. A single titer of >1:256 is considered diagnostic. About 50–60% of cases of legionellosis may have a positive direct fluorescent antibody test. Culture can have a sensitivity of 50%. All three methods may increase sensitivity to 90%. This test is species-specific. Polyvalent antiserum is needed to test for all serogroups and species. Urine *Legionella* antigen testing, in adjunct to cultures, may provide a rapid turnaround for results. The urine antigen test is very specific, but the sensitivity ranges from 70–90% because it detects primarily serogroup 1 infections. J Clin Microbiol 2002;40:3232. [PMID: 12202558] J Med Microbiol 2007;56(pt 1):94. [PMID: 17172523]

Leukemia/lymphoma phenotyping by flow cytometry		
Leukemia/lymphoma phenotyping by flow cytometry Blood, bone marrow aspirates, fine-needle aspirates, fresh tissue biopsies, body fluids. Lavender or yellow (blood), green (bone marrow) Specimen should be delivered within 24 hours. $$$$	Immunophenotyping by multiparameter flow cytometry is an integral part of the diagnosis and classification systems for leukemias and malignant lymphomas. The majority of immunophenotyping markers are the cluster of differentiation antigens, or CD antigens. Other commonly used markers include glycophorin A, HLA-DR, immunoglobulin (Ig), MPO (myeloperoxidase), and TdT (terminal deoxynucleotidyl transferase).	**Abnormal phenotype profile present in:** Acute myeloid leukemias, acute lymphoblastic leukemias, B- and T-cell non-Hodgkin lymphomas, plasma cell myeloma. **Markers expressed mainly in hematopoietic precursors:** HLA-DR, TdT, CD34; **B cells:** CD19, CD20, CD22, CD24, CD10, CD79, Ig heavy chains (γ, α, μ, δ), and light chains (κ, λ); **T cells:** CD3, CD7, CD5, CD2, CD4, CD8; **myeloid cells:** MPO, CD13, CD33, CD117. **Markers that suggest megakaryocytic differentiation:** CD41, CD42, CD61; **erythroid differentiation:** glycophorin, hemoglobin A; **monocytic differentiation:** CD14, CD15, CD64, CD68; **NK cells:** CD16, CD56; **hairy cell leukemia:** CD103.	Each leukemia/lymphoma has an unique diagnostic immunophenotype (Table 8–11). An interpretative report should be generated for each specimen analyzed. Multicolor analysis may be performed, allowing for an accurate definition of the surface and cytoplasmic antigen profile of specific cells. Two simultaneous hematologic malignancies may be detected within the same tissue site. Morphologic features remain the cornerstone of the evaluation of leukemia/lymphoma, but ancillary studies including immunophenotyping, cytogenetics, and/or molecular genetic testing are needed in most, if not all, cases. *WHO Classification of Tumors: Pathology and Genetics of Tumors of Hematopoietic and Lymphoid Tissues.* IARC Press 2001. Arch Pathol Lab Med 2004;128:1004. [PMID: 15335254]

	Lipase

Test/Range/Collection	Physiologic Basis	Interpretation	Comments
Lipase, serum 0–160 U/L [0–2.66 mckat/L] (laboratory-specific) SST $$	Lipases are responsible for hydrolysis of glycerol esters of long-chain fatty acids to produce fatty acids and glycerol. Lipases are produced in the liver, intestine, tongue, stomach, and many other cells. Assays are highly dependent on the substrate used.	**Increased in:** Acute, recurrent, or chronic pancreatitis, pancreatic pseudocyst, pancreatic malignancy, peritonitis, biliary disease, hepatic disease, diabetes mellitus (especially diabetic ketoacidosis), intestinal disease, gastric malignancy or perforation, cystic fibrosis, inflammatory bowel disease (Crohn disease and ulcerative colitis).	Serum lipase may be a more reliable test than serum amylase for the initial diagnosis of acute pancreatitis, due to an increased sensitivity in acute alcoholic pancreatitis and because lipase remains elevated longer than amylase. The specificity of lipase and amylase in acute pancreatitis is similar, though both are poor. Simultaneous measurement of serum amylase and lipase does not improve diagnostic accuracy. Measurement of serum lipase does not help in determining the severity or etiology of acute pancreatitis, and daily measurements are of no value in assessing the patient's clinical progress or ultimate prognosis. Test sensitivity is not very good for chronic pancreatitis or pancreatic cancer. Am J Gastroenterol 2002;97:1309. [PMID: 12094843] J Clin Gastroenterol 2002;34:459. [PMID: 11907364] Clin Chim Acta 2005;362:26. [PMID: 16024009]

	Luteinizing hormone		Lyme disease antibody
Luteinizing hormone, serum (LH) Male: 1–10 mIU/mL Female: (mIU/mL) Follicular 1–18 Luteal 0.4–20 Midcycle peak 24–105 Postmenopausal 15–62 (laboratory-specific) SST $$	LH is stimulated by the hypothalamic hormone gonadotropin-releasing hormone (GnRH). It is secreted from the anterior pituitary and acts on the gonads. LH is the principal regulator of steroid biosynthesis in the ovary and testis.	**Increased in:** Primary hypogonadism, polycystic ovary syndrome, postmenopause, endometriosis, after depot leuprolide injection; immunoassay result may be falsely elevated in pregnancy. **Decreased in:** Pituitary or hypothalamic failure, anorexia nervosa, bulimia, advanced prostate cancer, severe stress, malnutrition, Kallman syndrome (gonadotropin deficiency associated with anosmia). Drugs: digoxin, oral contraceptives, phenothiazines.	In male hypogonadism, serum LH and FSH levels can distinguish between primary (hypergonadotropic) and secondary (hypogonadotropic) hypogonadism. Hypogonadism associated with aging (andropause) may present a mixed picture, with low testosterone levels and low to low-normal gonadotropin levels. Repeated measurement may be required to diagnose gonadotropin deficiencies. Elevated serum LH levels are a common feature in polycystic ovary syndrome, but measurement of total testosterone is the test of choice to diagnose polycystic ovary syndrome. Endocr Res 2004;30:1. [PMID: 15098915] Hum Reprod 2004;19:41. [PMID: 14681154] Treat Endocrinol 2005;4:293. [PMID: 16185098]
Lyme disease antibody, serum ELISA: negative (<1:8 titer) Western blot: nonreactive SST $	Test detects the presence of antibody to *Borrelia burgdorferi*, the etiologic agent in Lyme disease, an inflammatory disorder transmitted by the ticks *Ixodes dammini, I pacificus,* and *I scapularis* in the northeastern and midwestern, western, and southeastern United States, respectively. Detects IgM antibody, which develops within 3–6 weeks after the onset of rash or IgG, which develops within 6–8 weeks after the onset of disease. IgG antibody may persist for months.	**Positive in:** Lyme disease, asymptomatic individuals living in endemic areas, immunization with recombinant outer-surface protein A (OspA) Lyme disease vaccine, syphilis (*Treponema pallidum*), tick-borne relapsing fever (*Borrelia hermsii*). **Negative in:** First 5 weeks of Borrelia infection or after antibiotic therapy.	Test is less sensitive in patients with only a rash. Because culture or direct visualization of the organism is difficult, serologic diagnosis (by ELISA) is indicated, although sensitivity and specificity and standardization of procedure between laboratories need improvement. Cross-reactions may occur with syphilis (should be excluded by RPR and treponemal antibody assays). Arch Intern Med 2001;161:2015. Med Clin North Am 2002;86:311. [PMID: 11982304] Clin Infect Dis 2006;43:1089. [PMID: 17029130] N Engl J Med 2006;354:2794. [PMID: 16807416]

	Magnesium

Test/Range/Collection	Physiologic Basis	Interpretation	Comments
Magnesium, serum (Mg^{2+}) 1.8–3.0 mg/dL [0.75–1.25 mmol/L] ***Panic:*** <0.5 or >4.5 mg/dL SST $	Magnesium is primarily an intracellular cation (second most abundant, 60% found in bone); it is a necessary cofactor in numerous enzyme systems, particularly ATPases. By regulating enzymes controlling intracellular calcium, Mg^{2+} affects smooth muscle vasoconstriction, important to the underlying pathophysiology of several critical illnesses. In extracellular fluid, it influences neuromuscular response and irritability. Magnesium concentration is determined by intestinal absorption, renal excretion, and exchange with bone and intracellular fluid.	**Increased in:** Dehydration, tissue trauma, renal failure, hypoadrenocorticism, hypothyroidism. Drugs: aspirin (prolonged use), lithium, magnesium salts, progesterone, triamterene. **Decreased in:** Chronic diarrhea, enteric fistula, starvation, chronic alcoholism, total parenteral nutrition with inadequate replacement, hypoparathyroidism (especially post parathyroid surgery), acute pancreatitis, chronic glomerulonephritis, hyperaldosteronism, diabetic ketoacidosis, CHF, critical illness, Gitelman syndrome (familial hypokalemia– hypomagnesemia– hypocalciuria), hereditary isolated magnesium wasting, induced hypothermia. Drugs: albuterol, amphotericin B, calcium salts, cisplatin, citrates (blood transfusion), cyclosporine, diuretics, ethacrynic acid.	Magnesium deficiency correlates with higher mortality and poorer clinical outcome in the ICU and is directly implicated in hypokalemia, hypocalcemia, tetany, and dysrhythmia. Hypomagnesemia is associated with tetany, weakness, disorientation, and somnolence. A magnesium deficit may exist with little or no apparent change in serum level. There is a progressive reduction in serum magnesium level during normal pregnancy (related to hemodilution). Eur J Heart Fail 2002;4:167. [PMID: 11959045] J Intensive Care Med 2005;20:3. [PMID: 15665255] J Natl Cancer Inst 2005;97:1221. [PMID: 16106027]

Mean corpuscular hemoglobin		
Mean corpuscular hemoglobin, blood (MCH) 26–34 pg Lavender $	MCH indicates the amount of hemoglobin per RBC in absolute units. MCH is calculated from measured values of hemoglobin (Hb) (g/dL) and RBC/L by the formula: $MCH = (Hb/RBC) \times 10$	**Increased in:** Macrocytosis, hemochromatosis. **Decreased in:** Microcytosis (iron deficiency), thalassemia, hypochromia (lead poisoning, sideroblastic anemia, anemia of chronic disease).	Low MCH can mean hypochromia or microcytosis or both. High MCH is evidence of macrocytosis. Pediatr Hematol Oncol 2002;19:569. [PMID: 12487832] Lab Hematol 2005;11:107. [PMID: 16024334] J Lab Clin Med 2006;147:191. [PMID: 16581347]

Test/Range/Collection	Physiologic Basis	Interpretation	Comments
Mean corpuscular hemoglobin concentration, blood (MCHC) 31–36 g/dL [310–360 g/L] Lavender $	MCHC is the average hemoglobin concentration in red blood cells. It is calculated from hemoglobin concentration of whole blood (Hb, g/dL) and hematocrit (MCV × RBC) in fL. MCHC equals $$\frac{Hb}{MCV \times RBC}$$	**Increased in:** Marked spherocytosis (hereditary spherocytosis or immune hemolysis). Spuriously increased in autoagglutination, hemolysis (with spuriously high Hb or low MCV or RBC), lipemia, cellular dehydration syndromes, xerocytosis. **Decreased in:** Hypochromic anemia (iron deficiency, thalassemia, lead poisoning), sideroblastic anemia, anemia of chronic disease. Spuriously decreased with high white blood cell count, low Hb, or high MCV or RBC.	The MCHC value may be misleading in the presence of a dimorphic population of RBCs. Pediatr Hematol Oncol 2002;19:569. [PMID: 12487832] Lab Hematol 2005;11:107. [PMID: 16024334]
Mean corpuscular volume, blood (MCV) 80–100 fL Lavender $	MCV is the average volume of the red cells, and it is measured by automated instrument (electrical impedance or light scatter).	**Increased in:** Liver disease (alcoholic and nonalcoholic), alcohol abuse, HIV/AIDS, hemochromatosis, megaloblastic anemia (folate, vitamin B_{12} deficiencies), reticulocytosis, newborns. Spurious increase in autoagglutination, high white blood cell count. Drugs: methotrexate, phenytoin, zidovudine. **Decreased in:** Iron deficiency, thalassemia, sideroblastic anemia, hereditary spherocytosis, and some anemia of chronic disease.	MCV can be normal in combined iron and folate deficiency. In patients with two red cell populations (macrocytic and microcytic), MCV may be normal. MCV is an insensitive test in the evaluation of anemia. It is not uncommon for patients with iron deficiency anemia or pernicious anemia to have a normal MCV. A low MCV can be used as an indication of iron depletion in frequent blood donors and thus a guide to phlebotomy therapy for hemochromatosis. See anemias (Figure 8–5; Tables 8–2, 8–3). Pediatr Hematol Oncol 2002;19:569. [PMID: 12487832] Lab Hematol 2005;11:107. [PMID: 16024334] J Lab Clin Med 2006;147:191. [PMID: 16581347]

	Mean corpuscular hemoglobin concentration	Mean corpuscular volume

Metanephrines, Free (Unconjugated), Plasma		
Metanephrines, free (unconjugated), plasma <0.56 pmol/L SST $$$	Catecholamines (norepinephrine and epinephrine), secreted in excess by pheochromocytomas, are metabolized within tumor cells by the enzyme catechol-*O*-methyltransferase to metanephrines (normetanephrine and metanephrine), and these can be detected in plasma. Measurement of plasma concentrations of free (unconjugated) metanephrines offers several advantages for the detection of pheochromocytoma: independence of short-term changes noted in catecholamine secretion in response to change of posture, exercise, or intraoperative stress; good correlation with tumor mass; and only minor interference from drugs. In diagnosis of pheochromocytoma, determination of plasma-free metanephrines is often more reliable and efficient than other biochemical tests.	**Increased in:** Pheochromocytoma (sensitivity ~100%, specificity 89–94%).	Plasma-free metanephrines has been recommended as one of the the first-line biochemical tests for the diagnosis of pheochromocytoma. (See Pheochromocytoma algorithm, Figure 8–17.) Sensitivity of plasma-free metanephrines (99%) is higher than that of urinary fractionated metanephrines (97%), plasma catecholamines (84%), and urinary vanillylmandelic acid (64%). Specificity of plasma-free metanephrines (89–94%) compares favorably to urinary vanillylmandelic acid (95%), urinary total metanephrines (93%), urinary catecholamines (88%), plasma catecholamines (81%), and urinary fractionated metanephrines (69%). JAMA 2002;287:1427. [PMID: 11903030] J Intern Med 2005;257:60. [PMID: 15606377] Horm Metab Res 2005;37:717. [PMID: 16372223] Med J Aust 2005;183:201. [PMID: 16097921]

	Metanephrines		
Test/Range/Collection	Physiologic Basis	Interpretation	Comments
Metanephrines, urine 0.3–0.9 mg/24 h [1.6–4.9 mcmol/24 h] Urine bottle containing hydrochloric acid $$$ Collect 24-hour urine.	Catecholamines (norepinephrine and epinephrine), secreted in excess by pheochromocytomas, are metabolized by the enzyme catechol-O-methyltransferase to metanephrines (normetaphrine and metanephrine), and these are excreted in the urine.	**Increased in:** Pheochromocytoma (98% sensitivity, 93% specificity), neuroblastoma, ganglioneuroma. Drugs: MAD inhibitors.	Urinary metanephrines are often the first-line biochemical tests for the diagnostic evaluation of pheochromocytoma. (see Pheochromocytoma algorithm, Figure 8–17). Because <0.1% of hypertensives have a pheochromocytoma, routine screening of all hypertensives would yield a positive predictive value of <10%. Avoid overutilization of tests. Do not order urine vanillylmandelic acid, urine catecholamines, and plasma metanephrines and catecholamines at the same time. Plasma catecholamine levels are often spuriously increased when drawn in the hospital setting. Curr Hypertens Rep 2004;6:477. [PMID: 15527694] J Intern Med 2005;257:60. [PMID: 15606377] Horm Metab Res 2005;37:717. [PMID: 16372223] Med J Aust 2005;183:201. [PMID: 16097921]

Methanol		
Methanol, whole blood Negative Green or lavender $$	Methanol is extensively metabolized by alcohol dehydrogenase to formaldehyde and by aldehyde dehydrogenase to formic acid, the major toxic metabolite. Serum methanol levels >20 mg/dL are toxic and levels >40 mg/dL are life-threatening.	**Increased in:** Methanol intoxication.	Methanol intoxication is associated with metabolic acidosis and an osmolal gap (see Table 8–14). Methanol is commonly ingested in its pure form or in cleaning and copier solutions. Acute ingestion causes an optic neuritis that may result in blindness. Methanol poisoning can be fatal. Fomepizole, a competitive alcohol dehydrogenase inhibitor, can be used to treat methanol poisoning and can obviate the need for hemodialysis. Quantitative measurement of the serum methanol level using gas chromatography is expensive, time-consuming, and not always available. Because methanol is osmotically active and measurement of serum osmolality is easily performed, the osmolal gap is often used as a screening test. See Table 8–14. Toxicol Rev 2004;23:189. [PMID: 15862085] Pediatr Emerg Care 2006;22:740. [PMID: 17110870]

Test/Range/Collection	Physiologic Basis	Interpretation	Comments
Methemoglobin, whole blood (MetHb) 0.15 g/dL [<23.25 mmol/L] or <1.15% of total Hb Blood gas syringe, Lavender or Green $$ Don't remove the stopper or cap, analyze promptly.	Methemoglobin has its heme iron in the oxidized ferric state and thus cannot combine with and transport oxygen. Methemoglobin can be assayed spectrophotometrically by measuring the decrease in absorbance at 630–635 nm due to the conversion of methemoglobin to cyanmethemoglobin with cyanide. CO-oximetry is useful for rapid quantitation of methemoglobin.	**Increased in:** Hereditary methemoglobinemia: structural hemoglobin variants (hemoglobin M) (rare), NADH-MetHb reductase (cytochrome b5 reductase) deficiency. Acquired methemoglobinemia: Oxidant drugs such as sulfonamides, dapsone, sulfasalazine, primaquine, isoniazid, nitrites, nitroglycerin, nitrates, aniline dyes, phenacetin, hydralazine, local anesthetics (eg, benzocaine, lidocaine), ifostamide chemotherapy, chloramine toxicity during hemodialysis, infants with diarrhea or urinary tract infections (due to oxidant stress).	Levels of 1.5 g/dL (about 10% of total Hb) result in visible cyanosis. The diagnosis can be suspected by the characteristic chocolate brown color of a freshly obtained blood sample. Patients with levels of about 35% have headache, weakness, and breathlessness (tachycardia, tachypnea). Levels in excess of 70% are usually fatal. Administration of methylene blue facilitates the reduction of MetHb to Hb in the enzyme deficiency and ameliorates the cyanosis. But it has no effect in reducing Hb M variants or in relieving the cyanosis that they cause. Blood 2002;100:3447. [PMID: 12028041] Clin Chem 2005;51:434. [PMID: 15514101] Pediatrics 2006;117:e806. [PMID: 16585290]

MTHFR mutation		
Methylenetetrahydrofolate reductase (MTHFR) mutation Blood Lavender $$$$	5,10-Methylenetetrahydrofolate reductase (MTHFR) plays a key role in folate metabolism. MTHFR enzyme deficiency leads to hyperhomocysteinemia and homocystinuria. Increased plasma homocysteine is a risk factor for arteriosclerotic vascular disease and deep-vein thrombosis. Two mutations in the human MTHFR gene, C667T and A1298C, result in moderate impairment of MTHFR activity.	**Positive in:** Individuals with MTHFR C677T and/or A1298C mutations (sensitivity and specificity approach 100%).	The MTHFR mutation assay is indicated for patients with early-onset arteriosclerotic vascular disease or thrombosis, particularly those with hyperhomocysteinemia or significant family histories. See recommended testing for venous thrombosis (Figure 8–24). Both C677T and A1298C mutations should be examined when assessing genetic risk factors for individuals with hyperhomocysteinemia. Only individuals homozygous for C677T mutation or compound heterozygous for the C677T/A1298C mutations have significantly elevated plasma homocysteine levels. Double homozygotes have not been reported. The assay is typically polymerase chain reaction (PCR) based. Mol Genet Metab 2005;86:91. [PMID: 16185908] Nutr Rev 2005;63:398. [PMID: 16370225]

	Methylmalonic acid

Test/Range/Collection	Physiologic Basis	Interpretation	Comments
Methylmalonic acid (MMA), serum 0–0.4 mcmol/L (0–4.7 mcg/dL) SST (also acceptable: lavender, green) $$	Elevation of serum methylmalonic acid (MMA) in cobalamin (B_{12}) deficiency results from impaired conversion of methylmalonyl-CoA to succinyl-CoA, a pathway involving methylmalonyl-CoA mutase as its enzyme and adenosylcobalamin as its coenzyme. Serum MMA is used to indirectly evaluate vitamin B_{12} status, mainly for confirming B_{12} deficiency in patients with low serum B_{12} levels.	**Increased in:** Vitamin B_{12} (cobalamin) deficiency (95%), pernicious anemia, renal insufficiency, pregnancy, elderly (5–15%).	Explanation of high frequency (5–15%) of increased serum MMA in the elderly with low or normal serum B_{12} is unclear. Only a small number have pernicious anemia confirmed. Normal levels can exclude vitamin B_{12} deficiency in the presence of low unexplained B_{12} levels found in lymphoid disorders. Test is usually normal in HIV patients who may have low vitamin B_{12} levels without actual vitamin B_{12} deficiency, these patients usually have low vitamin B_{12}-binding protein. In individuals with mildly elevated MMA levels (0.40–2.00 μmol/L), vitamin B_{12} treatment normalizes MMA level but has no significant effect on hemoglobin, MCV, or anemic, neurologic, or gastroenterologic symptoms, at least in the short term. Urine MMA (reference interval: 0–3.6 mmol/mol creatinine) test is also available for evaluating B_{12} status as well as monitoring patients with methylmalonic aciduria. Clin Chem 2003;49:2067. [PMID: 14633879] Clin Chem 2004;50:1482. [PMID: 15277369] Clin Chem 2006;52:754. [PMID: 16595826]

Metyrapone test (overnight)		
Metyrapone test (overnight), plasma or serum 8 AM cortisol: <10 mcg/dL [<280 nmol/L] 8 AM 11-deoxycortisol: >7 mcg/dL [>202 nmol/L] SST, lavender, or green $$$ Give 2.0–3.0 g of metyrapone orally (dependent upon body weight) at 12:00 midnight. Draw serum cortisol and 11-deoxycortisol levels at 8:00 AM.	The metyrapone stimulation test assesses both pituitary and adrenal reserve and is mainly used to diagnose secondary adrenal insufficiency (see Adrenocortical Insufficiency algorithm, Figure 8–3). Metyrapone is a drug that inhibits adrenal 11 β-hydroxylase and blocks cortisol synthesis. The consequent fall in cortisol increases release of ACTH and hence production of steroids formed proximal to the block (eg, 11-deoxycortisol).	**Decreased in:** An 8 AM 11-deoxycortisol level ≤7 mcg/dL indicates primary or secondary adrenal insufficiency.	The overnight metyrapone test assesses the integrity of the entire hypothalamic-pituitary-adrenal axis. It can be useful in assessing the HPA axis post-hypophysectomy, in diagnosing secondary adrenal insufficiency in AIDS patients, or in steroid-treated patients to assess the extent of suppression of the pituitary-adrenal axis. The use of an extended metyrapone test in the differential diagnosis of ACTH-dependent Cushing syndrome (pituitary versus ectopic) has been questioned. Test is not useful in panic disorder, posttraumatic stress disorder, or Fibromyalgia syndrome. Clin Endocrinol (Oxf) 2002;56:533. [PMID: 11966747] Neth J Med 2005;63:435. [PMID: 16397312]

Test/Range/Collection	Physiologic Basis	Interpretation	Comments
β₂-Microglobulin, serum (β₂-M) <0.2 mg/dL [<2.0 mg/L] SST $$$	β₂-Microglobulin is a low-molecular-weight protein that is the light chain of the class I MHC antigens. It is present on the surface of all nucleated cells and in all body fluids. It is almost totally reabsorbed and catabolized by the proximal renal tubules. It is increased in many conditions that are accompanied by high cell turnover and/or immune activation.	**Increased in:** Inflammatory conditions (eg, inflammatory bowel disease), infections (eg, HIV, CMV), graft rejection, autoimmune disorders, lymphoid malignancies, multiple myeloma, chronic renal failure, lymphoproliferative, myeloproliferative and myelodysplastic disorders.	Because of its accumulation with renal dysfunction and its ability to become glycosylated, form fibrils, and deposit in tissues, β₂-M is a cause of dialysis-associated amyloidosis. Of tests used to predict progression to AIDS in HIV-infected patients, CD4 cell number has the most predictive power, followed closely by β₂-M. Serum β₂-M levels are elevated in many hematological and lymphoid malignancies. An association has been found between serum β₂-M levels and tumor burden in some disorders, particularly multiple myeloma, making it a valuable prognostic marker in these conditions. J Commun Dis 2004;36:166. [PMID: 16509252] J Clin Oncol 2005;23:3412. [PMID: 15809451] Curr Opin Hematol 2006;13:266. [PMID: 16755224] Semin Dial 2006;19:105. [PMID: 16551286]

Microhemagglutination–*Treponema pallidum*		
Microhemagglutination- ***Treponema pallidum,*** serum (MHA-TP) Nonreactive Marbled $$	The MHA-TP test measures specific antibody against *T pallidum* in a patient's serum by agglutination of *T pallidum* antigen-coated erythrocytes. Antibodies to nonpathogenic treponemes are first removed by binding to nonpathogenic treponemal antigens.	**Increased in:** Syphilis: primary (64–87%), secondary (96–100%), late latent (96–100%), tertiary (94–100%); infectious mononucleosis, collagen-vascular diseases, hyperglobulinemia, and dysglobulinemia.	Test is used to confirm reactive serologic tests for syphilis (RPR or VDRL). Compared with FTA-ABS, MHA-TP is slightly less sensitive in all stages of syphilis and becomes reactive somewhat later in the disease. Because test usually remains positive for long periods of time regardless of therapy, it is not useful in assessing the effectiveness of therapy. In one study, 36 months after treatment of syphilis, 13% of patients had nonreactive MHA-TP tests. The MHA-TP, like the FTA-ABS, is not to be used as a screening test for syphilis and is not recommended for CSF specimens. Clin Microbiol Rev 1995;8:1. [PMID: 7704889] Murray PR et al (editors): *Manual of Clinical Microbiology,* 8th ed. ASM Press, 2003.

Test/Range/Collection	Physiologic Basis	Interpretation	Comments
			Mitochondrial antibody
Mitochondrial antibodies (AMA), serum Negative (<1.0 U) SST $$	Originally demonstrated using immunofluorescence approaches, antimitochondrial antibodies can now be detected using commercially available ELISAs. Although ELISAs are more practical, they are slightly less sensitive than immunofluorescence techniques. In AMA-negative patients with a high suspicion of primary biliary cirrhosis (PBC), antimitochondrial autoantibodies can be sought using recombinant autoantigens.	**Increased in:** Primary biliary cirrhosis (85–95%), chronic active hepatitis (25–28%), occasionally in CREST syndrome and other autoimmune diseases; lower titers in viral hepatitis, infectious mononucleosis, neoplasms, cryptogenic cirrhosis (25–30%).	Primarily used to distinguish PBC (antibody present) from extrahepatic biliary obstruction (antibody absent). The antigens recognized by AMA have been designated M1–M9. AMA from patients with PBC recognize the M2 antigen complex, which includes enzymes of the 2-pyruvate dehydrogenase (PDH-E2) and 2-oxoglutarate dehydrogenase. The titer or levels of AMA do not indicate disease activity or prognosis in patients with PBC. AMA subtype profiles do not predict prognosis in patients with PBC. Am J Gastroenterol 2002;97:999. [PMID: 12003438] N Engl J Med 2005;353:1261. [PMID: 16177252] Adv Clin Chem 2005;40:127. [PMID: 16177252] Semin Liver Dis 2005;25:337. [PMID: 16143949]

	Neutrophil cytoplasmic antibodies		Nuclear antibody
Neutrophil cytoplasmic antibodies (ANCA), serum Negative SST $$$	Measurement of autoantibodies in serum against cytoplasmic constituents of neutrophils. (See also Autoantibodies, Table 8–6.) Dual testing by standard indirect immunofluorescence for serum cytoplasmic ANCA (cANCA) and perinuclear ANCA (pANCA) and target antigen-specific assays (myeloperoxidase-ANCA or proteinase 3-ANCA) is often recommended.	**Positive in:** Wegener granulomatosis, systemic vasculitis, pauci-immune crescentic glomerulonephritis, paraneoplastic vasculitis, Churg-Strauss angiitis. microscopic polyangitis, drug-induced vasculitis, ulcerative colitis.	In the patient with systemic vasculitis, elevated ANCA levels imply active disease and high likelihood of recurrence. However, ANCA levels can be persistently elevated and should be used in conjunction with other clinical indices in treatment decisions. For ANCA-associated vasculitis, ANCA sensitivity, specificity, positive predictive value, and negative predictive value vary with method and population studied. Arch Intern Med 2002;162:1509. [PMID: 12090888] Clin Immunol 2002;103:196. [PMID: 12027425] Best Pract Res Clin Rheumatol 2005;19:263. [PMID: 15857795] Lancet 2006;368:404. [PMID: 16876669]
Nuclear antibody, serum (ANA) <1:20 SST $$	Heterogeneous antibodies to nuclear antigens (DNA and RNA, histone, and nonhistone proteins). Nuclear antibody is measured in serum by layering the patient's serum over human epithelial cells and detecting the antibody with fluorescein-conjugated polyvalent antihuman immunoglobulin.	**Elevated in:** Patients over age 65 (35–75%, usually in low titers), systemic lupus erythematosus (98%), drug-induced lupus (100%), Sjögren syndrome (80%), rheumatoid arthritis (30–50%), scleroderma (60%), mixed connective tissue disease (100%), Felty syndrome, mononucleosis, hepatic or biliary cirrhosis, hepatitis, leukemia, myasthenia gravis, dermatomyositis, polymyositis, chronic renal failure.	A negative ANA test does not completely rule out SLE, but alternative diagnoses should be considered. Pattern of ANA staining may give some clues to diagnoses, but because the pattern also changes with serum dilution, it is not routinely reported. Only the rim (peripheral) pattern is highly specific (for SLE). Not useful as a screening test. Should be used only when there is clinical evidence of a connective tissue disease. Curr Opin Rheumatol 2000;12:364. Am J Clin Pathol 2002;117:316. [PMID: 11863229] Scand J Immunol 2006;64:227. [PMID: 16918691]

	Oligoclonal bands	

Test/Range/Collection	Physiologic Basis	Interpretation	Comments
Oligoclonal bands, serum and CSF (OCBs) Negative SST and glass or plastic tube for CSF $$ Collect serum and CSF simultaneously.	Electrophoretic examination of IgG found in CSF may show oligoclonal bands not found in serum. This suggests local production in CSF of limited species of IgG. The pathogenesis of OCBs in MS is still obscure.	**Positive in:** Multiple sclerosis (sensitivity 81–95%; specificity 43%; positive predictive value 30%; negative predictive value 88%), CNS syphilis, subacute sclerosing panencephalitis, progressive multifocal leukoencephalopathy, Guillain-Barré syndrome, other CNS inflammatory diseases.	Test is indicated only when multiple sclerosis is suspected clinically. Test interpretation is very subjective. IgG index is a more reliable test analytically, but neither test is specific for multiple sclerosis. Quantification of OCBs in CSF is an insensitive prognostic indicator and should not be used to influence treatment decisions. J Neurol 2002;249:375. [PMID: 11967640] Adv Neurol 2006;98:147. [PMID: 16400832] Neurol Res 2006;28:236. [PMID: 16687047]

Osmolality, serum		

Osmolality, serum
(Osm)

285–293 mosm/kg H$_2$O
[mmol/kg H$_2$O]
Panic: <240 or >320
mosm/kg H$_2$O

SST
$$

Test measures the osmotic pressure of serum by the freezing point depression method.

Plasma and urine osmolality are more useful indicators of degree of hydration than BUN, hematocrit, or serum proteins.

Serum osmolality can be estimated by the following formula:

$$Osm = 2(Na^+) + \frac{BUN}{2.8}$$
$$+ \frac{Glucose}{18}$$

where Na$^+$ is in meq/L and BUN and glucose are in mg/dL.

Increased in: Diabetic ketoacidosis, nonketotic hyperosmolar hyperglycemic coma, hypernatremia secondary to dehydration (diarrhea, severe burns, vomiting, fever, hyperventilation, inadequate water intake, central or nephrogenic diabetes insipidus, or osmotic diuresis), hypernatremia with normal hydration (hypothalamic disorders, defective osmostat), hypernatremia with overhydration (iatrogenic or accidental excessive NaCl or NaHCO$_3$ intake), alcohol or other toxic ingestion (see Comments), hypercalcemia; tube feedings. Drugs: corticosteroids, mannitol, glycerin.

Decreased in: Pregnancy (third trimester), hyponatremia with hypovolemia (adrenal insufficiency, renal losses, diarrhea, vomiting, severe burns, peritonitis, pancreatitis), hyponatremia with normovolemia (SIADH), hyponatremia with hypervolemia (CHF, cirrhosis, nephrotic syndrome, postoperative state). Drugs: chlorthalidone, cyclophosphamide, thiazides.

If the difference between calculated and measured serum osmolality is greater than 10 mosm/kg H$_2$O, suspect the presence of a low-molecular-weight toxin (alcohol, methanol, isopropyl alcohol, ethylene glycol, acetone, ethyl ether, paraldehyde, or mannitol), ethanol being the most common. (See Table 8–14 for further explanation.)

Every 100 mg/dL of ethanol increases serum osmolality by 22 mosm/kg H$_2$O.

While the osmolal gap may overestimate the blood alcohol level, a normal serum osmolality excludes ethanol intoxication.

Measurement of serum osmolality is an important first step in the laboratory evaluation of the hyponatremic patient. The simultaneous measurement of plasma ADH (vasopressin) and plasma osmolality in a dehydration test is the most powerful diagnostic tool in the differential diagnosis of polyuria/polydipsia.

CMAJ 2002;166:1056. [PMID: 12002984]

	Osmolality, urine	
Test/Range/Collection	**Physiologic Basis**	**Interpretation**	**Comments**

Test/Range/Collection	Physiologic Basis	Interpretation	Comments
Osmolality, urine (Urine Osm) Random: 100–900 mosm/kg H_2O [mmol/kg H_2O] Urine container $$	Test measures renal tubular concentrating ability.	**Increased in:** Hypovolemia. Drugs: anesthetic agents (during surgery), carbamazepine, chlorpropamide, cyclophosphamide, metolazone, vincristine. **Decreased in:** Diabetes insipidus, primary polydipsia, exercise, starvation. Drugs: acetohexamide, demeclocycline, glyburide, lithium, tolazamide.	In the hypoosmolar state (serum osmolality <280 mom/kg), urine osmolality is used to determine whether water excretion is normal or impaired. A urine osmolality value of <100 mom/kg indicates complete and appropriate suppression of antidiuretic hormone secretion. With average fluid intake, normal random urine osmolality is 100–900 mosm/kg H_2O. After 12-hour fluid restriction, normal random urine osmolality is >850 mosm/kg H_2O. Am J Cardiol 2005;95:2B. [PMID: 15847851] Emerg Med Clin North Am 2005;23:749. [PMID: 15982544] Int J Biochem Cell Biol 2003;35:1495. [PMID: 12824060] Endocrinol Metab Clin North Am 2006;35:873. [PMID: 17127152]

Oxygen, partial pressure

Oxygen, partial pressure (Po_2), whole blood 83–108 mm Hg [11.04–14.36 kPa] Heparinized syringe $$$ Collect arterial blood in a heparinized syringe. Send to laboratory immediately on ice.	Test measures the partial pressure of oxygen (oxygen tension) in arterial blood. Partial pressure of oxygen is critical because it determines (along with hemoglobin and blood supply) tissue oxygen supply.	**Increased in:** Oxygen therapy. **Decreased in:** Ventilation/perfusion mismatching (asthma, COPD, atelectasis, pulmonary embolism, pneumonia, interstitial lung disease, airway obstruction by foreign body, shock); alveolar hypoventilation (kyphoscoliosis, neuromuscular disease, head injury, stroke); right-to-left shunt (congenital heart disease). Drugs: barbiturates, opioids.	% Saturation of hemoglobin (So_2) represents the oxygen content divided by the oxygen-carrying capacity of hemoglobin. % Saturation on blood gas reports is calculated, not measured. It is calculated from Po_2 and pH using reference oxyhemoglobin dissociation curves for normal adult hemoglobin (lacking methemoglobin, carboxyhemoglobin, etc). At Po_2 <60 mm Hg, the oxygen saturation (and content) cannot be reliably estimated from the Po_2. Therefore, oximetry should be used to determine % saturation directly. Emerg Med Clin North Am 1986;4:235. [PMID: 3084205] Br J Nurs 2004;13:522. [PMID: 15215728]

	Parathyroid hormone		
Test/Range/Collection	Physiologic Basis	Interpretation	Comments
Parathyroid hormone, serum (PTH) Intact PTH: 11–54 pg/mL [1.2–5.7 pmol/L] (laboratory-specific) SST $$$$ Fasting sample preferred; simultaneous measurement of serum calcium and phosphorus is also required.	PTH is secreted from the parathyroid glands. It mobilizes calcium from bone, increases distal renal tubular reabsorption of calcium, decreases proximal renal tubular reabsorption of phosphorus, and stimulates 1,25-hydroxy vitamin D synthesis from 25-hydroxy vitamin D by renal 1α-hydroxylase. The "intact" PTH molecule (84 amino acids) has a circulating half-life of about 5 minutes. Carboxyl terminal and mid-molecule fragments make up 90% of circulating PTH. They are biologically inactive, cleared by the kidney, and have half-lives of about 1–2 hours. The amino terminal fragment is biologically active and has a half-life of 1–2 minutes. Measurement of PTH by immunoassay depends on the specificity of the antibodies used. Intact PTH assays use two antibodies ("sandwich" immunoassay) are the standard assays. The second- and third-generation intact PTH assays are less prone to interference from large PTH fragments (eg, amino acids 7–84), and the enhanced assays measure only the biologically intact PTH molecule (amino acids 1–84).	**Increased in:** Primary hyperparathyroidism, secondary hyperparathyroidism due to renal disease, vitamin D deficiency. Drugs: lithium, furosemide, propofol, phosphates. **Decreased in:** Hypoparathyroidism, sarcoidosis, hyperthyroidism, hypomagnesemia, malignancy with hypercalcemia, nonparathyroid hypercalcemia.	PTH results must always be evaluated in light of concurrent serum calcium levels. PTH tests differ in sensitivity and specificity from assay to assay and from laboratory to laboratory. Carboxyl terminal antibody measures intact, carboxyl terminal and midmolecule fragments. It is 85% sensitive and 95% specific for primary hyperparathyroidism. Amino terminal antibody measures intact and amino terminal fragments. It is about 75% sensitive for hyperparathyroidism. Intact PTH assays are preferred because they detect PTH suppression in nonparathyroid hypercalcemia. Sensitivity of immunometric assays is 85–90% for primary hyperparathyroidism. Intraoperative quick PTH monitoring in patients undergoing parathyroidectomy can be used to confirm cure and predict long-term operative success in most cases. A low intraoperative PTH level during thyroid surgery is a predictor of postoperative hypocalcemia resulting from parathyroid gland ischemia. See diagnostic algorithms for hypercalcemia and hypocalcemia (Figures 8–12 and 8–13). Arch Surg 2002;137:186. [PMID: 11822958] Surgery 2002;131:515. [PMID: 12019404] Clin Chim Acta 2004;343:167. [PMID: 15115690] Semin Dial 2005; 18:296. [PMID: 16076352]

Parathyroid hormone-related protein		
Parathyroid hormone-related protein (PTHrP), plasma Assay-specific (pmol/L or undetectable) Tube containing anticoagulant and protease inhibitors; specimen drawn without a tourniquet. $$	Parathyroid hormone-related protein (PTHrP) is a 139- to 173-amino acid protein with amino terminal homology to PTH. The homology explains the ability of PTHrP to bind to the PTH receptor and have PTH-like effects on bone and kidney. PTHrP induces increased plasma calcium, decreased plasma phosphorus, and increased urinary cAMP. PTHrP is found in keratinocytes, fibroblasts, placenta, brain, pituitary gland, adrenal gland, stomach, liver, testicular Leydig cells, and mammary glands. Its physiologic role in these diverse sites is unknown. PTHrP is secreted by solid malignant tumors (lung, breast, kidney; other squamous tumors) and produces humoral hypercalcemia of malignancy. PTHrP can act as an oncoprotein to regulate the growth and proliferation of many common malignancies. PTHrP analysis is by immunoradiometric assay (IRMA). Assay of choice is amino terminal-specific IRMA. Two-site IRMA assays require sample collection in protease inhibitors because serum proteases destroy immunoreactivity.	**Increased in:** Humoral hypercalcemia of malignancy (80% of solid tumors).	Assays directed at the amino terminal portion of PTHrP are not influenced by renal failure. Increases in PTHrP concentrations are readily detectable with most current assays in the majority of patients with humoral hypercalcemia of malignancy. About 20% of patients with malignancy and hypercalcemia have low PTHrP levels because their hypercalcemia is caused by local osteolytic processes. Cancer 1994;73:2223. [PMID: 8156530] Endocrinol Metab Clin North Am 2000;29:629. [PMID: 11033764]

	Partial thromboplastin time	
Test/Range/Collection	Physiologic Basis	Interpretation	Comments

Test/Range/Collection	Physiologic Basis	Interpretation	Comments
Partial thromboplastin time, activated, plasma (aPTT) 25–35 seconds (range varies) ***Panic:*** ≥60 seconds (off heparin) Blue $$ Do not contaminate specimen with heparin.	The aPTT is a clot-based test in which phospholipid reagent, an activator substance, and calcium are added to the patient's plasma, and the time for a fibrin clot to form is measured. PTT evaluates the intrinsic and common coagulation pathways and adequacy of all coagulation factors except XIII and VII. PTT is usually abnormal if any factor level drops below 25–40% of normal, depending on the PTT reagent used. PTT is commonly used to monitor heparin therapy.	**Increased in:** Deficiency of any individual coagulation factor except Factors XIII and VII, presence of nonspecific inhibitor (eg, lupus anticoagulant), specific factor inhibitor, von Willebrand disease (PTT may also be normal), hemophilia A and B, DIC. Drugs: heparin, direct thrombin inhibitor (eg, hirudin, argatroban), warfarin. See evaluation of isolated prolongation of PTT (Figure 8–19) and bleeding disorders (Figure 8–7, Table 8–7). **Decreased in:** Hypercoagulable states (eg, increased factor VIII levels).	PTT cannot be used to monitor very high doses of heparin (eg, cardiac bypass surgery) because the clotting time is beyond the analytical measurement range of PTT. For patients with documented lupus anticoagulant, PTT can not be used to monitor heparin therapy. Patients receiving low molecular weight heparin usually have normal PTT values. PTT may be normal in patients with von Willebrand disease and chronic DIC. Heparin contamination is a very common cause of an unexplained prolonged PTT. Heparin neutralization with heparinase may be needed to rule out this possibility. PTT may be falsely prolonged if anticoagulant volume (eg, PV) or if the specimen tube is not fully filled. Chest 2004;126:188S. [PMID: 15383472] Thromb Haemost 2004;91:1137. [PMID: 15175800] Clin Lab Haematol 2006;28:105. [PMID: 16630214]

pH			
pH, whole blood Arterial: 7.35–7.45 Venous: 7.31–7.41 Heparinized syringe $$$ Specimen must be collected in heparinized syringe and immediately transported on ice to lab without exposure to air.	pH assesses the acid–base status of blood, an extremely useful measure of integrated cardiorespiratory function. The essential relationship between pH, P_{CO_2}, and bicarbonate (HCO_3^-) is expressed by the Henderson–Hasselbalch equation (at 37°C): $$pH = 6.1 + \log\left(\frac{HCO_3^-}{P_{CO_2} \times 0.03}\right)$$ Arteriovenous pH difference is 0.01–0.03 but is greater in patients with CHF and shock.	**Increased in:** *Respiratory alkalosis:* hyperventilation (eg, anxiety), sepsis, liver disease, fever, early salicylate poisoning, and excessive artificial ventilation. *Metabolic alkalosis:* Loss of gastric HCl (eg, vomiting), potassium depletion, excessive alkali administration (eg, bicarbonate, antacids), diuretics, volume depletion. **Decreased in:** *Respiratory acidosis:* decreased alveolar ventilation (eg, COPD, respiratory depressants), neuromuscular diseases (eg, myasthenia gravis). *Metabolic acidosis* (bicarbonate deficit): increased formation of acids (eg, ketosis [diabetes mellitus, alcohol, starvation], lactic acidosis); decreased H^+ excretion (eg, renal failure, renal tubular acidosis, Fanconi syndrome); increased acid intake (eg, ion-exchange resins, salicylates, ammonium chloride, ethylene glycol, methanol); and increased loss of alkaline body fluids (eg, diarrhea, fistulas, aspiration of gastrointestinal contents, biliary drainage).	The pH of a standing sample decreases because of cellular metabolism. The correction of pH (measured at 37°C), based on the patient's temperature, is not clinically useful. See acid–base disturbances (Figure 8–1; Table 8–1). Br J Nurs 2004;13:522. [PMID: 15215728] Dis Mon 2004;50:122. [PMID: 15069420]

Test/Range/Collection	Physiologic Basis	Interpretation	Comments
Phosphorus, serum 2.5–4.5 mg/dL [0.8–1.45 mmol/L] ***Panic:*** <1.0 mg/dL SST $ Avoid hemolysis.	The plasma concentration of inorganic phosphate is determined by parathyroid gland function, action of vitamin D, intestinal absorption, renal function, bone metabolism, and nutrition. Serum phosphorus concentrations have a circadian rhythm (highest level in late morning, lowest in evening) and are subject to rapid change secondary to environmental factors such as diet (carbohydrate), phosphate-binding antacids, and fluctuations in GH, insulin, and renal function. There is also a seasonal variation with maximum levels in May and June (low levels in winter). During first decade of menopause, values increase ~0.2 mg/dL (~0.06 mmol/L). Bedrest causes increase up to 0.5 mg/dL (0.16 mmol/L). Ingestion of food may cause a transient decrease in blood levels. Low values are also seen during menstruation.	**Increased in:** Renal failure, calcific uremic arteriolopathy (calciphylaxis), tumor lysis syndrome, massive blood transfusion, hypoparathyroidism, sarcoidosis, neoplasms, adrenal insufficiency, acromegaly, hypervitaminosis D, osteolytic metastases to bone, leukemia, milk-alkali syndrome, healing bone fractures, pseudohypoparathyroidism, diabetes mellitus with ketosis, malignant hyperpyrexia, cirrhosis, lactic acidosis, respiratory acidosis. Drugs: phosphate infusions or enemas, anabolic steroids, ergocalciferol, furosemide, hydrochlorothiazide, clonidine, verapamil, potassium supplements, and others. Thrombocytosis may cause spurious elevation of serum phosphate, but plasma phosphate levels are normal. **Decreased in:** Hyperparathyroidism, hypovitaminosis D (rickets, osteomalacia), malabsorption (steatorrhea), malnutrition, starvation or cachexia, refeeding syndrome, bone marrow transplantation, renal phosphate wasting due to autosomal dominant or X-linked dominant hypophosphatemic rickets, GH deficiency, chronic alcoholism, severe diarrhea, vomiting, nasogastric suction, acute pancreatitis, severe hypercalcemia (any cause), acute gout, osteoblastic metastases to bone, severe burns (diuretic phase), respiratory alkalosis, hyperalimentation with inadequate phosphate repletion, carbohydrate administration (eg, intravenous $D_{50}W$ glucose bolus), renal tubular acidosis and other renal tubular defects, diabetic ketoacidosis (during recovery), acid–base disturbances, hypokalemia, pregnancy, hypothyroidism, hemodialysis. Drugs: acetazolamide, phosphate-binding antacids, anticonvulsants, β-adrenergic agonists, catecholamines, estrogens, isoniazid, oral contraceptives, prolonged use of thiazides, glucose infusion, insulin therapy, salicylates (toxicity).	Maintenance of a normal serum phosphorus level depends chiefly upon regulation of phosphorus reabsorption by the kidney. The majority of this reabsorption (80%) occurs in the proximal tubule and is mediated by the sodium–phosphate cotransporter (NaPi-II). Parathyroid hormone, via a variety of intracellular signaling cascades leading to NaPi-IIa internalization and downregulation, is the main regulator of renal phosphate reabsorption. In renal insufficiency, phosphorus excretion declines and hyperphosphatemia develops. The body's homeostatic mechanisms cause secondary hyperparathyroidism and renal osteodystrophy. Shift of phosphorus from extracellular to intracellular compartments, decreased gastrointestinal absorption, and increased urinary losses, are the primary mechanisms of hypophosphatemia. Hypophosphatemia has been implicated as a cause of rhabdomyolysis, respiratory failure, hemolysis, and left ventricular dysfunction. Am J Health Syst Pharm 2005;62:2355. [PMID: 16278327] Nat Clin Pract Nephrol 2006;2:136. [PMID: 16932412]

Platelet antibodies

| **Platelet antibodies,** whole blood, plasma/serum

Negative

Lavender, yellow, or SST (methodology-dependent)
$$$$ | Clinically significant platelet antibodies (platelet-associated IgG) include autoimmune platelet antibodies that cause idiopathic thrombocytopenic purpura (ITP), platelet-specific alloantibodies that cause neonatal alloimmune thrombocytopenia (NATP) and posttransfusion purpura (PTP), and HLA alloantibodies that are associated with refractoriness to platelet transfusions. Platelet-specific alloantibodies are most commonly directed at the human platelet antigen referred to as HPA-1a (also known as PIA1), while ITP autoantibodies typically target platelet glycoproteins IIb/IIIa and/or Ib/IX. Several methods with variable sensitivity and specificity are available, and no method detects all antibodies. A combination of a sensitive binding assay such as a direct platelet immunofluorescence test along with an antigen capture immunoassay is recommended. ELISA kits are available that detect specific antibodies against platelet glycoproteins or HLA class I antigens. | **Positive in:** Chronic ITP (90–95%), NATP, PTP. Testing serum/plasma for NATP should be performed using a maternal sample. | Routine testing for platelet antibodies is generally not recommended. In selected cases (eg, refractory ITP, NATP, PTP), the testing may be of value. An assay for platelet-bound antibody (direct) is more informative than detection of unbound antibodies in plasma or serum (indirect). For patients who have repeatedly failed to respond to random donor platelet transfusions, detection and characterization of the specific HLA antibody may permit HLA-matched and cross-matched platelet transfusion.
Br J Haematol 2003;120:574. [PMID: 12588344]
Blood 2004;103:4562. [PMID: 14976036]
Haematologica 2005;90:247. [PMID: 15710579]
J Thromb Haemost 2005;3:74. [PMID: 15634268] |

Test/Range/Collection	Physiologic Basis	Interpretation	Comments
Platelet count, whole blood (Plt) 150–450 × 10³/mcL [× 10⁹/L] ***Panic:*** <25 × 10³/mcL Lavender $	Platelets are released from megakaryocytes in bone marrow and are important for normal hemostasis. Platelet counting is performed as part of the complete blood count (CBC) panel. It is typically obtained by automated hematology analyzer. An estimated platelet count may be obtained by multiplying the number of platelets per 100 × oil immersion field by 10,000.	**Increased in:** Myeloproliferative disorders (PV, chronic myeloid leukemia, essential thrombo-cythemia, myelofibrosis), acute blood loss, post-splenectomy, pre-eclampsia, reactive thrombocytosis secondary to inflammatory disorders, infection, tissue injury, iron deficiency, malignancies. **Decreased in:** Decreased production: bone marrow suppression or replacement/infiltration, chemotherapy, drugs, alcohol, infection (eg, HIV), congenital marrow failure (eg, Fanconi anemia, Wiskott-Aldrich syndrome, Thrombocytopenia with Absent Radius (TAR) syndrome, etc); increased destruction or excessive pooling: hypersplenism, DIC, platelet antibodies (idiopathic thrombocytopenic purpura, Evans' syndrome, posttransfusion purpura, neonatal isoimmune thrombocytopenia, drugs [eg, quinidine, cephalosporins, clopidogrel, HIT]).	Platelet counts are determined in patients with suspected bleeding disorders, purpura or petechiae, leukemia/lymphoma, DIC, in patients on chemotherapy, and to determine the response to platelet transfusions. There is little tendency to bleed until the platelet count falls below 20,000/mcL. Bleeding due to low platelet counts typically presents as petechiae, epistaxis, and gingival bleeding. For invasive procedures, platelet counts above 50,000/mcL are desirable. HIV infection may result in both decreased platelet production and decreased platelet survival. Please also see platelet antibodies, heparin-associated antibody, and complete blood cell count entries, as well as the diagnostic algorithms for thrombocytopenia and thrombocytosis (Figures 8–22 & 8–23). Blood Rev 2002;16:73. [PMID: 11914001] Br J Haematol 2005;131:588. [PMID: 16351634] Curr Opin Hematol 2005;12:499. [PMID: 16271169] Curr Hematol Rep 2006;5:55. [PMID: 16537047]

Platelet function		
Platelet function (FA-100 closure time), blood CEPI: 70–170 seconds CADP: 50–110 seconds (laboratory-specific) Blue $$ Specimen must be kept at room temperature and the test should be performed within 4 hours of collection.	The PFA (platelet function analyzer)-100 CT measures the time taken for blood to block a membrane aperture coated with collagen and epinephrine (CEPI) or collagen and ADP (CADP). The test is a combined measure of platelet adhesion and aggregation. PFA-100 CT serves as an alternative to the bleeding time in assessing primary hemostasis. Compared with bleeding time, the PFA-100 CT test is more reproducible, less invasive, rapid, and more technically appealing.	**Increased in:** Inherited or acquired abnormality of platelet function, von Willebrand disease (vWD), valvular heart disease, renal insufficiency, aspirin. **Increases in both CEPI CT and CADP CT:** Abnormal platelet function, vWD. **Increase in CEPI CT only:** Aspirin.	Normal PFA-100 CT can help exclude some severe platelet defects (eg, Glanzmann thrombasthenia and Bernard-Soulier syndrome) and moderate-severe vWD (eg, types 3, 2A, 2M, and severe type 1). It is less sensitive to mild platelet disorders such as primary secretion defects or dense granule deficiencies and mild type 1 vWD. There is no evidence that a preoperative PFA-100 CT test can predict bleeding during a surgical procedure. The role of PFA-100 CT in therapeutic monitoring (eg, DDAVP and factor concentrates in vWD) also remains to be established. Individuals with severe thrombocytopenia (platelets <100,000/mcL) and/or anemia (hematocrit <28%) may exhibit a prolonged PFA-100 CT. J Thromb Haemost 2006;4:312. [PMID: 16420557] J Thromb Haemost 2006;4:2099. [PMID: 16961628]

Test/Range/Collection	Physiologic Basis	Interpretation	Comments
Porphobilinogen, urine (PBG) Negative $$ Protect from light.	Porphyrias are characterized clinically by neurologic and cutaneous manifestations and chemically by overproduction of porphyrin and other precursors of heme production. PBG is a water-soluble precursor of heme whose urinary excretion is increased in symptomatic hepatic porphyrias. PBG is detected qualitatively by a color reaction with Ehrlich reagent and confirmed by extraction into chloroform (Watson-Schwartz test).	**Positive in:** Acute intermittent porphyria, variegate porphyria, coproporphyria, lead poisoning (rare). **Negative in:** 20–30% of patients with hepatic porphyria between attacks.	Positive qualitative urinary PBG tests should be followed up by quantitative measurements. Many labs report frequent false positives with the Watson-Schwartz test. A screening PBG test is insensitive, and a negative test does not rule out porphyria between attacks or in the carrier state. Specific porphyrias can be better defined by quantitative measurement of urine PBG, 5-aminolevulinic acid, and total porphyrin levels and by measurement of erythrocyte uroporphyrinogen-I-synthetase. Ann Intern Med 2005;142:439. [PMID: 15767622] Best Pract Res Clin Gastroenterol 2005;19:235. [PMID: 15833690]

Potassium			
Potassium, serum (K+) 3.5–5.0 meq/L [mmol/L] **Panic:** <3.0 or >6.0 meq/L SST $ Avoid hemolysis.	Potassium is predominantly an intracellular cation whose plasma level is regulated by renal excretion. Plasma potassium concentration determines neuromuscular irritability. Elevated or depressed potassium concentrations interfere with muscle contraction.	**Increased in:** Massive hemolysis, severe tissue damage, rhabdomyolysis, acidosis, dehydration, acute or chronic renal failure, Addison disease, renal tubular acidosis type IV (hyporeninemic hypoaldosteronism), hyperkalemic familial periodic paralysis, exercise (transient). Drugs: potassium salts, potassium-sparing diuretics (eg, spironolactone, triamterene, eplerenone), nonsteroidal anti-inflammatory drugs, β-blockers, ACE inhibitors, ACE-receptor blockers, high-dose trimethoprim-sulfamethoxazole. **Decreased in:** Low potassium intake, prolonged vomiting or diarrhea, renal tubular acidosis types I and II, hyperaldosteronism, Cushing syndrome, osmotic diuresis (eg, hyperglycemia), alkalosis, familial periodic paralysis, trauma (transient), subarachnoid hemorrhage, genetic hypokalemic salt-losing tubulopathies such as Gitelman syndrome (familial hypokalemia-hypocalciuria-hypomagnesemia). Drugs: adrenergic agents (isoproterenol), diuretics.	Spurious hyperkalemia can occur with hemolysis of sample, delayed separation of serum from erythrocytes, prolonged fist clenching during blood drawing, and prolonged tourniquet placement. Very high white blood cell or platelet counts may cause spurious elevation of serum potassium, but plasma potassium levels are normal. Emerg Med Clin North Am 2005;23:723. [PMID: 15982543] Expert Opin Drug Saf 2005;4:677. [PMID: 16011447] J Intensive Care Med 2005;20:272. [PMID: 16145218] Am Fam Physician 2006;73:283. [PMID: 16445274]

Test/Range/Collection	Physiologic Basis	Interpretation	Comments
Procalcitonin, serum >0.5 ng/mL SST $$$$	Procalcitonin is a 14-kDa protein encoded by the *Calc-1* gene along with calcitonin and katacalcin. It is reported to be selectively induced by severe bacterial infections, such as the systemic inflammatory response syndrome (SIRS), sepsis, or multi-organ dysfunction syndrome. Procalcitonin expression is only slightly induced, if at all, by viral infections, autoimmune disorders, neoplastic diseases, myocardial infarction, and surgical trauma. An elevated plasma procalcitonin level is found in nonleukopenic patients with severe bacterial infections and sepsis, and it appears to have greater specificity and sensitivity than acute-phase proteins such as C-reactive protein or nonspecific indicators such as leukocyte count.	**Increased in:** Severe bacterial infections (eg, pneumonia, meningitis) and systemic infections (SIRS, sepsis, septic shock).	Procalcitonin is a good biological marker for sepsis. Rapid determination of the plasma procalcitonin level can be useful in triage decisions in the emergency department and in treatment decisions in the critical care unit. Procalcitonin level has reduced sensitivity and specificity for sepsis in severely leukopenic (WBC <1.0 × 10⁹/L) and immunosuppressed patients. However, the test retains its utility in patients with renal failure. Am J Emerg Med 2002;20:202. [PMID: 11992340] Clin Infect Dis 2002;34:895. [PMID: 11880953] Crit Care Med 2002;30:757. [PMID: 11940741] Crit Care Med 2006;34:1996. [PMID: 16715031]

Prolactin		
Prolactin, serum (PRL) <20 ng/mL [mcg/L] SST $$$	Prolactin is a polypeptide hormone secreted by the anterior pituitary. It functions in the initiation and maintenance of lactation in the postpartum period. PRL secretion is inhibited by hypothalamic secretion of dopamine. Prolactin levels increase with renal failure, hypothyroidism, and drugs that are dopamine antagonists.	**Increased in:** Sleep, nursing, nipple stimulation, exercise, hypoglycemia, stress, hypothyroidism, pituitary tumors (prolactinomas and others), hypothalamic/pituitary stalk lesions, renal failure. HIV infection (21%), CHF, SLE, advanced multiple myeloma, Rathke cleft cyst. Drugs: phenothiazines, haloperidol, risperidone, reserpine, methyldopa, estrogens, opiates, cimetidine. **Decreased in:** Drugs: levodopa.	Serum PRL is used primarily in work-up of suspected pituitary tumor (60% of pituitary adenomas secrete PRL). Clinical presentation is usually amenorrhea and galactorrhea in women and impotence in men. (See Amenorrhea algorithm, Figure 8–4.) In patients with macroadenoma, PRL is frequently >1000 ng/mL; in microadenoma, PRL is usually >150 ng/mL. Only 4% of impotence is caused by hyperprolactinemia, and hyperprolactinemia is rare in the absence of low serum testosterone. Many patients with hyperprolactinemia (8–26%, depending on the population studied) have in fact normal amounts of circulating prolactin but falsely high values in commercial assays. This is caused by macromolecular prolactin (macroprolactin), a complex of prolactin with IgG antibodies leading to apparent hyperprolactinemia. Macroprolactinemia is a cause of hyperprolactinemia in patients with maintained fertility. PRL levels usually remain stable over time. HIV Clin Trials 2002;3:133. [PMID: 11976991] J Clin Endocrinol Metab 2002;87:581. [PMID: 11836289] J Clin Psychiatry 2002;63 (Suppl 4):56. [PMID: 11913677] Mayo Clinic Proc 2005;80:1050. [PMID: 16092584]

	Prostate-specific antigen

Test/Range/Collection	Physiologic Basis	Interpretation	Comments
Prostate-specific antigen, serum (PSA) 0–4 ng/mL [mcg/L] SST $$$	Prostate-specific antigen is a glycoprotein produced by cells of the prostatic ductal epithelium and is present in the serum of all men. It is absent from the serum of women.	**Increased in:** Prostate carcinoma (sensitivity ~44%; specificity ~94% at a 4.0 ng/mL cutoff), biochemical recurrence after localized treatment, benign prostatic hypertrophy (BPH), prostatitis. **Decreased in:** Metastatic prostate carcinoma treated with antiandrogen therapy, postprostatectomy, 5α-reductase inhibitor therapy.	PSA is used both for the early detection of prostate cancer and as a tumor marker to assess response and monitor recurrence of treated prostate cancer. There is still no consensus on whether PSA measurement should be used as a screening test for prostate cancer. Randomized trials of the benefits and risks of PSA testing for prostate cancer screening are underway. Decrease in mortality rates resulting from use for cancer screening is unproven, and the risks of early therapy are significant. The PSA nadir (the lowest PSA level achieved after therapeutic intervention) appears to correlate with the likelihood of remaining disease-free. Three consecutive PSA rises are interpreted as an indicator of treatment (biochemical) failure. PSA is often increased in BPH, and the positive predictive value in healthy older men is low. Use of the free/total PSA ratio or the complexed PSA test and prostate volume can improve the diagnostic accuracy for prostate cancer. Clin Lab 2005;51:1127. [PMID: 15819167] Curr Urol Rep 2005;6:307. [PMID: 15978235] Scand J Urol Nephrol Suppl 2005;(216):64. [PMID: 16019759] J Urol 2006;176:868. [PMID: 16890642] Urol Clin North Am 2006;33:147. [PMID: 16631453]

Protein C		
Protein C, plasma 70–170% (functional) 65–150% (antigenic) Blue $$$ Transport to lab on ice. Plasma must be separated and frozen in a polypropylene tube within 2 hours.	Protein C is a vitamin K-dependent proenzyme synthesized in the liver. It is activated at the endothelial surface when thrombin binds to thrombomodulin. In the presence of its cofactor protein S, activated protein C (APC) inactivates Va and VIIIa, thereby impeding further thrombin generation. The functional assay detects both quantitative (type I) and qualitative (type II) deficiency of protein C. The antigenic assay detects patients with quantitative protein C deficiency, but does not detect patients with qualitative abnormalities. Deficiency is inherited in an autosomal dominant fashion with incomplete penetrance or is acquired. Deficient patients may present with a hypercoagulable state, with recurrent thrombophlebitis or pulmonary embolism.	**Decreased in:** Congenital deficiency, liver disease, cirrhosis (13–25%), warfarin use (28–60%), vitamin K deficiency, DIC. **Interfering Factors:** Artifactually decreased functional protein C values may be seen in patients with abnormally elevated levels of factor VIII. Artifactually increased levels of functional protein C values may be seen in patients on heparin therapy.	Homozygous deficiency of protein C (<1% activity) is associated with fatal neonatal purpura fulminans and massive venous thrombosis at birth. Heterozygous patients (one in 200–300 of the population, with levels 25–50% of normal) may be at risk for venous thrombosis. Kindreds with dysfunctional protein C of normal quantity have been identified. Interpretation of an abnormally low protein C must be tempered by the clinical setting. Anticoagulant therapy, DIC, and liver disease must not be present. There is overlap between lower limits of normal values and values found in heterozygotes. Patients should be off oral anticoagulant therapy for two weeks for accurate measurement of functional protein C levels. See recommended testing for venous thrombosis (Table 8–24). J Thromb Haemost 2005;3:1428. [PMID: 15978099] J Thromb Haemost 2005;3:459. [PMID: 15748234] Haematologica 2006;91:695. [PMID: 16670075]

Protein electrophoresis

Test/Range/Collection	Physiologic Basis	Interpretation	Comments
Protein electrophoresis, serum Adults: Albumin: 3.3–5.7 g/dL α_1: 0.1–0.4 g/dL α_2: 0.3–0.9 g/dL β_2: 0.7–1.5 g/dL γ: 0.5–1.4 g/dL SST $$	Electrophoresis of serum separates serum proteins into albumin, α_1, α_2, β_2, and γ fractions. Albumin is the principal serum protein (see *Albumin*). The term *globulin* generally refers to the nonalbumin fraction of serum protein. The α_1 fraction contains α_1- antitrypsin (90%), α_1-lipoprotein, and α_1-acid glycoprotein. The α_2 fraction contains α_2-macroglobulin, haptoglobin, and ceruloplasmin. The β fraction contains transferrin, hemopexin, complement C3, and β-lipoproteins. The γ fraction contains immunoglobulins G, A, D, E, and M.	$\uparrow \alpha_1$: inflammatory states (α_1-antiprotease), pregnancy. $\uparrow \alpha_2$: nephrotic syndrome, inflammatory states, oral contraceptives, steroid therapy, hyperthyroidism. $\uparrow \beta$: hyperlipidemia, hemoglobinemia, iron deficiency anemia. $\uparrow \gamma$ polyclonal gammopathies (liver disease, cirrhosis [associated with β–γ "bridging"], chronic infections, autoimmune disease); monoclonal gammopathies (multiple myeloma, Waldenström macroglobulinemia, lymphoid malignancies, monoclonal gammopathy of undetermined significance). $\downarrow \alpha_1$: α_1-antiprotease deficiency. $\downarrow \alpha_2$: in vivo hemolysis, liver disease. $\downarrow \beta$: hypo-β-lipoproteinemias. $\downarrow \gamma$: immune deficiency.	Presence of "spikes" in α_2, β_2, or γ regions necessitates the use of IFE to verify the presence of a monoclonal gammopathy. If Bence Jones proteins (light chains) are suspected, UPEP followed by IFE needs to be done. Test is insensitive for detection of decreased levels of immunoglobulins and α_1-antitrypsin. Specific quantitation is required (see Immunoglobulins and α_1-Antitrypsin). If plasma is used, fibrinogen will be detected in the β–γ region. The acute-phase reactant protein pattern seen with acute illness, surgery, infarction, or trauma is characterized by an $\uparrow \alpha_2$ (haptoglobin) and $\uparrow \alpha_1$ (α_1-antitrypsin). Adv Clin Chem 2006;42:43. [PMID: 17131624]

	Protein S	**Protein, total**
Protein S (total anti-gen), plasma 55–155% Blue $$$ Transport to lab on ice. Plasma must be separated and frozen in a polypropylene tube within 2 hours.	Protein S is a vitamin K-dependent glycoprotein, synthesized in the liver. It has an anticoagulant function and acts as the cofactor of activated protein C (APC), with which it forms a stoichiometric complex. This complex inactivates Va and VIIIa. There are two forms of protein S: free and bound. Free protein S represents about 40% of the total and is the functional form that acts as the cofactor for APC. Bound protein S, attached to C4b-binding protein, does not possess any anticoagulant activity. Deficiency is associated with recurrent venous thrombosis before the age of 45.	**Decreased in:** Congenital protein S deficiency, liver disease, warfarin therapy, DIC, vitamin K deficiency, nephrotic syndrome.	This test measures the total protein S antigen, not biologic activity of protein S. Functional (activity) protein S assay and free protein S antigen assay are available to differentiate subtypes of congenital protein S deficiency (type I: decreased antigen and functional levels; type II: decreased functional levels, but normal antigen levels; type IIa: decreased functional and free antigen levels, but normal total antigen levels). Am J Clin Pathol 2005;123:778. [PMID: 15981819] Haematologica 2006;91:695. [PMID: 16670075] J Thromb Haemost 2006;4:186. [PMID: 16409468]
Protein, total, plasma or serum 6.0–8.0 g/dL [60–80 g/L] SST $ Avoid prolonged venous stasis during collection.	Plasma protein concentration is determined by nutritional state, hepatic function, renal function, hydration, and various disease states. Plasma protein concentration determines the colloidal osmotic pressure.	**Increased in:** Polyclonal or monoclonal gammopathies, marked dehydration. Drugs: anabolic steroids, androgens, corticosteroids, epinephrine. **Decreased in:** Protein-losing enteropathies, acute burns, nephrotic syndrome, severe dietary protein deficiency, chronic liver disease, malabsorption syndrome, agammaglobulinemia.	Serum total protein consists primarily of albumin and globulin. Serum globulin level is calculated as total protein minus albumin. Hypoproteinemia usually indicates hypoalbuminemia, because albumin is the major serum protein. Ann Thorac Surg 1999;67:236. [PMID: 10086560]

	Prothrombin time

Test/Range/Collection	Physiologic Basis	Interpretation	Comments
Prothrombin time, whole blood (PT) 11–15 seconds (laboratory specific) Blue $ Fill tube completely.	PT evaluates the extrinsic and common coagulation pathways. It is performed by adding calcium and tissue thromboplastin to a sample of citrated, platelet-poor plasma, and measuring the time required for fibrin clot formation. It is most sensitive to deficiencies in the vitamin K-dependent clotting factors II, VII, and X. It is also sensitive to deficiency of factor V. It is less sensitive to fibrinogen deficiency and heparin. PT is the most commonly used test for monitoring warfarin therapy. In addition to results reported in seconds, the International Normalized Ratio (INR) is calculated. INR = [Patient PT/Normal mean PT][ISI]	**Increased in:** Warfarin, liver disease, DIC, vitamin K deficiency, hereditary deficiency in factors VII, X, V and II, fibrinogen abnormality (eg, hypofibrinogenemia, afibrinogenemia, dysfibrinogenemia), circulating anticoagulant affecting the PT system (rarely lupus anticoagulant), massive transfusion.	Routine preoperative measurement of PT is unnecessary unless there is clinical history of a bleeding disorder (see Figure 8–7 and Table 8–7). The INR was introduced in the early 1980s to improve PT reporting and standardization. An International Sensitivity Index (ISI) is assigned to each thromboplastin by the reagent manufacture. The ISI is a measure of a reagent's respnsiveness to low levels of vitamin K-dependent factors compared with the WHO International Reference Preparation. Despite the improvement with INR reporting, significant variation in INR results between laboratories persists. These differences in INR reflect local variables (eg, reagent and/or instrument system). A high-sensitivity, low ISI thromboplastin reagent is recommended to improve precision and accuracy of the INR. Warfarin therapeutic range is INR 2.0–3.0. Bleeding has been reported to be three times more common in patients with INRs of 3.0–4.5 than in patients with INRs of 2.0–3.0. Thromb Haemost 2002;87:74. [PMID: 11848460] J Thromb Haemost 2006;4:967. [PMID: 16689743]

Q fever antibody		
Q fever antibody, serum <1:8 titer SST $$$ Submit paired sera, one collected within 1 week of illness and another 2–3 weeks later. Avoid hemolysis.	*Coxiella burnetii* is a rickettsial organism that is the causative organism for Q fever. Most likely mode of transmission is inhalation of aerosols from exposure to common reservoirs, sheep and cattle. Tick bites (ixodid ticks) may also be a mode of transmission. Antibodies to the organism can be detected by the presence of agglutinins, by complement fixation (CF), by immunofluorescent antibody testing (IFA), or by ELISA. Agglutinin titers are found 5–8 days after infection. IgM can be detected at 7 days (IFA, ELISA) and may persist for up to 32 weeks (ELISA). IgG (IFA, ELISA) appears after 7 days and peaks at 3–4 weeks. Phase I and phase II antibodies are produced in response to the organism, phase II antibodies appearing first and phase I antibodies weeks to months later. Diagnosis of Q fever is usually confirmed by serologic findings of anti–phase II antigen IgM titers of ≥1:50 and IgG titers of ≥1:200. The finding of elevated levels of both IgM and IgA by ELISA has both high sensitivity and high specificity for acute Q fever. In chronic Q fever, phase I antibodies, especially IgG and IgA, are predominant.	**Increased in:** Acute or chronic Q fever (CF antibodies are present by the second week in 65% of cases and by the fourth week in 90%; acute and convalescent titers [IFA or ELISA] detect infection with 89–100% sensitivity and 100% specificity), and recent vaccination for Q fever.	Clinical presentation is similar to that of severe influenza. Typically, there is no rash. Test acute and convalescent sera for evidence of current or recent *C burnetii* infection. Occasionally, titers do not rise for 4–6 weeks, especially if antimicrobial therapy has been given. Initial testing may not be helpful; treatment should be based on clinical and other laboratory assessment. As with any serologic procedure, demonstration of seroconversion or a fourfold increase in titer between acute and convalescent sera suggests current or recent infection. Patients with Q fever have a high prevalence of antiphospholipid antibody (81%), especially as measured by lupus anticoagulant test or measurement of antibodies to cardiolipin. These tests may be useful in diagnosing patients presenting with fever alone. Antibodies to Q fever do not cross-react with other rickettsial antibodies; a rise in titer is considered diagnostic for recent infection in the absence of prior vaccination. If chronic disease (endocarditis) suspected, order phase I antibodies; if acute disease suspected, order phase II antibodies. Murray PR et al (editors): *Manual of Clinical Microbiology,* 8th ed. ASM Press, 2003. J Clin Microbiol 2006;44:2283. [PMID: 16757641]

Test/Range/Collection	Physiologic Basis	Interpretation	Comments
Rapid plasma reagin, serum (RPR) Nonreactive Marbled $	Measures nontreponemal antibodies that are produced when *Treponema pallidum* interacts with host tissue. The card test is a flocculation test performed by using a cardiolipin-lecithin-cholesterol carbon-containing antigen reagent mixed on a card with the patient's serum. A positive test (presence of antibodies) is indicated when black carbon clumps produced by flocculation are seen by the naked eye.	**Increased in:** Syphilis: primary (78%), secondary (97%), symptomatic late (74%). Biologic false positives occur in a wide variety of conditions, including leprosy, malaria, intravenous drug abuse, aging, infectious mononucleosis, HIV infection (≤15%), autoimmune diseases (SLE, rheumatoid arthritis), pregnancy.	RPR is used as a screening test and in suspected primary and secondary syphilis. Because the test lacks specificity (false-positive rates 5–20%), positive tests should be confirmed with the FTA-ABS or MHA-TP test. RPR titers can be used to follow serologic response to treatment. (See Syphilis test, Table 8–22.) The incidence of syphilis has been on the rise and there is a high coinfection rate with HIV. Sex Transm Dis 1998;25:569. [PMID: 9858355] J Emerg Med 2000;18:361. [PMID: 10729677] Dermatol Clin 2006;24:497. [PMID: 17010778]
Red blood cell count (RBC, or erythrocyte count), whole blood 4.3–6.0 × 10⁶/mcL (male) 3.5–5.5 × 10⁶/mcL (female) [× 10¹²/L] Lavender $	Red blood cells (erythrocytes) are counted by automated instruments using electrical impedance or light scattering.	**Increased in:** Secondary polycythemia, hemoconcentration (dehydration), PV. Spurious increase with increased white blood cells. **Decreased in:** Anemia. Spurious decrease with autoagglutination (eg, cold agglutinins).	In patients with cold agglutinins, the spurious lowering of the RBC count is disproportionately greater than the false elevation of MCV, so the hematocrit is falsely depressed. N Engl J Med 1983;309:925. [PMID: 6888491] Mayo Clin Proc 2005;80:923. [PMID: 16007898]

Header above columns 3–4: **Rapid plasma reagin** | **Red blood cell count**

	Renin activity
Renin activity, plasma (PRA) Lavender $$	The renal juxtaglomerular apparatus generates renin, an enzyme that converts angiotensinogen to angiotensin I. The inactive angiotensin I is then converted to angiotensin II, which is a potent vasopressor. Renin activity is measured by the ability of patient's plasma to generate angiotensin I from substrate (angiotensinogen). Normal values depend on the patient's hydration, posture, and salt intake.	**Increased in:** Dehydration, some hypertensive states (eg, renal artery stenosis); edematous states (cirrhosis, nephrotic syndrome, CHF); hypokalemic states (gastrointestinal sodium and potassium loss, Bartter syndrome); adrenal insufficiency, chronic renal failure, left ventricular hypetrophy. Drugs: ACE inhibitors, estrogen, hydralazine, nifedipine, minoxidil, oral contraceptives. **Decreased in:** Hyporeninemic hypoaldosteronism, some hypertensive states (eg, primary aldosteronism, severe preeclampsia). Drugs: β-blockers, aspirin, clonidine, prazosin, reserpine, methyldopa, indomethacin.	The ratio of plasma aldosterone concentration to plasma renin activity is an effective screening test for primary aldosteronism (sensitivity 95%). It has a high negative predictive value even during antihypertensive therapy. Because of a low specificity of the ratio, autonomous aldosterone production must be confirmed by demonstration of high and autonomous secretion of aldosterone (using an aldosterone suppression test). Plasma renin activity is also useful in evaluation of hypoaldosteronism (low-sodium diet, patient standing) (see Aldosterone, plasma). Curr Cardiol Rep 2005;7.412. [PMID: 16256009] Methods Mol Biol 2006;324:187. [PMID: 16761379] Nat Clin Pract Nephrol 2006;2:198. [PMID: 16932426]

Test/Range/Collection	Physiologic Basis	Interpretation	Comments
Reptilase clotting time, plasma 13–19 seconds Blue $$	Reptilase is an enzyme derived from the venom of *Bothrops atrox* or *Bothrops jararaca*, South American pit vipers. Reptilase cleaves a fibrinopeptide from fibrinogen directly, bypassing the heparin-antithrombin system, and produces a fibrin clot. The reptilase time will be normal in heparin toxicity, even when the thrombin time is infinite.	**Increased in:** Hereditary decrease in or abnormal fibrinogen (hypofibrinogenemia, dysfibrinogenemia, afibrinogenemia), liver disease, DIC, paraproteinemia.	When the thrombin time is prolonged, the reptilase time is useful in distinguishing the presence of an antithrombin (normal reptilase time) from hypo- or dysfibrinogenemia (prolonged reptilase time). The reptilase time is normal when heparin is the cause of a prolonged thrombin time. The reptilase time is only slightly prolonged by fibrin degradation products. Arch Pathol Lab Med 2002;126:499. [PMID: 11900586]
Reticulocyte count, whole blood 33–137 × 10³/mcL [× 10⁹/L] Lavender $	Reticulocytes are immature red blood cells that contain cytoplasmic RNA. A reticulocyte count measures how rapidly reticulocytes are produced by the bone marrow and then released into the bloodstream.	**Increased in:** Hemolytic anemia, blood loss (before development of iron deficiency), recovery from iron, B₁₂ or folate deficiency or from drug-induced anemia. **Decreased in:** Iron deficiency anemia, aplastic anemia, anemia of chronic disease, megaloblastic anemia, sideroblastic anemia, pure red cell aplasia, renal disease, bone marrow suppression or infiltration, myelodysplastic syndrome.	This test is indicated in the evaluation of anemia to distinguish hypoproliferative from hemolytic anemia or blood loss. See anemia evaluation (Figure 8–5; Tables 8–2 & 8–3). The old method of measuring reticulocytes (manual staining and counting) has poor reproducibility. It has been replaced by automated methods (eg, flow cytometry), which are more precise and provide the absolute reticulocyte counts. Method-specific reference ranges must be used. Am J Clin Pathol 2002;117:871. [PMID: 12047138] Hematol Oncol Clin North Am 2002;16:373. [PMID: 12094477]

Column headers: Reptilase clotting time | Reticulocyte count

Rh(D) typing
Rh typing, red cells (Rh) Red $ Proper identification of specimen is critical.	The Rhesus blood group system is second in importance only to the ABO system for transfusion practice. Anti-Rh antibodies are the leading cause of hemolytic disease of the newborn and may also cause hemolytic transfusion reactions. Although there are other Rhesus anti-gens, only tests for the D antigen are performed routinely in pretransfusion testing because the D antigen is the most immunogenic. The terms Rh-positive and -negative refer to the presence or absence of the D antigen on the red cell surface. Persons whose red cells lack D do not regularly have anti-D in their serum. Formation of anti-D almost always results from exposure through transfusion or pregnancy to red cells possessing the D antigen.	83% of US non-Hispanic whites are Rh(D)-positive, 17% negative; 93% of Hispanic-Americans are Rh(D)-positive, 7% negative; 93% of African Americans are Rh(D)-positive, 7% negative; 98% of Asian Americans are Rh(D)-positive, 2% negative; 90% of North American Indians are Rh(D)-positive; 10% negative.	Of D-reactive+ persons receiving a single D-positive+ blood unit, 50–75% will develop anti-D. The blood of all donors and recipients is therefore routinely tested for D, so that D-negative recipients can be given D-negative blood. Donor bloods must also be tested for a weak form of D antigen, previously called D^u and must be labeled D-positive if "weak D" is detected. It is not required to test recipient blood specimen for weak D. *Technical Manual of the American Association of Blood Banks*, 15th ed. American Association of Blood Banks, 2005. Transfusion 2004;44:703. [PMID: 15104651]

		Rheumatoid factor		Ribonucleoprotein antibody
Test/Range/Collection	**Physiologic Basis**	**Interpretation**	**Comments**	

Test/Range/Collection	Physiologic Basis	Interpretation	Comments
Rheumatoid factor, serum (RF) Negative (<1:16) SST $	Rheumatoid factor (RF) consists of heterogeneous autoantibodies usually of the IgM class that react against the Fc region of human IgG. Most methods detect only IgM-class RF.	**Positive in:** Rheumatoid arthritis (75–90%), Sjögren syndrome (80–90%), scleroderma, dermatomyositis, SLE (30%), sarcoidosis, Waldenström macroglobulinemia. Drugs: methyldopa, others. Low-titers of RF (eg, ≤1:80) are questionable and can be found in healthy older patients (20%), in 1–4% of normal individuals, and in a variety of acute immune responses (eg, viral infections, including infectious mononucleosis and viral hepatitis), chronic bacterial infections (tuberculosis, leprosy, subacute infective endocarditis), and chronic active hepatitis.	Rheumatoid factor can be useful in differentiating rheumatoid arthritis from other chronic inflammatory arthritides. However, a positive RF test is only one of several criteria needed to make the diagnosis of rheumatoid arthritis. (See also Autoantibodies, Table 8–6.) RF must be ordered selectively because its predictive value is low (34%) if it is used as a screening test. The test has poor positive predictive value because of its lack of specificity. The subset of patients with seronegative rheumatic disease limits its sensitivity and negative predictive value. Clin Chem Lab Med 2006;44:138. [PMID: 16475897] Rheumatology (Oxford) 2006;45:379. [PMID: 16418203]
Ribonucleoprotein antibody, serum (RNP) Negative SST $$	This is an antibody to a ribonucleoprotein-extractable nuclear antigen.	**Increased in:** Scleroderma (20–30% sensitivity, low specificity), mixed connective tissue disease (MCTD) (95–100% sensitivity, low specificity), SLE (38–44%), Sjögren syndrome, rheumatoid arthritis (10%), discoid lupus (20–30%). Anti-RNP is present in 2.7% of patients with positive ANA.	A negative test essentially excludes MCTD. (See also Autoantibodies, Table 8–6.) Clin Dermatol 2006;24:374. [PMID: 16966019] Rheum Dis Clin North Am 2005;31:411. [PMID: 16084315]

Rubella antibody		
Rubella antibody, serum <1:8 titer SST $ For diagnosis of a recent infection, submit paired sera, one collected within 1 week of illness and another 2–4 weeks later.	Rubella (German measles) is a viral infection that causes fever, malaise, coryza, lymphadenopathy, fine maculopapular rash, and congenital birth defects when infection occurs in utero. Antibodies to rubella can be detected by hemagglutination inhibition (HI), complement fixation (CF), indirect hemagglutination (IHA), ELISA, or latex agglutination (LA). Tests can detect IgG and IgM antibody. Titers usually appear as rash fades (1 week) and peak at 10–14 days for HI and 2–3 weeks for other techniques. Baseline titers may remain elevated for life. Serological tests are used to determine the immune status of the individual, to diagnose postnatal rubella, and occasionally to support the diagnosis of rubella. IgM antibody disappears within 4–5 weeks; IgG antibody remains for life.	**Increased in:** Recent rubella infection, congenital rubella infection, previous rubella infection, or vaccination (immunity). Spuriously increased IgM antibody occurs in the presence of rheumatoid factor or by cross-reacting antibodies to other viral infections or autoimmune illnesses.	Rubella titers of ≤1:8 indicate susceptibility and need for immunization to prevent infection during pregnancy. Titers of >1:32 indicate immunity from prior infection or vaccination. Demonstration of a 4-fold rise in titer between acute and convalescent sera may be indicative of a recent infection. Single titers, even >1:256, cannot be interpreted as evidence of recent infection since they are more likely to indicate immune status. The recent resurgence of congenital rubella can largely be prevented with improved rubella testing and vaccination programs. Murray PR et al (editors): *Manual of Clinical Microbiology,* 8th ed. ASM Press, 2003. Epidemiol Rev 2006;28:81. [PMID: 16775038]

	Russell viper venom time (dRVVT)

Test/Range/Collection	Physiologic Basis	Interpretation	Comments
Russell viper venom time (dilute, dRVVT), plasma 24–37 seconds (laboratory-specific) Blue $$	Russell viper venom is extracted from a pit viper (*Vipera russelli*), which is common in Southeast Asia (especially Burma) and causes a rapidly fatal syndrome of consumptive coagulopathy with hemorrhage, shock, rhabdomyolysis, and renal failure. Approximately 70% of the protein content of the venom is phospholipase A₂, which activates factor X in the presence of phospholipid, bypassing factor VII. dRVVT is used in detection of antiphospholipid antibodies (so-called lupus anticoagulant, LAC). It should be noted that the 'anticoagulant' detected in vitro may be associated with vascular thrombosis and pregnancy-related morbidity in vivo.	**Increased in:** Circulating lupus anticoagulants (LAC) (sensitivity 96%; specificity 50–70%), severe fibrinogen deficiency (<50 mg/dL), deficiencies in prothrombin, factor V, factor X, and heparin therapy. **Normal in:** Factor VII deficiency and all intrinsic pathway factor deficiencies.	The test is sensitive to phospholipid and if heparin is not present, a prolonged dRVVT may indicate the presence of LAC (antiphospholipid antibodies). See Figure 8–19 for its use in evaluating isolated prolongation of PTT. Am J Clin Pathol 2005;124:894. [PMID: 16416739] Br J Biomed Sci 2005;62:127. [PMID: 16196459] Semin Thromb Hemost 2005;31:39. [PMID: 15706474]

Test / Specimen		Salicylate	Scleroderma-associated antibody

		Salicylate	**Scleroderma-associated antibody**
Salicylate, serum (aspirin) 20–30 mg/dL [200–300 mg/L] **Panic:** >35 mg/dL SST $$	At high concentrations, salicylate stimulates hyperventilation, uncouples oxidative phosphorylation, and impairs glucose and fatty acid metabolism. Salicylate toxicity is thus marked by respiratory alkalosis and metabolic acidosis.	**Increased in:** Acute or chronic salicylate intoxication.	The potential toxicity of salicylate levels after acute ingestion can be determined by using the salicylate toxicity nomogram (Figure 9–10). Nomograms have become less valid with the increasing popularity of enteric-coated slow-release aspirin preparations. Routine testing may not be required for fully conscious asymptomatic adult patients who deny ingesting salicylate. Pediatrics 1960;26:800. [PMID: 13723722] Eur J Emerg Med 2006;13:26. [PMID: 16374244]
Scleroderma-associated antibody (Scl-70 antibody), serum Negative SST $$	This antibody reacts with a cellular antigen (DNA topoisomerase 1) that is responsible for the relaxation of super-coiled DNA.	**Increased in:** Scleroderma (15–20% sensitivity, high specificity).	Predictive value of a positive test is >95% for scleroderma. Test has prognostic significance for severe digital ischemia in patients with Raynaud disease and scleroderma. (See also Autoantibodies, Table 8–6.) Am Fam Physician 2002;65:1073. [PMID: 11925083] Dermatology 2002;204:29. [PMID: 11834846] Ann N Y Acad Sci 2005;1050:217. [PMID: 16014537]

Test/Range/Collection	Physiologic Basis	Interpretation	Comments
Semen analysis, ejaculate Sperm count: >20 × 10⁶/mL [10⁹/L] Motility score: >60% motile Volume: 2–5 mL Normal morphology: >60% $$ Semen is collected in a urine container after masturbation following 3 days of abstinence from ejaculation. Specimen must be examined promptly.	Conventional semen analysis includes the determination of sperm count, semen volume, sperm motility (qualitative and quantitative), and sperm morphology. Sperm are viewed under the microscope for motility and morphology. In addition to sperm count, sperm morphology and motility may have the most predictive utility. Infertility can be associated with low counts or with sperm of abnormal morphology or decreased motility.	**Decreased in:** Primary or secondary testicular failure, cryptorchidism, following vasectomy, drugs.	A low sperm count should be confirmed by sending two other appropriately collected semen specimens for evaluation. The usefulness of conventional semen analysis parameters as predictor of fertility is somewhat limited. Therefore, alternative tests based on more functional aspects (sperm penetration, capacitation, acrosome reaction) have been developed. Flow cytometer-based Sperm Chromatin Structure Assay (SCSA) can provide an assessment of DNA integrity as another parameter of sperm quality. Int J Androl 2002;25:306. [PMID: 12270029] Adv Clin Chem 2005;40:317. [PMID: 16355926] Gynecol Obstet Invest 2005;59:86. [PMID: 15572878]
Smith (anti-Sm) antibody, serum Negative SST $$	This antibody to Smith antigen (an extractable nuclear antigen) is a marker antibody for SLE.	**Positive in:** SLE (30–40% sensitivity, high specificity).	A positive test substantially increases posttest probability of SLE. Test rarely needed for the diagnosis of SLE. (See also Autoantibodies, Table 8–6.) South Med J 2005;98:704. [PMID: 16108239]

Smooth muscle antibodies		Sodium

Smooth muscle antibodies, serum

Negative

SST
$$

Antibodies against smooth muscle proteins are found in patients with chronic active hepatitis and primary biliary cirrhosis.

Positive in: Autoimmune chronic active hepatitis (40–70%, predominantly IgG antibodies), lower titers in primary biliary cirrhosis (50%, predominantly IgM antibodies), viral hepatitis, infectious mononucleosis, cryptogenic cirrhosis (28%), HIV infection, vitiligo (25%), endometriosis, Behçet disease (<2% of normal individuals).

The presence of high titers of smooth muscle antibodies (>1:80) is useful in distinguishing autoimmune chronic active hepatitis from other forms of hepatitis.
Adv Clin Chem 2005;40:127. [PMID: 16355922]

Sodium, serum
(Na⁺)

135–145 meq/L [mmol/L]
Panic: <125 or >155 meq/L

SST
$

Sodium is the predominant extracellular cation. The serum sodium level is primarily determined by the volume status of the individual. Hyponatremia can be divided into hypovolemia, euvolemia, and hypervolemia categories. (See Hyponatremia algorithm, Figure 8–14.)
Sodium is commonly measured by ion-selective electrode.

Increased in: Dehydration (excessive sweating, severe vomiting, or diarrhea), polyuria (diabetes mellitus, diabetes insipidus), hyperaldosteronism, inadequate water intake (coma, hypothalamic disease). Drugs: steroids, licorice, oral contraceptives.
Decreased in: CHF, cirrhosis, vomiting, diarrhea, exercise, excessive sweating (with replacement of water but not salt, eg, marathon running), salt-losing nephropathy, adrenal insufficiency, nephrotic syndrome, water intoxication, SIADH, AIDS. Drugs: thiazides, diuretics, ACE inhibitors, chlorpropamide, carbamazepine, antidepressants (selective serotonin reuptake inhibitors), antipsychotics.

Spurious hyponatremia may be produced by severe lipemia or hyperproteinemia if sodium analysis involves a dilution step.
The serum sodium falls about 1.6 meq/L for each 100 mg/dL increase in blood glucose.
Hyponatremia in a normovolemic patient with urine osmolality higher than plasma osmolality suggests the possibility of SIADH, myxedema, hypopituitarism, or reset osmostat.
Treatment of disorders of sodium balance relies on clinical assessment of the patient's extracellular fluid volume rather than the serum sodium.
Emerg Med Clin North Am 2005;23:749. [PMID: 15982544]
QJM 2005;98:529. [PMID: 15955797]
Am J Med 2006;119:S74. [PMID: 16843089]
Am J Med 2006;119:S30. [PMID: 16843082]
Endocr Pract 2006;12:446. [PMID: 16901803]

Test/Range/Collection	Physiologic Basis	Interpretation	Comments
		SS-A/Ro antibody	**SS-B/La antibody**
SS-A/Ro antibody, serum Negative SST $$	Antibodies to Ro (SSA) cellular ribo-nucleoprotein complexes are found in connective tissue diseases such as Sjögren syndrome (SS), SLE, rheumatoid arthritis (RA), and vasculitis.	**Increased in:** Sjögren syndrome (60–70% sensitivity, low specificity), SLE (30–40%), RA (10%), subacute cutaneous lupus, vasculitis.	Useful in counseling women of childbearing age with known connective tissue disease, because a positive test is associated with a small but real risk of neonatal SLE and congenital heart block. The few (<10%) patients with SLE who do not have a positive ANA commonly have antibodies to SS-A. (See also Autoantibodies, Table 8–6.) Autoimmunity 2004;37:305. [PMID: 15518047] Autoimmunity 2005;38:55. [PMID: 15804706] Lupus 2005;14:660. [PMID: 16218462] Arch Med Res 2006;37:921. [PMID: 17045106]
SS-B/La antibody, serum Negative SST $$	Antibodies to La (SSB) cellular ribo-nucleoprotein complexes are found in Sjögren syndrome and appear to be relatively more specific for Sjögren syndrome than are antibodies to SSA. They are quantitated by immunoassay.	**Increased in:** Sjögren syndrome (50% sensitivity, higher specificity than anti-SSA), SLE (10%).	Direct pathogenicity and usefulness of autoanti-body test in predicting disease exacerbation not proved. (See also Autoantibodies, Table 8–6.) Autoimmunity 2004;37:305. [PMID: 15518047] Autoimmunity 2005;38:55. [PMID: 15804706] Lupus 2005;14:660. [PMID: 16218462] Arch Med Res 2006;37:921. [PMID: 17045106]

T-cell receptor gene rearrangement		
T-cell receptor (TCR) gene rearrangement Whole blood, bone marrow, frozen or paraffin-embedded tissue Lavender $$$	In general, the percentage of T lymphocytes with identical T-cell receptors is very low; in malignancies, however, the clonal expansion of one population leads to a large number of cells with identical T-cell receptor gene rearrangement. T-cell clonality can be assessed by restriction fragment Southern blot hybridization and polymerase chain reaction (PCR).	**Positive in:** T-cell neoplasms such as T-cell prolymphocytic leukemia, Sézary syndrome, peripheral T-cell lymphoma (monoclonal T-cell proliferation).	The diagnostic sensitivity and specificity are heterogeneous and laboratory- and method-specific. Results of the test must always be interpreted in the context of morphologic and other relevant data (eg, flow cytometry), and should not be used alone for a diagnosis of malignancy. The test is not intended to detect minimal residual disease. Arch Dermatol 2005;141:1107. [PMID: 16172307] Methods Mol Med 2005;115:197. [PMID: 15998969]

Testosterone

Test/Range/Collection	Physiologic Basis	Interpretation	Comments
Testosterone, serum Males: 3.0–10.0 Females: 0.3–0.7 ng/mL [Males: 10–35 Females: 1.0–2.4 nmol/L] SST $$$	Testosterone is the principal male sex hormone, produced by the Leydig cells of the testes. Dehydroepiandrosterone (DHEA) is produced in the adrenal cortex, testes, and ovaries and is the main precursor for serum testosterone in women. In normal males after puberty, the testosterone level is twice as high as all androgens in females. In serum, it is largely bound to albumin (38%) and to a specific steroid hormone-binding globulin (SHBG) (60%), but it is the free hormone (2%) that is physiologically active. The total testosterone level measures both bound and free testosterone in the serum (by immunoassay). Free or bioavailable testosterone may be calculated or measured.	**Increased in:** [Idiopathic sexual precocity (in boys, levels may be in adult range), adrenal hyperplasia (boys), adrenocortical tumors, trophoblastic disease during pregnancy, idiopathic hirsutism, virilizing ovarian tumors, arrhenoblastoma, virilizing luteoma, testicular feminization (normal or moderately elevated), cirrhosis (through increased SHBG), hyperthyroidism. Drugs: anticonvulsants, barbiturates, estrogens, oral contraceptives (through increased SHBG). **Decreased in:** Hypogonadism (primary and secondary), orchidectomy, Klinefelter syndrome, uremia, hemodialysis, hepatic insufficiency, ethanol [men]. Drugs: digoxin, spironolactone, acarbose.	The diagnosis of male hypogonadism is based on clinical symptoms and signs plus laboratory confirmation of low AM total serum testosterone levels on two different occasions. Levels below 3.0 ng/mL should be treated. **Free testosterone** should be measured in symptomatic patients with normal total testosterone levels. Obtain serum luteinizing hormone and FSH levels to distinguish between primary (hypergonadotropic) and secondary (hypogonadotropic) hypogonadism. Hypogonadism associated with aging (andropause) may present a mixed picture, with low testosterone levels and low to low-normal gonadotropin levels. In men, there is a diurnal variation in serum testosterone with a 20% elevation in levels in the evenings. Treat Endocrinol 2005;4:293. [PMID: 16185098] Ann Clin Biochem 2006;43(Pt 1):3. [PMID: 16390603] Best Pract Res Clin Endocrinol Metab 2006;20:177. [PMID: 16772150]

Thrombin time		
Thrombin time, plasma 17–23 seconds (laboratory-specific) Blue $	The thrombin time (TT) is a clot-based assay that measures the conversion of fibrinogen to fibrin. The TT is therefore affected by the level of fibrinogen and the presence of thrombin inhibitor and/or fibrin degradation products (FDPs). Because it bypasses all other coagulation reactions, it is not influenced by deficiencies of other coagulation factors.	**Increased in:** Low fibrinogen (<50 mg/dL), abnormal fibrinogen (dysfibrinogenemia), increased FDPs (eg, DIC), heparin, fibrinolytic agents (streptokinase, urokinase, tissue plasminogen activator), liver disease.	The thrombin time (TT) is very sensitive to heparin and has been used to monitor unfractionated heparin therapy. Heparin contamination is a common cause of an unexplained significantly prolonged TT. If suspected, heparin neutralization or a reptilase time can be performed (reptilase time is not affected by heparin). See evaluation for bleeding disorders (Figure 8–7 and Table 8–7). Arch Pathol Lab Med 2002;126:499. [PMID: 11900586]

	Thyroglobulin		
Test/Range/Collection	**Physiologic Basis**	**Interpretation**	**Comments**
Thyroglobulin, serum 3–42 ng/mL [mcg/L] SST $$$	Thyroglobulin is a large protein specific to the thyroid gland from which thyroxine is synthesized and cleaved. Highly sensitive immunoradiometric assays (IRMAs) have minimal interference from autoantibodies.	**Increased in:** Hyperthyroidism, subacute thyroiditis, untreated thyroid carcinomas (except medullary carcinoma): follicular cancer (sensitivity 72%, specificity 81%), Hürthle cell cancer (sensitivity 56%, specificity 84%). **Decreased in:** Factitious hyperthyroidism, presence of thyroglobulin autoantibodies, after (>25 days) total thyroidectomy.	Follow-up of patients with differentiated thyroid cancers who are apparently disease-free after surgery and radioiodine therapy involves periodic measurement of serum thyroglobulin (Tg). Patients with detectable serum Tg during TSH suppression by thyroxine therapy or Tg that rises above 2 ng/mL after TSH stimulation are highly likely to harbor residual tumor. Undetectable serum Tg during TSH suppressive therapy does not exclude persistent disease. Therefore, serum Tg should be measured after TSH stimulation achieved either by thyroxine withdrawal or administration of recombinant human TSH (rhTSH). Results are equivalent in detecting recurrent thyroid cancer, but use of rhTSH helps to avoid symptomatic hypothyroidism. Serum Tg levels during TSH stimulation are usually well correlated with the results of (I^{131}) whole body scanning for local or distant metastases. Thus, rh-TSH-stimulated Tg levels may be the only necessary test to differentiate patients with persistent disease from disease-free patients. These recommendations do not apply when Tg antibodies are present in the serum. Minerva Endocrinol 2004;29:161. [PMID: 15765026] Curr Treat Options Oncol 2005;6:323. [PMID: 15967085] Med Sci Monit 2005;11:RA368. [PMID: 16319807] Semin Nucl Med 2005;35:257. [PMID: 16150246]

Thyroglobulin antibody	Thyroperoxidase antibody
Thyroglobulin antibody, serum <1:10 (highly method-dependent) SST $$	Antibodies against thyroglobulin are produced in autoimmune diseases of the thyroid and other organs. Ten percent of the normal population have slightly elevated titers (especially women and the elderly).	**Increased in:** Hashimoto thyroiditis (>90%), thyroid carcinoma (45%), thyrotoxicosis, pernicious anemia (50%), SLE (20%), subacute thyroiditis, Graves disease. **Not increased in:** Multinodular goiter, thyroid adenomas, and some carcinomas.	The thyroperoxidase antibody test is more sensitive than the thyroglobulin antibody test in autoimmune thyroid disease. (See Thyroperoxidase Antibody, below.) There is little indication for this test except in monitoring of patients with thyroid carcinoma after treatment. (See Thyroglobulin.) Ann Clin Biochem 2006;43(Pt 3):173. [PMID: 16704751]
Thyroperoxidase antibody (TPO), serum Negative SST $$	TPO is a membrane-bound glycoprotein. This enzyme mediates the oxidation of iodide ions and incorporation of iodine into tyrosine residues of thyroglobulin. Its synthesis is stimulated by thyroid-stimulating hormone (TSH). TPO is the major antigen involved in thyroid antibody-dependent cell-mediated cytotoxicity. Antithyroperoxidase antibody assays are performed by ELISA or radioimmunoassay.	**Increased in:** Hashimoto thyroiditis (>99%), idiopathic myxedema (>99%), Graves disease (75–85%), Addison disease (50%), and Riedel thyroiditis. Low titers are present in approximately 10% of normal individuals and patients with nonimmune thyroid disease.	Thyroperoxidase antibody is an antibody to the main autoantigenic component of microsomes and is a more sensitive and specific test than hemagglutination assays for microsomal antibodies in the diagnosis of autoimmune thyroid disease. Thyroperoxidase antibody testing alone is almost always sufficient to detect autoimmune thyroid disease. TPO antibody titers correlate with TSH levels; their presence may herald impending thyroid failure. See thyroid function tests and thyroid disorders (Table 8–24, Figures 8–26 and 8–27.) Best Pract Res Clin Endocrinol Metab 2005;19:1. [PMID: 15826919] Ann Clin Biochem 2006;43(Pt 3):173. [PMID: 16704751]

	Thyroid-stimulating hormone		
Test/Range/Collection	**Physiologic Basis**	**Interpretation**	**Comments**
Thyroid-stimulating hormone, serum (TSH; thyrotropin) 0.4–6 mcU/mL [mU/L] SST $$	TSH is an anterior pituitary hormone that stimulates the thyroid gland to produce thyroid hormones. Secretion is stimulated by thyrotropin-releasing hormone from the hypothalamus. There is negative feedback on TSH secretion by circulating thyroid hormone.	**Increased in:** Hypothyroidism. Mild increases in recovery phase of acute illness. Subclinical hypothyroidism defined as a mild increase in serum TSH and normal free thyroxine and triiodothyronine levels occurs in 4–8.5% of the population. **Decreased in:** Hyperthyroidism, acute medical or surgical illness, pituitary hypothyroidism. Drugs: dopamine, high-dose corticosteroids. Subclinical hyperthyroidism defined as a mild decrease in serum TSH and normal free thyroxine and triiodothyronine levels occurs in ~2% of the population.	Newer sensitive TSH assays are useful in the diagnosis of both hyperthyroidism and hypothyroidism. Measurement of serum TSH is the best initial laboratory test of thyroid function. It should be followed by measurement of free thyroxine if the TSH value is low and by measurement of anti-thyroperoxidase antibody if the TSH value is high. Most experts recommend against routine screening of asymptomatic patients, but screening is recommended for high-risk populations. See also Thyroid function tests and thyroid disorders (Table 8–24; Figures 8–26 and 8–27). Test is useful for following patients taking thyroid medication. Neonatal and cord blood levels are 2–4 times higher than adult levels. Am Fam Physician 2005;72:623. [PMID: 16127951] Am Fam Physician 2005;72:1517. [PMID: 16273818] Clin Chem 2005;51:1480. [PMID: 15961550] Eur J Endocrinol 2006;154:633. [PMID: 16645008]

Thyroid-stimulating hormone receptor antibody, serum (TSH-R [stim] Ab) <130% basal activity of adenylyl cyclase SST $$$$	The thyroid-stimulating hormone receptor (TSH-R) is a G protein-linked, 7-transmembrane domain receptor. It is also a primary antigen in autoimmune thyroid disease. Test detects heterogeneous IgG antibodies directed against the TSH receptor on thyroid cells. Frequently, they cause excess release of hormone from the thyroid. Test measures antibodies indirectly by their stimulation of adenylyl cyclase to produce cAMP.	**Increased in:** Graves disease, transient neonatal thyrotoxicosis.	Although TSH-R [stim] Ab is a marker of Graves disease, the test is not necessary for the diagnosis in most cases. Test is very rarely indicated but may be helpful in: (1) pregnant women with a history of Graves disease, because TSH-R [stim] Ab may have some predictive value for neonatal thyrotoxicosis; and (2) patients presenting with exophthalmos who are euthyroid, to confirm Graves disease. High titers of TSH-R Ab are associated with relapse of hyperthyroidism at the end of a course of anti-thyroid drugs. Endocrinol Metab Clin North Am 2000;29:339. [PMID: 10874533] Horm Metab Res 2005;37:745. [PMID: 16372228] Horm Metab Res 2005;37:741. [PMID: 16372227] J Clin Invest 2005;115:1972. [PMID: 16075037] Treat Endocrinol 2005;4:31. [PMID: 15649099]

Test/Range/Collection	Physiologic Basis	Interpretation	Comments
Thyroxine, total, serum (T4) 5.0–11.0 mcg/dL [64–142 nmol/L] SST $	Total T4 is a measure of thyroid gland secretion of T4, bound and free, and thus is influenced by serum thyroid hormone-binding activity.	**Increased in:** Hyperthyroidism, increased thyroid-binding globulin (TBG) (eg, pregnancy, drug). Drugs: amiodarone, high-dose β-blockers (especially propranolol). **Decreased in:** Hypothyroidism, low TBG due to illness or drugs, congenital absence of TBG. Drugs: phenytoin, carbamazepine, androgens.	Total T4 should be interpreted with the TBG level or as part of a free thyroxine index. Clin Chem 2005;51:1480. [PMID: 15961550] Drugs Aging 2005;22:23. [PMID: 15663347] Pediatrics 2006;117:2290. [PMID: 16740880]
Thyroxine, free, serum (FT4) Varies with method SST $$	FT4 (if done by equilibrium dialysis or ultrafiltration method) is a more direct measure of the free T4 hormone concentration (biologically available hormone) than the free T4 index. FT4 done by a two-step immunoassay is similar to the free thyroxine index. The presence of rheumatoid factor or drug treatment with furosemide, intravenous heparin, and subcutaneous low-molecular-weight heparin may interfere with newer assays for free thyroxine.	**Increased in:** Hyperthyroidism, non-thyroidal illness, especially psychiatric. Drugs: amiodarone, β-blockers (high dose). **Decreased in:** Hypothyroidism, non-thyroidal illness. Drugs: phenytoin.	FT4 is functionally equivalent to the FT4I (see below). The free thyroxine and sensitive TSH assays have similar sensitivities for detecting clinical hyperthyroidism and hypothyroidism. The TSH assay detects subclinical dysfunction and monitors thyroxine treatment better; the free thyroxine test detects central hypothyroidism and monitors rapidly changing function better. Arch Intern Med 1998;158:266. [PMID: 9472207] Lancet 2001;357:619. [PMID: 11558500]

Thyroxine index, free		
Thyroxine index, free, serum (FT_4I) 6.5–12.5 SST $$	Free thyroxine index is expressed as total $T_4 \times T_3$ (or T_4) resin uptake and provides an estimate of the level of free T_4, since the T_3 (or T_4) resin uptake (ie, thyroid hormone binding ratio) is an indirect estimate of the TBG concentration (TBG binds 70% of circulating thyroid hormone). The unbound form of circulating T_4, normally 0.03% of total serum T_4, determines the amount of T_4 available to cells.	**Increased in:** Hyperthyroidism, non-thyroidal illness, especially psychiatric. Drugs: amiodarone, β-blockers (high dose). **Decreased in:** Hypothyroidism, non-thyroidal illness. Drugs: phenytoin.	Calculation of the FT_4I has largely been replaced by measurement of the FT_4 (see above). Lancet 2001;357:619. [PMID: 11558500] Clin Chem 2005;51:1480. [PMID: 15961550]

	***Toxoplasma* antibody**		
Test/Range/Collection	**Physiologic Basis**	**Interpretation**	**Comments**

***Toxoplasma* antibody,** serum or CSF (Toxo)
 	
IgG: <1:16
IgM:
   Infant <1:2
   Adult <1:8 titer
 	
SST or CSF
$$$
 	
Submit paired sera, one collected within 1 week of illness and another 2–3 weeks later.
	Toxoplasma gondii is an obligate intracellular protozoan that causes human infection via ingestion, transplacental transfer, blood products, or organ transplantation. Cats are the definitive hosts of *T gondii* and pass oocysts in their feces. Human infection occurs through ingestion of sporulated oocysts or via the transplacental route.
	
	In the immunodeficient host, acute infection may progress to lethal meningoencephalitis, pneumonitis, or myocarditis.
	
	In acute primary infection, IgM antibodies develop 1–2 weeks after onset of illness, peak in 6–8 weeks, and then decline. IgG antibodies develop on a similar time-course but persist for years.
	
	In adult infection, the disease usually represents a reactivation, not a primary infection. Therefore, the IgM test is less useful.
	
	Approximately 30% of all US adults have antibodies to *T gondii*.
		Increased in: Acute or congenital toxoplasmosis (IgM), previous toxoplasma exposure (IgG), and false-positive (IgM) reactions (SLE, HIV infection, rheumatoid arthritis).	Single IgG titers of >1:256 are considered diagnostic of active infection; titers of >1:128 are suspicious. Titers of 1:16–1:64 may merely represent past exposure. If titers subsequently rise, they probably represent early disease.
			IgM titer >1:16 is very important in the diagnosis of congenital toxoplasmosis.
			High titer IgG antibody results should prompt an IgM test. IgM, however, is generally not found in adult AIDS patients because the disease usually represents a reactivation.
			Some recommend ordering baseline toxoplasma IgG titers in all asymptomatic HIV-positive patients because a rising toxoplasma titer can help diagnose CNS toxoplasmosis in the future.
			Culture of the *T gondii* organism is difficult, and most laboratories are not equipped for the procedure.
			(See also Brain abscess.)
			Br J Biomed Sci 2002;59:4. [PMID: 12000186]
			J Infect Dis 2002;185 (Suppl 1):S73. [PMID: 11865443]
			Trans R Soc Trop Med Hyg 2002;96 (Suppl 1): S205. [PMID: 12055840]
			Murray PR et al (editors): *Manual of Clinical Microbiology*, 8th ed. ASM Press, 2003.
			Clin Perinatol 2005;32:705. [PMID: 16085028]

Transferrin

| Transferrin (Tf), serum

200–400 mg/dL

SST
$ | Transferrin is the major plasma transport protein for iron. Only a small amount of transferrin is required for normal homeostasis. The presence of moderate amounts of unsaturated transferrin may be important in control of infections and infestations by iron-requiring organisms.

Immunochemical assays of transferrin are more accurate than chemical assays of total iron-binding capacity (TIBC). Assuming a molecular weight for transferrin of 89,000 daltons, 1 mg of transferrin binds 1.25 mcg of iron. Therefore a serum transferrin level of 300 mg/dL is equal to a TIBC of 375 mcg/dL. | **Increased in:** Pregnancy, oral contraceptives, iron deficiency.
Decreased in: Inherited atransferrinemia (rare), disorders associated with inflammation or necrosis, chronic inflammation or malignancy, generalized malnutrition, nephrotic syndrome, iron overload states. | Indications for transferrin quantitation include screening for nutritional status and differential diagnosis of anemia. To control for effects of estrogens and acute-phase responses, other acute-phase reactant proteins should be assayed at the same time. Iron deficiency and iron overload are best diagnosed using assays of serum levels of iron, transferrin, and ferritin in combination. Transferrin in CSF appears in its desialated form, the Tau protein (β_2-transferrin). This form can be identified electrophoretically by immunofixation with antitransferrin antibody. The clinical application for identification of the Tau protein is in the investigation of rhinorrhea or otorrhea suspected to be of CSF origin.
Clin Chem 1992;38:2078. [PMID: 1394993] |

	Transferrin receptor, soluble

Test/Range/Collection	Physiologic Basis	Interpretation	Comments
Transferrin receptor, soluble (sTfR), serum or plasma Male 2.2–5 mg/L Female 1.9–4.4 mg/L (laboratory-specific) SST or green $$	The transferrin receptor (TfR) is expressed on the surface of human cells that require iron and acts as an iron transporting molecule. The expression of TfR depends on the concentration of iron in the cellular cytoplasm. The concentration of soluble TfR (sTfR) has been reported to be proportional to the total amount of cell-associated TfR.	**Increased in:** Iron deficiency anemia, conditions of high red cell turnover (eg, hemolytic anemia).	sTfR level increases in iron deficiency and is usually unaffected by chronic disease states. An sTfR level may be useful in combination with other tests of iron status in differentiating iron deficiency anemia from anemia of chronic disease. A diagnostic algorithm that combines the results of ferritin and sTfR has been proposed. A patient with a ferritin of ≤10 μg/L is considered iron deficient in all cases regardless of sTfR level. A patient with ferritin ≥220 μg/L is not considered iron deficiency. For ferritin values between 10 and 220 μg/L, levels of sTfR may be used to identify iron-deficient patients. When assessing iron deficiency, the combination of both ferritin and sTfR levels minimizes false positives due to hemolytic anemia that elevates sTfR and false negatives due to acute-phase elevation of ferritin. Ann Hematol 2005;84:358. [PMID: 15789229]

Triglycerides		
Triglycerides, serum (TG) <165 mg/dL [<1.65 g/L] SST $ Fasting specimen required.	Dietary fat is hydrolyzed in the small intestine, absorbed and resynthesized by mucosal cells, and secreted into lacteals as chylomicrons. Triglycerides in the chylomicrons are cleared from the blood by tissue lipoprotein lipase. Endogenous triglyceride production occurs in the liver. These triglycerides are transported in association with β-lipoproteins in very low density lipoproteins (VLDL).	**Increased in:** Hypothyroidism, diabetes mellitus, nephrotic syndrome, chronic alcoholism (fatty liver), biliary tract obstruction, stress, familial lipoprotein lipase deficiency, familial dysbetalipoproteinemia, familial combined hyperlipidemia, obesity, the metabolic syndrome, viral hepatitis, cirrhosis, pancreatitis, chronic renal failure, gout, pregnancy, glycogen storage diseases types I, III, and VI, anorexia nervosa, dietary excess. Drugs: β-blockers, cholestyramine, corticosteroids, diazepam, diuretics, estrogens, oral contraceptives. **Decreased in:** Tangier disease (α-lipoprotein deficiency), hypo- and abetalipoproteinemia, malnutrition, malabsorption, parenchymal liver disease, hyperthyroidism, intestinal lymphangiectasia. Drugs: ascorbic acid, clofibrate, nicotinic acid, gemfibrozil.	If serum is clear, the serum triglyceride level is generally <350 mg/dL. Elevated triglycerides are now considered an independent risk factor for coronary artery disease, and a major risk factor for acute pancreatitis, particularly when serum triglyceride levels are >1000 mg/dL. Triglycerides >1000 mg/dL can be seen when a primary lipid disorder is exacerbated by alcohol or fat intake or by corticosteroid or estrogen therapy. Am J Med Sci 2005;330:343. [PMID: 16355020] Am J Med Sci 2005;330:295. [PMID: 16355014] Curr Med Res Opin 2005;21:665. [PMID: 15969866] J Fam Pract 2006;55:S1. [PMID: 16822443]

Test/Range/Collection	Physiologic Basis	Interpretation	Comments
Triiodothyronine			
Triiodothyronine, total, serum (T_3) 95–190 ng/dL [1.5–2.9 nmol/L] SST $$	T_3 reflects the metabolically active form of thyroid hormone and is influenced by thyroid hormone-binding activity.	**Increased in:** Hyperthyroidism (some), increased thyroid-binding globulin. **Decreased in:** Hypothyroidism, nonthyroidal illness, decreased thyroid-binding globulin. Drugs: amiodarone.	T_3 may be increased in approximately 5% of hyperthyroid patients in whom T_4 is normal (T_3 toxicosis). Therefore, test is indicated when hyperthyroidism is suspected and T_4 value is normal. Test is of no value in the diagnosis of hypothyroidism. Lancet 2001;357:619. [PMID: 11558500] Am Fam Physician 2005;72:1517. [PMID: 16273818] Clin Chem 2005;51:1480. [PMID: 15961550]

Troponin-I, cardiac		
Troponin-I, cardiac, serum (cTnI) <1.5 ng/mL (method-dependent) SST $$	Troponin is the contractile regulatory protein of striated muscle. It contains three subunits: T, C, and I. Subunit I consists of three forms, which are found in slow-twitch skeletal muscle, fast-twitch skeletal muscle, and cardiac muscle, respectively. Troponin I is predominantly a structural protein and is released into the circulation after cellular necrosis. Cardiac troponin I is expressed only in cardiac muscle, throughout development and despite pathology, and thus its presence in serum can distinguish between myocardial injury and skeletal muscle injury. cTnI is measured by immunoassay using monoclonal antibodies.	**Increased in:** Myocardial infarction (sensitivity 50% at 4 hours, 97% at 6 hours; specificity 95%), cardiac trauma, cardiac surgery, myocardial damage following PTCA, and other cardiac interventions, nonischemic dilated cardiomyopathy, prolonged supraventricular tachycardia, acute dissection of the ascending aorta. Slight elevations noted in patients with recent aggravated unstable angina, muscular disorders, CNS disorders, HIV infection, chronic renal failure, cirrhosis, sepsis, lung diseases, and endocrine disorders. **Not increased in:** Skeletal muscle disease (myopathy, myositis, dystrophy), external electrical cardioversion, noncardiac trauma or surgery, rhabdomyolysis, severe muscular exertion, chronic renal failure.	Cardiac troponin I is a more specific marker for myocardial infarction than CK-MB with roughly equivalent sensitivity early in the course of infarction (4–36 hours). Sensitivity and specificity for peak concentrations of cTnI (100%; 96%) are equivalent to or better than those for CK-MB (88%; 93%) and total CK (73%; 85%). cTnI appears in serum approximately 4 hours after onset of chest pain, peaks at 8–12 hours, and persists for 5–7 days. This prolonged persistence gives it much greater sensitivity than CK-MB for diagnosis of myocardial infarction beyond the first 36–48 hours. Given its utility in detection of acute coronary syndromes, the serum troponin is important in the evaluation and stratification of patients with chest pain in the emergency room. However, there is no benefit in obtaining a routine admission troponin level in ICU patients when an acute coronary event is not suspected. Minor elevations of cardiac troponin I should be interpreted with caution. Cardiol Rev 2002;10:306. [PMID: 12215194] J Intensive Care Med 2005;20:334. [PMID: 16280406] QJM 2005;98:365. [PMID: 15820969] Clin Biochem 2006;39:692. [PMID: 16580659]

Tularemia agglutinins			

Test/Range/Collection	Physiologic Basis	Interpretation	Comments
Tularemia agglutinins, serum <1:80 titer SST $$	*Francisella tularensis* is an organism of wild rodents (rabbits and hares) that infects humans (eg, trappers and skinners) via contact with animal tissues, by the bite of certain ticks and flies, and by consumption of undercooked meat or contaminated water. Agglutinating antibodies appear in 10–14 days and peak in 5–10 weeks. A four-fold rise in titers is typically needed to prove acute infection. Titers decrease over years.	**Increased in:** Tularemia; cross-reaction with brucella antigens and proteus OX-19 antigen (but at lower titers).	Single titers of >1:160 are indicative of infection. Maximum titers are >1:1280. A history of exposure to rabbits, ticks, dogs, cats, or skunks is suggestive of, but not a requirement for, the diagnosis. Most common presentation is a single area of painful lymphadenopathy with low-grade fever. Initial treatment should be empiric. Culture of the organism is difficult, requiring special media, and hazardous to laboratory personnel. Serologic tests are the mainstay of diagnosis. Clin Microbiol Rev 2002;15:631. [PMID: 12364373] Murray PR et al (editors): *Manual of Clinical Microbiology*, 8th ed. ASM Press, 2003.

Type and cross-match		
Type and cross-match (T/C), serum and red cells (type and cross) Red $$ Specimen label must be signed by the person drawing the blood. A second "check" specimen is needed at some hospitals.	A type and cross-match involves ABO and Rh typing, antibody screen, and cross-match. (Compare with Type and Screen, below.) A major cross-match involves testing recipient serum (or plasma) against donor cells. It uses antihuman globulin (AHG) to detect recipient's antibodies on donor red cells. If the recipient's serum contains a clinically significant alloantibody by antibody screen or by history, a cross-match including the AHG phase is required. If no clinically significant antibodies are detected in current screen and there is no record of previous detection of such antibodies, only a method to detect ABO incompatibility, such as an immediate- spin or computer cross-match, is required.	See Type and Screen below.	A type and screen is adequate preparation for operative procedures unlikely to require transfusion. Unnecessary type and cross-match orders reduce blood availability and add to labor and reagent costs. A preordering system should be in place, indicating the number of units of blood likely to be needed for each operative procedure. Genotyping is a powerful adjunct to serologic testing and in the future could enable electronic selection of units with antigen matched to recipients at multiple blood group loci and could therefore improve transfusion outcomes. *Technical Manual of the American Association of Blood Banks*, 15th ed. American Association of Blood Banks, 2005. Curr Opin Hematol 2006;13:471. [PMID: 17053461]

Test/Range/Collection	Physiologic Basis	Interpretation	Comments
Type and screen (T/S), serum and red cells Red or lavender $$ Specimen label must be signed by the person drawing the blood. A second "check" specimen is needed at some hospitals.	Type and screen includes ABO and Rh typing and antibody screen. (Compare with Type and cross-match, above.) This is a procedure in which the patient's blood sample is tested for ABO, Rh(D), and unexpected antibodies, then stored in the transfusion service for future cross-match if a unit is needed for transfusion.	A negative antibody screen implies that a recipient can receive un-cross-matched type-specific blood with minimal risk. If the recipient's serum contains a clinically significant alloantibody by antibody screen, a cross-match is required if transfusion is needed.	Type and screen is indicated for patients undergoing operative procedures unlikely to require transfusion. However, in the absence of preoperative indications, routine preoperative blood type and screen testing is not cost-effective and may be eliminated for some procedures, such as laparoscopic cholecystectomy, expected vaginal delivery, and vaginal hysterectomy. *Technical Manual of the American Association of Blood Banks,* 15th ed. American Association of Blood Banks, 2005.

Type and screen

Uric acid		
Uric acid, serum Males: 2.4–7.4 Females 1.4–5.8 mg/dL [Males: 140–440 Females: 80–350 mcmol/L] SST $	Uric acid is an end product of nucleo-protein metabolism and is excreted by the kidney. An increase in serum uric acid con-centration occurs with increased nucleoprotein synthesis or catabolism (blood dyscrasias, therapy of leu-kemia) or decreased renal uric acid excretion (eg, thiazide diuretic therapy or renal failure).	**Increased in:** Renal failure, gout, myeloproliferative disorders (leuke-mia, lymphoma, myeloma, P), pso-riasis, glycogen storage disease (type I), Lesch-Nyhan syndrome (X-linked hypoxanthine-guanine phosphori-bosyltransferase deficiency), lead nephropathy, hypertensive diseases of pregnancy [pre-eclampsia and eclampsia], menopause, syndrome X (obesity, insulin resistance, hyperten-sion, hyperuricemia, dyslipidemia). Drugs: antimetabolite and chemo-therapeutic agents, diuretics, ethanol, nicotinic acid, salicylates (low dose), theophylline. **Decreased in:** SIADH, xanthine oxidase deficiency, low-purine diet, Fanconi syndrome, neoplastic disease (various, causing increased renal excretion), liver disease. Drugs: salicylates (high dose), allopurinol (xanthine oxidase inhibitor).	Sex, age, and renal function affect uric acid levels. The incidence of hyperuricemia is greater in some ethnic groups (eg, Filipinos) than others (whites). Whether uric acid level is an independent risk fac-tor for for heart disease is controversial. Serum uric acid is a poor predictor of maternal and fetal complications in women with preeclampsia. Curr Opin Rheumatol 2002;14:281. [PMID: 11981327] Clin Chim Acta 2005;356:35. [PMID: 15936302] Semin Nephrol 2005;25:43. [PMID: 15660334] BJOG 2006;113:369. [PMID: 16553648] Curr Opin Rheumatol 2006;18:199. [PMID: 16462529]

Test/Range/Collection	Physiologic Basis	Interpretation	Comments
Vanillylmandelic acid, urine (VMA) 2–7 mg/24 h [10–35 mcmol/d] Urine bottle containing hydrochloric acid $$ Collect 24-hour urine.	Catecholamines secreted in excess by pheochromocytomas are metabolized by the enzymes monoamine oxidase and catechol-O-methyltransferase to VMA, which is excreted in urine.	**Increased in:** Pheochromocytoma (64% sensitivity, 95% specificity), neuroblastoma, ganglioneuroma, generalized anxiety. **Decreased in:** Drugs: monoamine oxidase.	Because of its low sensitivity, test is no longer recommended for the diagnosis of pheochromocytoma. A urine or plasma free metanephrine level is the recommended test. (See also Pheochromocytoma algorithm, Figure 8–17.) The ratio of urinary VMA to urinary creatinine (VMA/Cr) is the most accurate biochemical test in the diagnosis of neuroblastoma. JAMA 2002;287:1427. [PMID: 11903030] Ann Clin Biochem 2006;43(Pt 4):300. [PMID: 16824281]
Venereal Disease Research Laboratory test, serum (VDRL) Nonreactive SST $	This syphilis test measures non-treponemal antibodies that are produced when *Treponema pallidum* interacts with host tissues. The VDRL usually becomes reactive at a titer of >1:32 within 1–3 weeks after the genital chancre appears.	**Increased in:** Syphilis: primary (59–87%), secondary (100%), late latent (79–91%), tertiary (37–94%); collagen-vascular diseases (rheumatoid arthritis, SLE), infections (mononucleosis, leprosy, malaria), pregnancy, drug abuse.	VDRL is used as a syphilis screening test and in suspected cases of primary and secondary syphilis. Positive tests should be confirmed with an FTA-ABS or MHA-TP test. The VDRL has sensitivity and specificity similar to the RPR. Am Fam Physician 2003;68:283. [PMID: 12892348]

VDRL test, CSF		
Venereal Disease Research Laboratory test, CSF (VDRL) Nonreactive $$ Deliver in a clean plastic or glass tube.	The CSF VDRL test measures non-treponemal antibodies that develop in the CSF when *Treponema pallidum* interacts with the central nervous system.	**Increased in:** Tertiary neurosyphilis (10–27%).	The quantitative VDRL is the test of choice for CNS syphilis. Because the sensitivity of CSF VDRL is very low, a negative test does not rule out neurosyphilis. Clinical features, CSF white cell count, and CSF protein should be used together to make the diagnosis (see CSF profiles, Table 8–8). Because the specificity of the CSF VDRL test is high, a positive test confirms the presence of neurosyphilis. Patients being screened for neurosyphilis with CSF VDRL testing should have a positive serum RPR, VDRL, FTA-ABS, MHA-TP test, or other evidence of infection. Repeat testing may be indicated in HIV-infected patients in whom neurosyphilis is suspected. When the CSF VDRL is negative but suspicion of CNS syphilis is high, other commonly used laboratory tests (CSF FTA-ABS, serum FTA-ABS, CSF *Treponema pallidum* hemagglutination [TPHA], serum TPHA, and CSF cells) can, in combination, identify 87% of patients with neurosyphilis with 94% specificity. Gen Hosp Psychiatry 1995;17:305. [PMID: 7590195] Sex Transm Dis 1996;23:392. [PMID: 8885070] Int J Psychiatry Med 1998;28:333. [PMID: 9844837] Psychosomatics 2001;42:453. [PMID: 11815679]

	Vitamin B₁₂		
Test/Range/Collection	Physiologic Basis	Interpretation	Comments
Vitamin B₁₂, serum

140–820 pg/mL
[100–600 pmol/L]

SST
$$

Serum vitamin B₁₂ specimens should be frozen if not analyzed immediately. | Vitamin B₁₂ is a necessary cofactor for three important biochemical processes: conversion of methylmalonyl-CoA to succinyl-CoA and methylation of homocysteine to methionine and demethylation of methyltetrahydrofolate to tetrahydrofolate (THF). Consequent deficiency of folate coenzymes derived from THF is probably the crucial lesion caused by B₁₂ deficiency.
All vitamin B₁₂ comes from ingestion of foods of animal origin.
Vitamin B₁₂ in serum is protein bound, 70% to transcobalamin I (TC I) and 30% to transcobalamin II (TC II). The B₁₂ bound to TC II is physiologically active; that bound to TC I is not. | **Increased in:** Leukemia (acute myelocytic, chronic myelocytic, chronic lymphocytic, monocytic), marked leukocytosis, PV. (Increased B₁₂ levels are not diagnostically useful.)
Decreased in: Pernicious anemia, gastrectomy, gastric carcinoma, malabsorption (sprue, celiac disease, steatorrhea, regional enteritis, fistulas, bowel resection, *Diphyllobothrium latum* [fish tapeworm] infestation, small bowel bacterial overgrowth), pregnancy, dietary deficiency, HIV infection (with or without malabsorption), chronic high-flux hemodialysis, Alzheimer disease, drugs (eg, omeprazole, metformin, carbamazepine).
Using a cutoff of 150 pmol/L, this test has sensitivity 90%, specificity 60% for B₁₂ deficiency. | The previously used Schilling test is being utilized less frequently in the assessment of pernicious anemia. New testing algorithms have been developed using B₁₂, methylmalonic acid (MMA), intrinsic factor blocking antibodies, parietal cell autoantibodies, and serum gastrin analysis. However, further study is needed to validate this new strategy.
The commonly available competitive protein binding assay measures total B₁₂. It is insensitive to significant decreases in physiologically significant B₁₂ bound to TC II.
Low B₁₂ levels warrant treatment; intermediate levels should be followed by the serum methylmalonic acid test (see Methylmalonic acid entry). Neuropsychiatric disorders caused by low serum B₁₂ level can occur in the absence of anemia or macrocytosis.
Clin Lab Med 2002;22:435. [PMID: 12134470]
Haematologica 2006;91:1506. [PMID: 17043022] |

Vitamin D₃, 25-hydroxy			
Vitamin D₃, 25-hydroxy, serum or plasma (25[OH]D₃) 10–50 ng/mL [25–125 nmol/L] SST or green $$$	The vitamin D system functions to maintain serum calcium levels. Vitamin D is a fat-soluble steroid hormone. Two molecular forms exist: D₃ (cholecalciferol), synthesized in the epidermis, and D₂ (ergocalciferol), derived from plant sources. To become active, both need to be further metabolized. Two sequential hydroxylations occur: in the liver to 25(OH)D₃ and then, in the kidney, to 1,25[OH]₂D₃. Plasma levels increase with sun exposure.	**Increased in:** Heavy milk drinkers (up to 64 ng/mL), vitamin D intoxication, sun exposure. **Decreased in:** Dietary deficiency, malabsorption, rickets, osteomalacia, biliary and portal cirrhosis, nephrotic syndrome, renal failure, lack of sun exposure, age, primary hyperparathyroidism. Drugs: phenytoin, phenobarbital.	Measurement of 25(OH)D₃ is the best indicator of both vitamin D deficiency and toxicity. It is indicated in hypocalcemic disorders associated with increased PTH levels, in children and adults with rickets and in adults with osteomalacia. Inadequate intake of vitamin D causes nutritional rickets; type I vitamin D-dependent rickets results from abnormalities in the gene coding for 25(OH)D3-1-α-hydroxylase, and type II results from defective vitamin D receptors. The vitamin D-resistant types are familial hypophosphatemic rickets and hereditary hypophosphatemic rickets with hypercalciuria. Other causes of rickets include renal disease, medications, and malabsorption syndromes. In hypercalcemic disorders, 25(OH)D₃ is useful in disorders associated with decreased PTH levels, or possible vitamin D overdose (hypervitaminosis D). Low plasma 25(OH)D₃ may also enhance the risk of primary hyperparathyroidism or modify its severity. Vitamin D toxicity is manifested by hypercalcemia, hyperphosphatemia, soft tissue calcification, and renal failure. Am Fam Physician 2005;71:299. [PMID: 15686300] Clin Endocrinol (Oxf) 2005;63:506. [PMID: 16268801] Clin Nephrol 2005;64:288. [PMID: 16240900] Eur J Endocrinol 2006;155:237. [PMID: 16868136] Drug Ther Bull 2006;44:25. [PMID: 16617932] Joint Bone Spine 2006;73:249. [PMID: 16563839] J Endocrinol Invest 2006;29:511. [PMID: 16840828]

	Vitamin D₃, 1,25-dihydroxy		
Test/Range/Collection	Physiologic Basis	Interpretation	Comments
Vitamin D₃, 1,25-dihydroxy, serum or plasma (1,25[OH]₂D₃) 20–76 pg/mL SST or green $$$$	1,25-Dihydroxy vitamin D₃ is the most potent form of vitamin D. The main actions of vitamin D are the acceleration of calcium and phosphate absorption in the intestine and stimulation of bone resorption.	**Increased in:** Primary hyperparathyroidism, idiopathic hypercalciuria, sarcoidosis, some lymphomas, 1,25(OH)₂D₃-resistant rickets, normal growth (children), pregnancy, lactation, vitamin D toxicity. **Decreased in:** Chronic renal failure, anephric patients, hypoparathyroidism, pseudohypoparathyroidism, 1-α-hydroxylase deficiency, postmenopausal osteoporosis.	Test is rarely needed. Measurement of 1,25(OH)₂D₃ is only useful in distinguishing 1-α-hydroxylase deficiency from 1,25(OH)₂D₃-resistant rickets or in monitoring vitamin D status of patients with chronic renal failure. Test is not useful for assessment of vitamin D intoxication because of efficient feedback regulation of 1,25(OH)₂D₃ synthesis. Parathyroid tissue expresses the vitamin D receptor and it is thought that circulating 1,25(OH)₂D₃ participates in the regulation of parathyroid cell proliferation, differentiation, and secretion. Primary hyperparathyroidism is usually associated with increased plasma 1,25(OH)₂D₃. Clin Lab Med 2000;20:569. [PMID: 10986622] Eur J Endocrinol 2006;155:237. [PMID: 16868136]

von Willebrand factor		
von Willebrand factor (vWF), plasma Blue Antigen (vWFAg by ELISA) Activity (ristocetin cofactor) 50–180% $$$	The vWF is an endothelium-derived multimeric plasma protein with two important functions in hemostasis: (1) promoting platelet adhesion at the site of injury; and (2) transporting and stabilizing factor VIII in plasma. von Willebrand disease (vWD) is caused by hereditary quantitative (types 1 and 3) or qualitative (type 2A, 2B, 2M, 2N) defects of the vWF. Acquired vWD can occur but is rare.	**Increased in:** Inflammatory states (acute-phase reactant). **Decreased in:** Hereditary or acquired von Willebrand disease (vWD): type 1, decreased antigen and activity levels; type 3, undetectable antigen and activity; type 2, antigen level may be normal, but activity is impaired.	In vWD, the platelet count and morphology are generally normal and the bleeding time is usually prolonged (markedly prolonged by aspirin). The PTT may not be prolonged if factor VIII coagulant level is >30%. Diagnosis of vWD is suggested by bleeding symptoms and family history. Initial tests for vWD (bleeding time or PFA-100 CT, platelet count, PTT) are typically followed by the diagnostic tests: vWF antigen and activity. Further tests may be necessary to distinguish the subtypes of vWD, such as vWF multimer analysis, factor VIII assay, and platelet aggregation studies (low-dose ristocetin). N Engl J Med 2003;349:343. [PMID: 12878741] N Engl J Med 2004;351:683. [PMID: 15306670] Semin Thromb Hemost 2006;32:456. [PMID: 16862518]

Test/Range/Collection	Physiologic Basis	Interpretation	Comments
White blood cell count (WBC) and differential, blood Reference ranges are age- and laboratory-specific Adult ranges: WBC $4.5–11.0 \times 10^3$/mcL; differential: segmented neutrophils 50–70%; band neutrophils 0–5%; lymphocytes 20–40%; monocytes 2–6%; eosinophils 1–4%; basophils 0–1%. ***Panic:*** $<1.5 \times 10^3$/mcL Lavender $	The WBC count and differential determine the number of white blood cells and the percentage of each type of white cell in a blood sample. It is typically generated by an automated laboratory hematology analyzer as part of the CBC panel. The basic principles used for WBC count and differential are instrument-dependent (eg, Beckman Coulter, Bayer, Abbott, Sysmex). Manual differential is also routinely obtained by examing a blood smear under a microscope.	**Increased in:** Acute infections, inflammatory disorders, acute and chronic leukemias, myeloproliferative disorders, circulating lymphoma, tissue injury/necrosis, various drugs, corticosteroids, allergies, hypersensitivity reactions, stress, smoking. **Decreased in:** Infections, constitutional and acquired myeloid hypoplasia, myelosuppression (eg, chemotherapy, radiation, various drugs), myelodysplasia, collagen vascular diseases, hypersplenism, cyclic neutropenia, autoimmune neutropenia, alcoholism.	There are five types of white cells, each with different functions: neutrophils, lymphocytes, monocytes, eosinophils, and basophils. Absolute counts for individual cell populations can be calculated from a combination of the WBC count and the percentage of each cell type from the differential. It is important to perform a manual differential in certain conditions such as presence of blasts, immature granulocytes, nucleated red blood cells, leukemia or lymphoma cells, plasma cells, or dysplasia. Lab Hematol 2005;11:62. [PMID: 15790554] Mayo Clin Proc 2005;80:923. [PMID: 16007898] Arch Pathol Lab Med 2006;130:596. [PMID: 16663868] Lab Hematol 2006;12:15. [PMID: 16513543]

D-Xylose absorption test		
D-Xylose absorption test, urine >5 g per 5-hour urine (>20% excreted in 5 hours) $$$ Fasting patient is given D-xylose, 25 g in two glasses of water, followed by four glasses of water over the next 2 hours. Urine is collected for 5 hours and refrigerated.	Xylose is normally easily absorbed from the small intestine. Measuring xylose in serum or its excretion in urine after ingestion evaluates the carbohydrate absorption ability of the proximal small intestine.	**Decreased in:** Intestinal malabsorption (eg, celiac sprue), small intestinal bacterial overgrowth, renal insufficiency, small intestinal HIV enteropathy, cryptosporidiosis, cytotoxic therapy-related malabsorption.	Test can be helpful in distinguishing intestinal malabsorption (decreased D-xylose absorption) from pancreatic insufficiency (normal D-xylose absorption). Urinary xylose excretion may be spuriously decreased in renal failure, thus limiting the specificity and usefulness of the test. In this case, a serum xylose level (gray-top tube) obtained 1 hour after administration of a 25-g dose of D-xylose can be used to evaluate xylose absorption. The normal level should be >29 mg/dL (1.9 mmol/L). J Clin Gastroenterol 2001;33:36. [PMID: 11418788] Clin Gastroenterol Hepatol 2005;3:679. [PMID: 16206501]

4

Therapeutic Drug Monitoring: Principles and Test Interpretation

Diana Nicoll, MD, PhD, MPA

UNDERLYING ASSUMPTIONS

The basic assumptions underlying therapeutic drug monitoring (Table 4–1) are that drug metabolism varies from patient to patient and that the plasma level of a drug is more closely related to the drug's therapeutic effect or toxicity than is the dosage.

INDICATIONS FOR DRUG MONITORING

Drugs with a **narrow therapeutic index** (where therapeutic drug levels do not differ greatly from levels associated with serious toxicity) should be monitored. *Example:* Lithium.

Patients who have **impaired clearance of a drug with a narrow therapeutic index** are candidates for drug monitoring. The clearance mechanism of the drug involved must be known. *Example:* Patients with renal failure have decreased clearance of gentamicin and therefore are at a higher risk for gentamicin toxicity.

Drugs whose **toxicity is difficult to distinguish from a patient's underlying disease** may require monitoring. *Example:* Theophylline in patients with chronic obstructive pulmonary disease.

Drugs whose efficacy is **difficult to establish clinically** may require monitoring of plasma levels. *Example:* Phenytoin.

SITUATIONS IN WHICH DRUG MONITORING MAY NOT BE USEFUL

Drugs that can be given in extremely high doses before toxicity is apparent are not candidates for monitoring. *Example:* Penicillin.

If there are better means of assessing drug effects, drug level monitoring may not be appropriate. *Example:* Warfarin is monitored by prothrombin time and International Normalized Ratio (INR) determinations, not by serum levels.

Drug level monitoring to assess compliance is limited by the inability to distinguish noncompliance from rapid metabolism without direct inpatient scrutiny of drug administration.

Drug toxicity cannot be diagnosed with drug levels alone; it is a clinical diagnosis. Drug levels within the usual therapeutic range do not rule out drug toxicity in a given patient. *Example:* Digoxin, where other physiologic variables (eg, hypokalemia) affect drug toxicity.

In summary, therapeutic drug monitoring may be useful to guide dosage adjustment of certain drugs in certain patients. Patient compliance is essential if drug monitoring data are to be correctly interpreted.

OTHER INFORMATION REQUIRED FOR EFFECTIVE DRUG MONITORING

Reliability of the Analytic Method

The analytic **sensitivity** of the drug monitoring method must be adequate. For some drugs, plasma levels are in the nanogram per milliliter range. *Example:* Tricyclic antidepressants, digoxin.

The **specificity** of the method must be known, because the drug's metabolites or other drugs may interfere. Interference by metabolites—which may or may not be pharmacologically active—is of particular concern in immunologic assay methods using antibodies to the parent drug.

The **precision** of the method must be known to assess whether changes in levels are caused by method imprecision or by clinical changes.

Reliability of the Therapeutic Range

Establishing the therapeutic range for a drug requires a reliable clinical assessment of its therapeutic and toxic effects, together with plasma drug level measurements by a particular analytic method. In practice, as newer, more specific analytic methods are introduced, the therapeutic ranges for those methods are estimated by comparing the old and new methodologies—without clinical correlation.

Pharmacokinetic Parameters

Five pharmacokinetic parameters that are important in therapeutic drug monitoring include:

1. *Bioavailability.* The bioavailability of a drug depends in part on its formulation. A drug that is significantly metabolized as it first passes through the liver exhibits a marked "first-pass effect," reducing the effective oral absorption of the drug. A reduction in this first-pass effect (eg, because of decreased hepatic blood flow in heart failure) could cause a clinically significant increase in effective oral drug absorption.

2. *Volume of distribution and distribution phases.* The volume of distribution of a drug determines the plasma concentration reached after a loading dose. The distribution phase is the time taken for a drug to distribute from the plasma to the periphery. Drug levels drawn before completion of a long distribution phase may not reflect levels of pharmacologically active drug at sites of action. *Examples:* Digoxin, lithium.

3. *Clearance.* Clearance is either renal or nonrenal (usually hepatic). Whereas changes in renal clearance can be predicted on the basis of serum creatinine or creatinine clearance, there is no routine liver function test for assessment of hepatic drug metabolism. For most therapeutic drugs measured, clearance is independent of plasma drug concentration, so that a change in dose is reflected in a similar change in plasma level. If, however, clearance is dose dependent, dosage adjustments produce disproportionately large changes in plasma levels and must be made cautiously. *Example:* Phenytoin.

4. *Half-life.* The half-life of a drug depends on its volume of distribution and its clearance and determines the time taken to reach a steady state level. In three or four half-lives, the drug level will be 87.5–93.75% of the way to steady state. Patients with decreased drug clearance and therefore increased drug half-lives will take longer to reach a higher steady-state level. In general, because non–steady-state drug levels are potentially misleading and can be difficult to interpret, it is recommended that most clinical monitoring be done at steady state.

5. *Protein binding of drugs.* All routine drug level analysis involves assessment of both protein-bound and free drug. However, pharmacologic activity depends on only the free drug level. Changes in protein binding (eg, in uremia or hypoalbuminemia) may significantly affect interpretation of reported levels for drugs that are highly protein-bound. *Example:* Phenytoin. In such cases, where the ratio of free to total measured drug level is increased, the usual therapeutic range based on total drug level will not apply.

Drug Interactions

For patients receiving several medications, the possibility of drug interactions affecting drug elimination must be considered. *Example:* Quinidine, verapamil, and amiodarone decrease digoxin clearance.

Time to Draw Levels

In general, the specimen should be drawn after steady state is reached (at least three or four half-lives after a dosage adjustment) and just before the next dose (trough level).

Peak and trough levels may be indicated to evaluate the dosage of drugs whose half-lives are much shorter than the dosing interval. *Example:* Gentamicin.

REFERENCE

Winter ME. *Basic Clinical Pharmacokinetics,* 4th ed. Lippincott Williams & Wilkins, 2004. ISBN 0-7817-4147-5.

TABLE 4-1. THERAPEUTIC DRUG MONITORING.

Drug	Effective Concentrations	Half-Life (hours)	Dosage Adjustment	Comments
Amikacin	Peak: 10–30 mcg/mL Trough: <10 mcg/mL	2–3 ↑ in uremia	↓ in renal dysfunction	Concomitant kanamycin or tobramycin therapy may give falsely elevated amikacin results by immunoassay.
Amitriptyline	95–250 ng/mL	9–46		Drug is highly protein bound. Patient-specific decrease in protein binding may invalidate quoted range of effective concentration.
Carbamazepine	4–12 mg/mL	15		Induces its own metabolism. Metabolite 10,11-epoxide exhibits 13% cross-reactivity by immunoassay. Toxicity: diplopia, drowsiness, nausea, vomiting, and ataxia.
Cyclosporine	150–400 ng/mL (mcg/L) whole blood	6–12	Need to know specimen and methodology used	Cyclosporine is lipid soluble (20% bound to leukocytes; 40% to erythrocytes; 40% in plasma, highly bound to lipoproteins). Binding is temperature dependent, so whole blood is preferred to plasma or serum as specimen. High-performance liquid chromatography or monoclonal fluorescence polarization immunoassay measures cyclosporine reliably. Polyclonal fluorescence polarization immunoassays cross-react with metabolites, so the therapeutic range used with those assays is higher. Anticonvulsants and rifampin increase metabolism. Erythromycin, ketoconazole, and calcium channel blockers decrease metabolism.
Desipramine	100–250 ng/mL	13–23		Drug is highly protein bound. Patient-specific decrease in protein binding may invalidate quoted range of effective concentration.

(continued)

TABLE 4–1. THERAPEUTIC DRUG MONITORING. (*CONTINUED*)

Drug	Effective Concentrations	Half-Life (hours)	Dosage Adjustment	Comments
Digoxin	0.8–2.0 ng/mL	42 ↑ in uremia, CHF, hypothyroidism; ↓ in hyperthyroidism	↓ in renal dysfunction, CHF, hypothyroidism; ↑ in hyperthyroidism	Bioavailability of digoxin tablets is 50–90%. Specimen must not be drawn within 6 hours of dose. Dialysis does not remove a significant amount. Hypokalemia potentiates toxicity. Digitalis toxicity is a clinical and *not* a laboratory diagnosis. Digibind (digoxin-specific antibody) therapy of digoxin overdose can interfere with measurement of digoxin levels depending on the digoxin assay. Elimination is reduced by quinidine, verapamil, and amiodarone.
Ethosuximide	40–100 mg/L	Child: 30 Adult: 50		Levels used primarily to assess compliance. Toxicity is rare and does not correlate well with plasma concentrations.
Gentamicin	Peak: 4–8 mcg/mL Trough: <2 mcg/mL	2–5 ↑ in uremia (7.3 on dialysis)	↓ in renal dysfunction	Draw peak specimen 30 minutes after end of infusion. Draw trough just before next dose. In uremic patients, carbenicillin may reduce gentamicin half-life from 46 to 22 hours. If a once-daily regimen (5 mg/kg) is used to maximize bacterial killing by optimizing the peak concentration/MIC ratio and to reduce the potential for toxicity, dosage should be reduced if trough concentration is >1 mcg/mL (1 mg/L). Measurement of peak concentrations is not recommended with this drug.
Imipramine	180–350 ng/mL	10–16		Drug is highly protein bound. Patient-specific decrease in protein binding may invalidate quoted range of effective concentration.
Lidocaine	1–5 mcg/mL	1.8 ↔ in uremia, CHF; ↑ in cirrhosis	↓ in CHF, liver disease	Levels increased with cimetidine therapy. CNS toxicity common in the elderly.

Drug	Therapeutic Range			Comments
Lithium	0.7–1.5 mmol/L	22 ↑ in uremia	↓ in renal dysfunction	Thiazides and loop diuretics may increase serum lithium levels.
Methotrexate		8.4 ↑ in uremia	↓ in renal dysfunction	7-Hydroxymethotrexate cross-reacts 1.5% in immunoassay. To minimize toxicity, leucovorin should be continued if methotrexate level is >0.1 mcmol/L at 48 hours after start of therapy. Methotrexate >1 mcmol/L at >48 hours requires an increase in leucovorin rescue therapy.
Nortriptyline	50–140 ng/mL	18–44		Drug is highly protein bound. Patient-specific decrease in protein binding may invalidate quoted range of effective concentration.
Phenobarbital	10–40 mcg/mL	86 ↑ in cirrhosis	↓ in liver disease	Metabolized principally by the hepatic microsomal enzyme system. Many drug–drug interactions.
Phenytoin	10–20 mcg/mL ↓ in uremia, hypoalbuminemia	Dose dependent		Metabolite cross-reacts 10% in immunoassay. Metabolism is capacity limited. Increase dose cautiously when level approaches therapeutic range, because new steady-state level may be disproportionately higher. Drug is very highly protein bound, and when protein binding is decreased in uremia and hypoalbuminemia, the usual therapeutic range does not apply. In this situation, use a reference range of 5–10 mcg/mL.
Primidone	5–10 mcg/mL	8		Phenobarbital cross-reacts 0.5%. Metabolized to phenobarbital. Primidone/phenobarbital ratio >1:2 suggests poor compliance.
Procainamide	4–8 mcg/mL	3 ↑ in uremia	↓ in renal dysfunction	Thirty percent of patients with plasma levels of 12–16 mcg/mL have ECG changes; 40% of patients with plasma levels of >16 mcg/mL have severe toxicity. Metabolite *N*-acetylprocainamide is active.

(continued)

TABLE 4–1. THERAPEUTIC DRUG MONITORING. (CONTINUED)

Drug	Effective Concentrations	Half-Life (hours)	Dosage Adjustment	Comments
Quinidine	1–4 mcg/L	7 ↔ in CHF; ↑ in liver disease	↓ in liver disease, CHF	Effective concentration is lower in chronic liver disease and nephrosis where binding is decreased.
Salicylate	150–300 mcg/mL (15–30 mg/dL)	Dose dependent		See Figure 9–10 for nomogram of salicylate toxicity.
Sirolimus (Rapamune, Rapamycin)	Trough: 4–12 ng/mL when used in combination with cyclosporine A; 12–20 ng/mL if used alone.	62	↓ in liver dysfunction and drugs affecting CYP3A4 activity	Sirolimus, a macrocyclic lactone, is an immunosuppressant used in combination with cyclosporine and corticosteroids for prophylaxis of organ rejection after kidney transplantation. It has also been used in liver and heart transplantation. Side effects include anemia, thrombocytopenia, hyperlipidemia, and hypertension. When used in combination with cyclosporine, careful monitoring of renal function is required because this combination has been associated with increases in serum creatinine. Because of the long half-life of sirolimus, dosage adjustments would ideally be based on trough levels obtained more than 5–7 days after initiation of therapy or dosage change. Once the initial dose titration is complete, monitoring sirolimus trough concentrations weekly for the first month and every 2 weeks for the second month appears to be appropriate.
Tacrolimus (Prograf)	Trough: 5–20 ng/mL	8.7–11.3	↓ in liver dysfunction and drugs affecting CYP3A4 activity	Tacrolimus is a macrolide compound with potent immunosuppressant properties. It is used for prophylaxis of organ rejection in adult patients undergoing liver or kidney transplantation and in pediatric patients undergoing liver transplantation. It has also been used to prevent rejection in heart, small bowel, and allogeneic bone marrow transplant patients and to treat autoimmune diseases.

Theophylline	5–20 mcg/mL	↓ in CHF, cirrhosis, and with cimetidine	Side effects include nausea, vomiting, diarrhea, headache, tremor, and renal dysfunction. Antacid or sucralfate administration should be separated from tacrolimus by at least 2 hours.
	9		Caffeine cross-reacts 10%. Elimination is increased 1.5–2 times in smokers. 1,3-Dimethyl uric acid metabolite increased in uremia and because of cross-reactivity may cause an apparent slight increase in serum theophylline.
Tobramycin	Peak: 5–10 mcg/mL Trough: <2 mcg/mL	↓ in renal dysfunction	Tobramycin, kanamycin, and amikacin may cross-react in immunoassay. If a once-daily regimen is used to maximize bacterial killing by optimizing the peak concentration/MIC ratio and to reduce the potential for toxicity, dosage should be reduced if trough concentration is >1 mcg/mL (1 mg/L). Measurement of peak concentrations is not recommended with this drug.
	2–3 ↑ in uremia		
Valproic acid	55–100 mcg/mL		Ninety-five percent protein-bound. Reduced binding in uremia and cirrhosis.
	13–19		
Vancomycin	Trough: 5–15 mcg/mL	↓ in renal dysfunction	Toxicity in uremic patients leads to irreversible deafness. Keep peak level 30–40 mcg/mL to avoid toxicity.
	6 ↑ in uremia		

↔ = unchanged; ↑ = increased; ↓ = decreased; CHF = congestive heart failure.

5

Microbiology: Test Selection

Jane Jang, BS, MT (ASCP) SM

HOW TO USE THIS SECTION

This section displays information about clinically important infectious diseases in tabular form. Included in these tables are the *Organisms* involved in the disease/syndrome listed; *Specimens/Diagnostic Tests* that are useful in the evaluation; and *Comments* regarding the tests and diagnoses discussed. Topics are listed by body area/organ system: Central Nervous System, Eye, Ear, Sinus, Upper Airway, Lung, Heart and Vessels, Abdomen, Genitourinary, Bone, Joint, Muscle, Skin, and Blood.

Thereafter is a short section on emerging and re-emerging pathogens (viral and bacterial) and antibiotic resistance in bacterial pathogens.

Organisms

This column lists organisms that are known to cause the stated illness. Scientific names are abbreviated according to common usage (eg, *Streptococcus pneumoniae* as *S pneumoniae* or pneumococcus). Specific age or risk groups are listed in order of increasing age or frequency (eg, Infant, Child, Adult, HIV).

When bacteria are listed, Gram stain characteristics follow the organism name in parentheses—eg, "*S pneumoniae* (GPDC)." The following abbreviations are used:

AFB	Acid-fast bacilli	**GPC**	Gram-positive cocci
GPDC	Gram-positive diplococci	**GPCB**	Gram-positive coccobacilli
GPR	Gram-positive rods	**GVCB**	Gram-variable coccobacilli
GNC	Gram-negative cocci	**GNDC**	Gram-negative diplococci
GNCB	Gram-negative coccobacilli	**GNR**	Gram-negative rods

When known, the frequency of the specific organism's involvement in the disease process is also provided in parentheses-eg, "*S pneumoniae* (GPDC) (50%)."

Specimen Collection/Diagnostic Tests

This column describes the collection of specimens, laboratory processing, useful radiographic procedures, and other diagnostic tests. Culture or test sensitivities with respect to the diagnosis in question are placed in parentheses immediately following the test when known—eg, "Gram stain (60%)." Pertinent serologic tests are also listed. Keep in mind that few infections can be identified by definitive diagnostic tests and that clinical judgment is critical to making difficult diagnoses when test results are equivocal.

Comments

This column includes general information about the utility of the tests and may include information about patient management. Appropriate general references are also listed.

Syndrome Name/Body Area

In the last two columns, the syndrome name and body area are placed perpendicular to the rest of the table to allow for quick referencing.

COMMON INFECTIONS WITH ESTABLISHED PATHOGENS/INFECTIOUS AGENTS.

		CENTRAL NERVOUS SYSTEM
		Brain abscess
Organism	**Specimen/Diagnostic Tests**	**Comments**
Brain abscess	Blood for bacterial and fungal cultures.	Occurs in patients with otitis media and sinusitis; cyanotic congenital heart disease and right-to-left shunting (eg, tetralogy of Fallot) or arteriovenous vascular abnormalities of the lung (eg, Osler-Weber-Rendu).
Usually polymicrobial	Brain abscess aspirate for Gram stain (82%), bacterial (88%), AFB, fungal cultures, and cytology.	
Child: anaerobes (40%), S aureus (GPC), S pneumoniae (GPDC), S pyogenes (GPC in chains), viridans streptococci (GPC in chains), less common, Enterobacteriaceae (GNR), P aeruginosa (GNR), H influenzae (GNCB), N meningitidis (GNDC).	Lumbar puncture is dangerous and contraindicated. Sources of infection in the ears, sinuses, lungs, or bloodstream should be sought for culture when brain abscess is found.	
Adults: Viridans streptococci, anaerobic streptococci, S pneumoniae, S milleri, Rhodococcus sp. Group B streptococci (GPC in chains) (60–70%), bacteroides (GNR) (10–30%), Enterobacteriaceae (GNR) (23–33%), S aureus (GPC) (10–15%), N meningitidis, Listeria sp., other anaerobes (10–20%) including prevotella (GNR), fusobacterium (GNR), Eubacterium (GNR), and propionibacterium (GPC), nocardia (GPR), actinomyces (GPR), T solium (cysticerci), Entamoeba histolytica, Shistosoma japonicium and fungi (1%).	CT scan and MRI are the most valuable imaging procedures (see Chapter 6) and can guide brain biopsy if a specimen is needed. Serum toxoplasma antibody in HIV-infected patients may not be positive at initiation of presumptive therapy. If negative or if no response to empiric therapy, biopsy may be needed to rule out lymphoma, fungal infection, or tuberculosis. Biopsy material should be sent for toxoplasma antigen (detected by direct fluorescent antibody, DFA).	Majority of toxoplasmosis abscesses are multiple and are seen on MRI in the basal ganglia, parietal and frontal lobes. [99m]Technetium brain scan is a very sensitive test for abscess and becomes the test of choice if CT and MRI are unavailable. Infect Dis Clin north Am 2001;15:2. [PMID: 11447718] Infect Dis Clin North Am 2001;15:4. [PMID: 11780274] Clin Neurol Neurosurg 2002;105:60. [PMID: 12445926]
Immunocompromised: T gondii, C neoformans, nocardia (GPR), Listeria sp., mycobacteria (AFB), C albicans, Cryptococcus, coccidioides, mucor, cytomegalovirus (CMV), herpes simplex (HSV), varicella-zoster (VZV), E histolytica.	Detection of toxoplasma DNA in blood or CSF samples by PCR techniques is now available from specialized or reference laboratories. A positive PCR result must be interpreted in the context of the clinical presentation. Active or recent infection is indicated by a positive IgM antibody test.	N Engl J Med 2003;348:2125. [PMID: 12761369] Clin Infect Dis 2004;38:206 [PMID: 11780274] J Infect 2006;53:821. [PMID: 16436297]
Posttraumatic: S aureus (GPC), viridans streptococci (GPC in chains), Enterobacteriaceae (GNR), coagulase-negative staphylococci (GPC), P acnes (GPR).	(See also Toxoplasma antibody, Chapter 6)	

	CENTRAL NERVOUS SYSTEM
	Encephalitis

Organism	Specimen/Diagnostic Tests	Comments
Encephalitis Arboviruses (California group, St. Louis, eastern and western equine, and West Nile virus in summer and fall), enteroviruses (coxsackie, echo, polio), HSV (10–20%), *B henselae*, lymphocytic choriomeningitis, mumps, tick-borne encephalitis virus, postinfectious (following influenza in winter and spring, measles, mumps, rubella, VZV), rabies, Creutzfeldt-Jakob, *B burgdorferi*. Postvaccination: Rabies, pertussis. Immunocompromised: CMV, toxoplasmosis, papovavirus, fungi.	CSF for pressure (elevated), cell count (WBCs elevated but variable [10–2000/mcL], mostly lymphocytes), protein (elevated, especially IgG fraction), glucose (normal), RBCs (suggestive of herpesvirus or other necrotizing virus). Repeat examination of CSF after 24 hours often useful. (See CSF [enteroviruses, HSV-2, mumps] profiles, Table 8–8. CSF cultures for viruses, bacteria, fungi, and mycobacteria (low yield). CSF PCR for CMV (33%), HSV (98%), VZV, enterovirus and West Nile virus. Identification of HSV DNA in CSF by PCR techniques is now the definitive diagnostic test. Throat swab for enterovirus, mumps. Stool culture for enterovirus, which is frequently shed for weeks (especially in children). Urine culture for mumps. Culture of both skin biopsy from hairline and saliva for rabies. Single serum for *Bartonella* (cat-scratch disease) IgM and IgG. Single serum for West Nile virus IgM antibody, MAC-ELISA. Paired sera for arboviruses, mumps, or rabies should be drawn acutely and after 1–3 weeks of illness. Urine PCR and/or serum PCR are options for diagnosis of enteroviruses.	MRI with gadolinium (most sensitive) or CT scan with contrast (50% sensitive) showing temporal lobe lesions) suggests herpes simplex. Polyradiculopathy is highly suggestive of CMV in AIDS. MMWR Recomm Rep 2000;49:714. [PMID: 10902834] Ann Intern Med 2002;137:173. [PMID: 12160365] Clin Infect Dis 2002;35:254. [PMID: 12115090] Clin Infect Dis 2002;35(Suppl 2):5173. [PMID: 12353203] Lancet 2002;359:507. [PMID: 11853816] Clin Infect Dis 2003;36:731. [PMID: 15841069]

CENTRAL NERVOUS SYSTEM		
Aseptic meningitis		
Aseptic meningitis Acute: Enteroviruses (coxsackie, echo, polio) (90%), mumps, HSV, HIV (primary HIV sero-conversion), VZV, lymphocytic choriomeningitis virus, adenovirus, bunyavirus, parainfluenza virus 3, West Nile, St. Louis and California encephalitis viruses (rare). Recurrent: HSV-2 (Mollaret syndrome).	CSF for pressure (elevated), cell count (WBCs 10–100/mcL, PMNs early, lymphocytes later), protein (normal or slightly elevated), and glucose (normal). On repeat CSF after 24–48 hours, an increase in lymphocytes is seen. (See CSF profiles, Table 8–8.) CSF viral culture can be negative despite active viral infection. Enteroviruses can be isolated from the CSF in the first few days after onset (positive in 40–80%) but only rarely after the first week. Detection of enteroviral RNA in CSF by PCR in specialized or reference laboratories. Urine viral culture for mumps. Vesicle (DFA) or culture for HSV or VZV. Paired sera for viral titers: poliovirus, mumps, and VZV. Not practical for other organisms unless actual isolate known and then only useful epidemiologically. Detection of VZV or HSV in CSF by PCR. CT or MRI of head should be performed prior to lumbar puncture to evaluate for mass lesions or hydrocephalus if focal neurologic signs or papilledema are present.	Aseptic meningitis is acute meningeal inflammation in the absence of pyogenic bacteria or fungi. Diagnosis is usually made by examination of the CSF and by ruling out other infectious causes (eg, toxoplasmosis, Lyme disease, syphilis, tuberculosis, Rocky Mountain spotted fever, ehrlichiosis, fungi, and angiostrongyliasis). Consider nonsteroidal anti-inflammatory drugs as a noninfectious cause. Enteroviral aseptic meningitis is rare after age 40. Patients with deficiency of the complement regulatory protein factor I may have recurrent aseptic meningitis. Semin Neurol 2000;20:277. [PMID: 11051293]

	CENTRAL NERVOUS SYSTEM
	Bacterial meningitis

Organism	Specimen/Diagnostic Tests	Comments
Bacterial meningitis Neonate: Group B streptococci (GPC) (70%), *L monocytogenes* (GPR) (10%), *S pneumoniae* (GPC) (10%), *E coli* (GNR) and *Klebsiella sp* (GNR) (1%), and other streptococci. Infant: *S pneumoniae* (GPC) (47%), *N meningitidis* (GNDC) (30%), group B streptococci (GPC) (18%), *Listeria monocytogenes* (GPR), *H influenzae* (GNCB) (5%). Child: *N meningitidis* (60%), *S pneumoniae* (25%), *H influenzae* (8%), and other streptococci. Adult: *S pneumoniae* (60%), *N meningitidis* (20%), *L monocytogenes* (6%), group B streptococci (4%), other *Hemophilus* sp., and staphylococci (1%). Postneurosurgical: *S aureus* (GPC), *S pneumoniae*, *P acnes* (GPR), coagulase-negative staphylococci (GPC), pseudomonas (GNR), *E coli* (GNR), other Enterobacteriaceae, acinetobacter (GNR). Alcoholic patients and the elderly: In addition to the adult organisms, Enterobacteriaceae, pseudomonas, *H influenzae*.	CSF for pressure (>180 mm H_2O), cell count (WBCs 1000–100,000/mcL, >50% PMNs), protein (150–500 mg/dL), glucose (<40% of serum). (See CSF profiles, Table 8–8.) CSF for Gram stain of cytocentrifuged material (positive in 70–80%). CSF culture for bacteria. Blood culture positive in 40–60% of patients with pneumococcal, meningococcal, and *H influenzae* meningitis. CSF antigen tests are no longer considered useful because of their low sensitivity and false-positive results.	The first priority in the care of the patient with suspected acute meningitis is therapy, then diagnosis. Antibiotics should be started within 30 minutes of presentation. The death rate for meningitis is about 50% for pneumococcal, less for others. With recurrent *N meningitidis* meningitis, suspect a terminal complement component deficiency. With other recurrent bacterial meningitides, suspect a CSF leak. *S pneumoniae* is most likely pathogen. Treat with 3rd generation cephalosporin plus vancomycin until culture results return. This will also cover *H influenzae*. Therapy can be altered once the susceptibility is determined. If the gram stain of CSF yields a gram negative rod, add an aminoglycoside. For *S pneumoniae*, there is an increase in prevalence of penicillin resistance and multidrug (ie, cephalosporins, macrolides, carbapenems, TMP-SMX) resistance. Medicine (Baltimore) 2000;79:360. [PMID: 11144034] J Infect Dis 2002;186(Suppl 2):S225. [PMID: 12424705] Clin Infect Dis 2004;39:1267. [PMID: 15494903] N Engl J Med 2004;351:1849. [PMID: 15509815]

CENTRAL NERVOUS SYSTEM		
Fungal meningitis		
Fungal meningitis *C neoformans* (spherical, budding yeast), *C immitis* (spherules), *H capsulatum.* Immunocompromised: *Aspergillus* sp., *P boydii*, *Candida* sp., sporothrix, blastomyces.	CSF for pressure (normal or elevated), cell count (WBCs 50–1000/mcL, mostly lymphocytes), protein (elevated), and glucose (decreased). Serum cryptococcal antigen (CrAg) for *C neoformans* (99%). For other fungi, collect at least 5 mL of CSF for fungal culture. Initial cultures are positive in 40% of *C neoformans* cases and 27–65% of histoplasma cases. Repeat cultures are frequently needed. Culture of bone marrow, skin lesions, or other involved organs if clinically indicated. CSF India ink preparation for cryptococcus is not recommended. Serum coccidioidal serology is a concentrated serum immunodiffusion test for the organism (75–95%). CSF serologic testing is rarely necessary. (See Coccidioides serology, Chapter 3) Complement fixation test for histoplasma is available from public health department laboratories (see Chapter 4). Histoplasma antigen can be detected in urine (90%), blood (70%), or CSF in 61% of cases of histoplasma meningitis.	The clinical presentation of fungal meningitis in immunocompromised patients is that of an indolent chronic meningitis. Prior to AIDS, cryptococcal meningitis was seen both in patients with cellular immunologic deficiencies and in patients who lacked obvious defects (about 50% of cases). In AIDS patients, cryptococcus is the most common cause of meningitis nd may present with normal CSF findings. Titer of CSF CrAg can be used to monitor therapeutic success (falling titer) or failure (unchanged or rising titer) or to predict relapse during suppressive therapy (rising titer) in immunocompetent patients, though not in patients with AIDS. Clin Infect Dis 2002;16:837. [PMID: 12512184] Clin Infect Dis 2003;36:337. [PMID: 12539076] Trends Microbiol 2003;11:488. [PMID: 14557032] Clin Infect Dis 2005;40:844. [PMID: 15736018]

	CENTRAL NERVOUS SYSTEM
	Spirochetal meningitis/neurologic diseases

Organism	Specimen/Diagnostic Tests	Comments
Spirochetal meningitis/neurologic diseases *B burgdorferi* (neuro-borreliosis), *T pallidum* (neurosyphilis), leptospira, other borreliae.	**Neuroborreliosis:** CSF for pressure (normal or elevated), cell count (WBCs elevated, mostly lymphocytes), protein (may be elevated), and glucose (normal). Serum and CSF for serologic testing by ELISA or IFA. False-positive serologic tests may occur. Western blots should be used to confirm borderline or positive results. CSF serology for anti-*B burgdorferi* IgM (90%). PCR is very specific for detecting *Borrelia* DNA, but sensitivity is variable owing to stage of disease and type of body fluid tested. PCR is more sensitive than culture in chronic disease. (See Lyme disease serologies, Chapter 3). **Acute syphilitic meningitis:** CSF for pressure (elevated), cell count (WBCs 25–2000/mcL, mostly lymphocytes), protein (elevated), and glucose (normal or low). (See CSF profiles, Table 8–8). Serum VDRL. (See VDRL, serum, Chapter 3) CSF VDRL is the preferred test (see Chapter 3), but is only 66% sensitive for acute syphilitic meningitis. **Neurosyphilis:** CSF for pressure (normal), cell count (WBCs normal or slightly increased, mostly lymphocytes), protein (normal or elevated), glucose (normal), and CSF VDRL. Serum VDRL, FTA-ABS, or MHA-TP should be done. **Leptospirosis:** CSF cell count (WBCs <500/mcL, mostly monocytes), protein (slightly elevated), and glucose (normal). Urine for dark-field examination of sediment. Blood and CSF dark-field examination only positive in acute phase prior to meningitis. Serum for serology for IgM by EIA (93% specificity) and ELISA.	Neurosyphilis is a late stage of infection and can present with meningovascular (hemiparesis, seizures, aphasia), parenchymal (general paresis, tabes dorsalis), or asymptomatic (latent) disease. Because there is no single highly sensitive or specific test for neurosyphilis, the diagnosis must depend on a combination of clinical and laboratory data. Therapy of suspected neurosyphilis should not be withheld on the basis of a negative CSF VDRL if clinical suspicion is high. In HIV neurosyphilis, treatment failures may be common. Lyme disease can present as a lymphocytic meningitis, facial palsy, or painful radiculitis. Leptospirosis follows exposure to rats. N Engl J Med 2001;345:115. [PMID: 11450660] Med Clin North Am 2002;86:311. [PMID: 11982304] Med Clin North Am 2002;86:261. [PMID: 11982031]

CENTRAL NERVOUS SYSTEM		
Parasitic meningoencephalitis		

Parasitic meningo-encephalitis

T gondii, E chaffeensis (human monocytic ehrlichiosis) (HME), *E equis* (HME), *E canis* (HME), and other species of human granulocytic ehrlichiosis (*E phagocytophila, E ewingii*) (HGE), *E histolytica, N fowleri, T solium* (cysticerci), *Acanthamoeba* (GAE), *Balamuthia* sp. (GAE), *Angiostrongylus* (eosinophilic meningoen-cephalitis), *Trypanosoma sp.*

CSF for pressure (normal or elevated), cell count (WBCs 100–1000/mcL, chiefly monocytes, lymphocytes), protein (elevated), glucose (normal to low). Serology as for brain abscess.

Toxoplasmosis: CSF: wet mount, culture, PCR, neuroimaging.

Ehrlichiosis: White blood cell count low (1300–4000/mcL), platelets low (50,000–140,000/mcL), elevated hepatic aminotransferases (tenfold above normal). Buffy coat for Giemsa (1% in HME, 18–80% in HGE), PCR of blood (50–90% sensitive, depending on prior therapy). Serum IgG and IgM usually not positive until the third week.

Naegleria: CSF wet mount, culture, and Giemsa stain. Serological tests not helpful.

Cysticercosis: Characteristic findings on CT and MRI are diagnostic. Serology is less sensitive.

Balamuthia: Culture not helpful.

Angiostrongyliasis: CSF pressure (normal or elevated), cell count (WBC eosinophilic pleocytosis), protein (elevated), glucose (normal). CSF wet mount, ELISA serology.

Trypanosomiasis: Blood Giemsa stain on thick and thin smears. CSF wet mount. Serologic tests by ELISA, IFA have 93–98% sensitivity and 99% specificity in acute stages. Serologic tests may be negative in chronic stages; PCR and DNA methods sometimes helpful.

Naegleria follows exposure to warm fresh and polluted water (eg, swimming pools, sewers. Ehrlichia follows exposure to horses and ticks. Lancet Infect Dis 2001;1:92. [PMID: 11871482]

Chin Med J (Engl) 2002;115:1312. [PMID: 12411101]

Clin Infect Dis 2002;34:22. [PMID: 11731941]

Emerg Infect Dis 2002;8:398. [PMID: 11971774]

Med Clin North Am 2002;86:375. [PMID: 11982308]

Clin Microbiol Rev 2003;16:273. [PMID: 12692099]

Microb Pathog 2003;34:277. [PMID: 12782480]

	CENTRAL NERVOUS SYSTEM
	Tuberculous meningitis

Organism	Specimen/Diagnostic Tests	Comments
Tuberculous meningitis *M tuberculosis* (MTb), *M avium* (AFB)	CSF for pressure (elevated), cell count (WBCs 100–500/mcL, PMNs early, lymphocytes later), protein (elevated), glucose (decreased). (See CSF profiles, Table 8–8.) CSF for AFB stain. Stain is positive in only 30%; culture may be negative in 15–25% of cases. Cytocentrifugation and repeat smears increase yield. CSF for AFB culture (positive in <70%). Repeated sampling of the CSF during the first week of therapy is recommended; ideally, 3 or 4 specimens of 5–10 mL each should be obtained (87% yield with 4 specimens). PCR available but not yet validated. DNA probes are available for rapid confirmation from mycobacterial growth.	Tuberculous meningitis is usually secondary to rupture of a subependymal tubercle from pulmonary focus or may be a consequence of miliary tuberculosis rather than blood-borne invasion. Because CSF stain and culture are not sensitive for tuberculosis, diagnosis and treatment should be based on a combination of clinical and microbiologic data. Evidence of inactive or active extrameningeal tuberculosis, especially pulmonary, is seen in 75% of patients. MMWR Recomm Rep 2000;49(RR-6):1. [PMID: 10881762] Am J Respir Crit Care Med 2000;161:1376. [PMID: 10764337] Lancet 2002;360:1287. [PMID: 12414204]

EYE		
Conjunctivitis		
Conjunctivitis Neonate (ophthalmia neonatorum): *C trachomatis* (15–50%), *N gonorrhoeae* (GNDC), HSV Children and adults: adenovirus, staphylococci (GPC), HSV, *H influenzae* (GNCB), *S pneumoniae* (GPDC), *S pyogenes* (GPC), VZV, *N gonorrhoeae* (GNDC), *M lacunata* (GNCB), *M catarrhalis, Bartonella* sp. (Parinaud oculoglandular syndrome). Adult inclusion conjunctivitis/trachoma: *C trachomatis.* Acute hemorrhagic conjunctivitis (acute epidemic keratoconjunctivitis): enterovirus, coxsackievirus.	Conjunctival Gram stain is especially useful if gonococcal infection is suspected. Bacterial culture for severe cases (routine bacterial culture) or suspected gonococcal infection. Conjunctival scrapings or smears by direct immunofluorescent monoclonal antibody staining for *C trachomatis.* Cell culture for chlamydia. Detection of chlamydial DNA on ocular swabs by PCR techniques. Ocular HSV and VZV PCR available in reference laboratories.	The causes of conjunctivitis change with the season. Adenovirus occurs mainly in the fall, *H influenzae* in the winter. Gonococcal conjunctivitis is an ophthalmologic emergency. Cultures are usually unnecessary unless chlamydia or gonorrhea is suspected or the case is severe. Consider noninfectious causes (eg, allergy, contact lens deposits, trauma). BMJ 2003;327:789. [PMID: 14525879] Semin Pediatr Infect Dis 2005;16:258. [PMID: 16210106] Semin Pediatr Infect Dis 2005;16:235. [PMID: 16210104] *Color Atlas & Textbook of Diagnostic Microbiology,* 16th ed. Lippincott Williams & Wilkins, 2006. Pediatr Clin North Am 2006;53(Suppl 1):7. [PMID: 16898650]

	EYE
	Keratitis
Organism	**Specimen/Diagnostic Tests**	**Comments**

Organism	Specimen/Diagnostic Tests	Comments
Keratitis Bacteria: *P aeruginosa* (GNR), staphylococci (GPC), *S pneumoniae* (GPDC), *Moraxella* sp. Virus: HSV (dendritic pattern on fluorescein slit-lamp examination), VZV. Contact lens: Acanthamoeba, Enterobacteriaceae (GNR). Fungus: Candida, fusarium, aspergillus, rhodotorula, other filamentous fungi. Parasite: *O volvulus* (river blindness), microsporidia (HIV).	Corneal scrapings for Gram stain, KOH, and culture. Routine bacterial culture is used for most bacterial causes, viral culture for herpes, and special media for acanthamoeba (can be detected with trichrome or Giemsa stain of smears). Treatment depends on Gram stain appearance and culture. Corneal biopsy may be needed if initial cultures are negative. Ocular viral DFA for HSV and VZV.	Prompt ophthalmologic consultation is mandatory. Acanthamoeba infection occurs in soft contact (extended-wear) lens wearers and may resemble HSV infection on fluorescein examination (dendritic ["branching"] ulcer). Bacterial keratitis is usually caused by contact lens use or trauma. Fungal (ie, *Fusarium* sp.) keratitis is usually caused by trauma. Increased resistance noted among all bacterial isolates (eg, coagulase-negative staphylococci) to ciprofloxacin (20–38%) and cefazolin (19–40%). Resistance to bactracin, trimethoprim–sulfamethoxazole and vancomycin remains unchanged. Am Fam Physician 2002;66:173. [PMID: 12449270] Br J Opthalmol 2003;87:834. [PMID: 12812878] Eye 2003;17:919. [PMID: 14631397] Arch J Ophthalmol 2006;142:212. [PMID: 16876498] JAMA 2006;296:953. [PMID: 16926355] MMWR Morb Mortal Wkly Rep 2006;55:563. [PMID: 16723968]

EYE		
Endophthalmitis		
Endophthalmitis Spontaneous or postoperative: coagulase-negative staphylococci (70%) (GPC), S aureus (10%) (GPC), viridans group strep- tococci (5%) (GPC in chains), S pneumoniae (5%) (GPDC), gram-negative rods (6%) (eg, E coli, Klebsiella sp.. Pseudomonas sp.), and other gram-positive organisms (4%) (eg, group B streptococci, Listeria sp.). Trauma: Bacillus sp. (GPR), fungi, coagulase- negative staphylococci (GPC), streptococci (GPC), and gram-negative rods. Postfiltering bleb: Viridans groupstreptococci (57%) (GPC in chains), S pneumoniae (GPDC), H influenzae (GNCB), M catarrhalis (GNCB), S aureus (GPC), S epidermidis (GPC), enterococci (GPC), gram-negative rods. IV drug abuse: Add Bacillus cereus.	Culture material from anterior chamber, vitreous cavity, and wound abscess for bacteria, mycobacteria, and fungi. Traumatic and postoperative cases should have aqueous and vitreous aspiration for culture and smear (56%). Conjunctival cultures are inadequate and misleading.	Endophthalmitis refers to bacterial or fungal infections and is an inflammatory process of the ocular cavity and adjacent structures. Rapid diagnosis is critical, because vision may be compromised. Bacterial endophthalmitis usually occurs as a consequence of ocular surgery, 75% within first postoperative week. Prophylactic antibiotic use is of unproved benefit, though topical antibiotics are widely used. Also consider retinitis in immunocompro- mised patients, caused by CMV, HSV, VZV, and toxoplasma (retinochoroiditis), which is diagnosed by retinal examination. Clin Infect Dis 2000;30:662. [PMID: 10770728] Clin Microbiol Rev 2002;15:111. [PMID: 11781270] Diagnostic Microbiology, 11th ed. Mosby, 2002. Surv Ophthalmol 2003;48:403. [PMID: 12850229]

	EAR	
	Otitis media	
Organism	**Specimen/Diagnostic Tests**	**Comments**
Otitis media Infant, child, and adult: *S pneumoniae* (30%) (GPDC), *H influenzae* (57%) (GNCB), *M catarrhalis* (2–15%) (GNDC), *S aureus* (GPC), *S pyogenes* (GPC in chains), viruses (eg, respiratory syncytial virus [RSV], influenza virus, rhinovirus, adenovirus, human metapneumovirus). *M pneumoniae, C pneumoniae,* "sterile," anaerobes, fungi (eg, *Blastomyces dermatitidis, Candida* sp., *Aspergillus* sp.). Neonate: Same as above plus Enterobacteriaceae (GNR), group B streptococcus (GPC). Endotracheal intubation: *Pseudomonas* sp. (GNR), klebsiella (GNR), Enterobacteriaceae (GNR). Chronic: *S aureus* (GPC), *P aeruginosa* (GNR), anaerobes, *M tuberculosis* (AFB).	Tympanocentesis aspirate for Gram stain and bacterial culture in the patient who has a toxic appearance. Otherwise, microbiologic studies of effusions are so consistent that empiric treatment is acceptable. CSF examination if clinically indicated. Nasopharyngeal swab may be substituted for tympanocentesis. Blood culture in the toxic patient.	Peak incidence of otitis media occurs in the first 3 years of life, especially between 6 and 24 months of age. In neonates, predisposing factors include cleft palate, hypotonia, mental retardation (Down syndrome). Tympanocentesis is indicated if the patient fails to improve after 48 hours or develops fever. It may hasten resolution and decrease sterile effusion. Persistent middle ear effusion may require placement of ventilating or tympanostomy tubes. Bullous myringitis suggests mycoplasma. Emerging antibiotic resistance should be considered in choice of empiric antibiotic therapy. There is emerging resistance of *S pneumoniae* to macrolides to erythromycin (eg, 56% resistance) and to penicillin (50% resistance). *M catarrhalis* organisms produce β-lactamase (90%), as do *H influenzae* organisms (~33–50%). Bluestone CE et al. Otitis Media in Infants and Children in *Microbiology*, 3rd ed. Saunders, 2001. Clin Pediatr 2002;41:373. [PMID: 12166789] Ear Nose Throat J 2002;81(8 Suppl 1):21. [PMID: 12199185] Pediatr Infect Dis J 2003;22:623. [PMID: 12867838] Pediatr Infect Dis J 2004;23:824. [PMID: 15361720] Am Fam Physician 2006;74:956. [PMID: 17002029] Clin Ther 2006;28:118. [PMID: 16490585]

EAR	
Otitis externa	

Otitis externa		
Acute localized: *S aureus* (15%) (GPC), anaerobes (32%), *S pyogenes* (GPC in chains), *H influenzae*, other gram-positive cocci. "Swimmer's ear": *Pseudomonas* sp. (40%) (GNR), Enterobacteriaceae (GNR), vibrio (GNR), fungi (6%) (eg, *Aspergillus* sp., *Candida* sp.). Chronic: Usually secondary to seborrhea or eczema. Diabetes mellitus. AIDS ("malignant otitis externa"): *P aeruginosa* (GNR), aspergillus, *Candida* sp. Furuncle of external canal: *S aureus*.	Ear drainage for Gram stain and bacterial culture, especially in malignant otitis externa. CT or MRI can aid in diagnosis by demonstrating cortical bone erosion or meningeal enhancement.	Infection of the external auditory canal is similar to infection of skin and soft tissue elsewhere. If malignant otitis externa is present, exclusion of associated osteomyelitis and surgical drainage may be required. Am Fam Physician 2006;74:956. [PMID: 17002029] Otolaryngol Head Neck Surg 2006;134(4 Suppl)S4. [PMID: 16638473]

	SINUS	
	Sinusitis	
Organism	**Specimen/Diagnostic Tests**	**Comments**
Sinusitis	Nasal aspirate for bacterial culture is not usually helpful due to respiratory flora contamination of aerobes and anaerobes. Maxillary sinus aspirate for bacterial culture may be helpful in severe or atypical cases.	Diagnosis and treatment of sinusitis is usually based on clinical and radiologic features. Microbiologic studies can be helpful in severe or atypical cases.
Acute: S pneumoniae (GPC) (20–43%), H influenzae (GNCB) (21–35%), M catarrhalis (GNDC) (2–10%), other streptococci (3–9%) (GPC), anaerobes (1–9%), viruses (4%) (adenovirus, influenza, parainfluenza), S aureus (GPC) (1–8%).		Sinus CT scan (or MRI) is better than plain x-ray for diagnosing sinusitis, particularly if sphenoid sinusitis is suspected. However, sinus CT scans should be interpreted cautiously, because abnormalities are also seen in patients with the common cold.
Chronic (child): Viridans and anaerobic streptococci (GPC in chains) (23%), S aureus (19%), S pneumoniae, H influenzae, M catarrhalis, P aeruginosa (GNR) in cystic fibrosis.		Acute and chronic sinusitis occur frequently in HIV-infected patients, may be recurrent or refractory, and may involve multiple sinuses (especially when the CD4 cell count is <200/mcL).
Chronic (adult): Coagulase-negative staphylococci (GPC) (36%), S aureus (GPC) (25%), viridans streptococci (GPC in chains) (8%), corynebacteria (GPR) (5%), anaerobes (6%), including Bacteroides sp., Prevotella sp. (GNR), peptostreptococcus (GPC), Fusobacterium sp. (GNR).		Acute sinusitis often results from bacterial superinfection following viral upper respiratory infection. Ann Otol Rhinol Laryngol 2002;111:1002. [PMID: 12450174]
Hospitalized with nasogastric tube or nasotracheal intubation: Enterobacteriaceae (GNR), Pseudomonas sp. (GNR).		Arch Otolaryngol Head Neck Surg Am Fam Physician 2004;70:1685. [PMID: 15554486] N Engl J Med 2004;351:902. [PMID: 15329428]
Fungal: Zygomycetes (rhizopus), aspergillus, P boydii, other dematiaceous mold.		
Immunocompromised: P aeruginosa (GNR), CMV, Aspergillus sp. and other filamentous fungi plus microsporidia, Cryptosporidium parvum, acanthamoeba in HIV-infected patients.		

UPPER AIRWAY		
Pharyngitis		

Pharyngitis

Exudative: *S pyogenes* (GPC) (15–30%), viruses (rhinovirus, coronavirus, adenovirus) (30%), group C and G streptococci (GPC) (5%), herpes simplex virus (HSV) (4%), parainfluenza and influenza virus A and B (2–4%), Epstein-Barr virus (mononucleosis) (1%), HIV (1%) *N gonorrhoeae* (GNDC) (1%), *C diphtheriae* (GPR) (≤1%), *Arcanobacterium hemolyticum* (GPR) (≤1%) *M pneumoniae*, *C pneumoniae*.
Membranous: *C diphtheriae* (GPR), *C pseudodiphtheriticum* (GPR), Epstein-Barr virus.

Throat swab for culture. Place in sterile tube or transport medium. If *N gonorrhoeae* suspected, use chocolate agar or Thayer-Martin media. If *C diphtheriae* suspected, use Tinsdale or blood agar. Throat swabs are routinely cultured for group A streptococcus only. If other organisms are suspected, this must be stated.
Throat culture has about 70–90% sensitivity and 95% specificity for group A streptococcus.
"Rapid" tests for group A streptococcus can speed diagnosis and aid in the treatment of family members. However, false-negative results may lead to underdiagnosis and failure to treat.

Controversy exists over how to evaluate patients with sore throat. Some authors suggest culturing all patients and then treating only those with positive cultures.
In patients with compatible histories, be sure to consider pharyngeal abscess or epiglottitis, both of which may be life-threatening. Complications include pharyngeal abscess and Lemierre syndrome (infection with *Fusobacterium* sp.), which can progress to sepsis and multi-organ failure.
J Clin Microbiol 2000;38:279. [PMID: 10618101]
Ann Intern Med 2001;134:506. [PMID: 11255529]
Clin Infect Dis 2002;35:113. [PMID: 12087516]
Am Fam Physician 2004;69:1465. [PMID: 15053411]

UPPER AIRWAY		
Laryngitis		
Organism	**Specimen/Diagnostic Tests**	**Comments**
Laryngitis Virus (90%) (influenza, rhinovirus, adenovirus, parainfluenza, Epstein-Barr virus), *S pyogenes* (GPC) (10%), *M catarrhalis* (GNDC), *H influenzae* (GNCB), *M tuberculosis*, fungus (cryptococcosis, histoplasmosis). Immunocompromised: *Candida* sp., CMV, HSV.	Diagnosis is made by clinical picture of upper respiratory infection with hoarseness.	Laryngitis usually occurs with common cold or influenzal syndromes. Fungal laryngeal infections occur most commonly in immunocompromised patients (AIDS, cancer, organ transplants, corticosteroid therapy, diabetes mellitus). Chronic laryngitis is associated with one or more chronic irritants such as gastric acid, chronic sinusitis, chronic alcohol use, inhaled toxins. J Laryngol Otol 2004;118:379. [PMID: 15165317] Int J Pediatr Otorhinolaryngol 2007;71:341. [PMID: 17126415]

UPPER AIRWAY		
Laryngotracheobronchitis		
Laryngotracheobronchitis Infant/child: RSV (50–75%) (bronchiolitis), adenovirus, parainfluenza virus (HPIV types 1, 2, 3) (15%) (croup), *B pertussis* (GNCB) (whooping cough), other viruses, including rhinovirus, coronavirus, influenza. Adolescent/adult: Usually viruses, *M pneumoniae*, *C pneumoniae*, *B pertussis*. Chronic adult: *S pneumoniae* (GPDC), *H influenzae* (GNCB), *M catarrhalis* (GNDC), klebsiella (GNR), other Enterobacteriaceae (GNR), viruses (eg, influenza), aspergillus (allergic bronchopulmonary aspergillosis). Chronic obstructive airway disease: Viral (25–50%), *S pneumoniae* (GPC), *H influenzae* (GNCB), *S aureus* (GPC), Enterobacteriaceae (GNR), anaerobes (<10%).	Nasopharyngeal aspirate for respiratory virus DFA, for viral culture (rarely indicated), and for PCR for *B pertussis*. PCR for pertussis is test of choice; culture and DFA are less sensitive. Cellular examination of early morning sputum will show many PMNs in chronic bronchitis. Sputum Gram stain and culture for ill adults. In chronic bronchitis, mixed flora are usually seen with oral flora or colonized *H influenzae* or *S pneumoniae* on culture. Paired sera for viral, mycoplasmal, and chlamydial titers can help make a diagnosis retrospectively in infants and children but are not clinically useful except for seriously ill patients.	Chronic bronchitis is diagnosed when sputum is coughed up on most days for at least 3 consecutive months for more than 2 successive years. Bacterial infections are usually secondary infections of initial viral or mycoplasma-induced inflammation. Airway endoscopy can aid in the diagnosis of bacterial tracheitis in children. Pediatr Infect Dis J 2000;19:893. [PMID: 11001119] Pediatr Infect Dis J 2002;21:76. [PMID: 11791108] Am Fam Physician 2004;69:535. [PMID: 14971835]

UPPER AIRWAY
Epiglottitis

Organism	Specimen/Diagnostic Tests	Comments
Epiglottitis Child: *H influenzae* type B (GNCB). *H parainfluenzae* (GCNB), *S pneumoniae* (GPC), *S aureus* (GPC), other streptococci (Groups A, B, C) Adult: *S pyogenes* (GPC), *S pneumoniae* (GPC), *Klebsiella* sp. (GNR), *H influenzae* (GNCB), *Pseudomonas* sp. (GNR), HSV, viruses (parainfluenza and influenza). HIV: Candida (fungi) and *Pseudomonas* sp. (GNR)	Blood for bacterial culture: positive in 50–100% of children with *H influenzae*. Lateral neck x-ray may show an enlarged epiglottis but has a low sensitivity (31%).	Acute epiglottitis is a rapidly moving cellulitis of the epiglottis and represents an airway emergency. Epiglottitis can be confused with croup, a viral infection of gradual onset that affects infants and causes inspiratory and expiratory stridor. Airway management is the primary concern, and an endotracheal tube should be placed or tracheostomy performed as soon as the diagnosis of epiglottitis is made in children. A tracheostomy set should be at the bedside for adults. Am J Otolaryngol 2001;22:268. [PMID: 11464324] Am J Otolaryngol 2003;24:374. [PMID: 14608569] Lancet 2003;361:39. [PMID: 12573380] Respir Care 2003;48:248. [PMID: 12667275]

LUNG

Community-acquired pneumonia

Community-acquired pneumonia

Neonate: *E coli* (GNR), group A or B streptococcus (GPC), *S aureus* (GPC), *Pseudomonas* sp (GNR), *C trachomatis*.

Infant/child (<5 years): Virus, *S pneumoniae* (GPC), *H influenzae* (GNCB), *S aureus*.

Age 5–40 years: Virus, *M pneumoniae, C pneumoniae* (formerly known as TWAR strain), *S aureus, C psittaci, S pneumoniae, Legionella* sp.

Age >40 without other disease: *S pneumoniae* (GPDC), *H influenzae* (GNCB), *S aureus* (GPC), *M catarrhalis* (GNDC), *C pneumoniae, Legionella* sp. (GNR), *C pseudodiphtheriticum* (GPR), *S pyogenes* (GPC), *K pneumoniae* (GNR), Enterobacteriaceae (GNR), *N meningitidis* (GNDC), viruses (eg. influenza).

Cystic fibrosis: *P aeruginosa* (GNR), *Burkholderia cepacia.*

Elderly: *S pneumoniae* (GPDC), *H influenzae* (GNCB), *S aureus* (GPC), Enterobacteriaceae (GNR), *M catarrhalis* (GNDC), group B streptococcus (GPC), legionella (GNR), nocardia (GPR), influenza.

Aspiration: *S pneumoniae* (GPDC), *K pneumoniae* (GNR), Enterobacteriaceae (GNR), *Bacteroides* sp. and other oral anaerobes.

Fungal: *H capsulatum, C immitis, B dermatitidis*

Exposure to birthing animals, sheep: *C burnetii* (Q fever), rabbits: *F tularensis* (tularemia), deer mice: hantavirus, birds: *C psittaci.*

Sputum for Gram stain desirable; culture, if empiric therapy fails or patient is seriously ill. An adequate specimen should have <10 epithelial cells and >25 PMNs per low-power field. Special sputum cultures for legionella are available. DFA for *Legionella* sp. has a sensitivity of 25–70% and a specificity of 95%. (Positive predictive value is low in areas of low disease prevalence.)

Blood for bacterial cultures (2 sets) obtain before antibiotic treatment, especially in ill patients.

Pleural fluid for bacterial culture if significant effusion is present.

Bronchoalveolar lavage or brushings for bacterial, fungal, and viral antigen tests and AFB culture in immunocompromised patients and atypical cases.

Paired sera for *M pneumoniae* complement fixation testing can diagnose infection retrospectively.

Serologic tests for *C pneumoniae, C psittaci* strains, and Q fever are available. Serologic tests and PCR for hantavirus (IgM and IgG) are available.

Other special techniques (bronchoscopy with telescoping plugged catheter or protected brush, transtracheal aspiration, transthoracic fine-needle aspiration, or, rarely, open-lung biopsy) can be used to obtain specimens for culture in severe cases, in immunocompromised patients, or in cases with negative conventional cultures and progression despite empiric antibiotic therapy.

PCR for *M pneumoniae*, legionella, and *C pneumoniae* are available.

About 60% of cases of community-acquired pneumonia have an identifiable microbial cause. Pneumatoceles suggest *S aureus* but are also associated with pneumococcus, group A streptococcus, *H influenzae*, and Enterobacteriaceae (in neonates).

An "atypical pneumonia" presentation (diffuse pattern on chest x-ray with lack of organisms on Gram stain of sputum) should raise suspicion of mycoplasma, legionella, or chlamydial infection. Consider hantavirus pulmonary syndrome if symptoms follow afebrile illness.

Aspirations are most commonly associated with stroke, alcoholism, drug abuse, sedation, and periodontal disease.

Am J Med 2001;111(Suppl 9A):4S. [PMID: 11755437]

Am J Respir Crit Care Med 2001;163:1703. [PMID: 11401897]

N Engl J Med 2002;347:2039. [PMID: 1240686]

Ann Intern Med 2003;138:109. [PMID: 12529093]

Clin Infect Dis 2003;37:1405. [PMID: 14614663]

Emerg Infect Dis 2006;12:958. [PMID: 16707052]

Organism	Specimen/Diagnostic Tests	Comments
LUNG		
Anaerobic pneumonia		
Anaerobic pneumonia/lung abscess Usually polymicrobial: *Bacteroides* sp. (15% *B fragilis*), *Peptostreptococcus prevotella* sp., *Porphyromonas* sp., *Fusobacterium* sp., microaerophilic streptococcus, veillonella, *S aureus*, *P aeruginosa* type 3 *S pneumoniae* (rare), klebsiella (rare), *H influenzae* type B, legionella, nocardia, actinomyces, fungi, parasites.	Sputum Gram stain and culture for anaerobes are of little value because of contaminating oral flora. Bronchoalveolar sampling (brush or aspirate) for Gram stain will usually make an accurate diagnosis. As contamination is likely with a bronchoscope alone, a Bartlett tube should be used. Percutaneous transthoracic needle aspiration may be useful for culture and for cytology to demonstrate coexistence of an underlying carcinoma. Blood cultures are usually negative (80%).	Aspiration is the most important background feature of lung abscess. Without clear-cut risk factors such as alcoholism, coma, or seizures, bronchoscopy is often performed to rule out neoplasm. N Engl J Med 2001;344:481. [PMID: 11172189] Thorax 2001;56:379. [PMID: 11312407]
Hospital-acquired pneumonia		
Hospital-acquired pneumonia *P aeruginosa* (GNR), klebsiella (GNR), *S aureus* (GPC), acinetobacter (GNR), Enterobacteriaceae (GNR), *S pneumoniae* (GPDC), *H influenzae* (GNCB), influenza virus, RSV, parainfluenza virus, adenovirus, legionella (GNR), oral anaerobes, *S maltophilia* (GNR), *B cepacia* (GNR). Mendelson syndrome (see Comments): No organisms initially, then pseudomonas, Enterobacteriaceae, *S aureus*, *S pneumoniae*.	Sputum Gram stain and culture for bacteria (aerobic and anaerobic) and fungus (if suspected). Blood cultures for bacteria are often negative (80%). Endotracheal aspirate or bronchoalveolar sample for bacterial and fungal culture in selected patients.	Most cases are related to aspiration. Hospital-acquired aspiration pneumonia is associated with intubation and the use of broad-spectrum antibiotics. A strong association between aspiration pneumonia and swallowing dysfunction is demonstrable by videofluoroscopy. Mendelson syndrome is due to acute aspiration of gastric contents (eg, during anesthesia or drowning). Hospital-acquired pneumonia is the second most common nosocomial infection, accounting for 25% of all ICU infections. Moreover, there has been a dramatic increase in multi-drug-resistant bacteria. Am J Respir Crit Care Med 2005;171:388. [PMID: 15699079] Chest 2005;128:3854. [PMID: 16354854] Clin Infect Dis 2005;41:848. [PMID: 16107985]

LUNG		
Pneumonia in immunocompromised host		
Pneumonia in the immunocompromised host Child with HIV infection: Lymphoid interstitial pneumonia (LIP). AIDS: *M avium* (31%), *P jiroveci* (13%), CMV (11%), *H capsulatum* (7%), *S pneumoniae* (GPDC), *H influenzae* (GNCB), *P aeruginosa* (GNR), Enterobacteriaceae (GNR), *C neoformans, C pseudodiphtheriticum* (GPR), *M tuberculosis* (AFB), other mycobacteria, *C immitis, P marneffei, Rhodococcus equi* (GPR). Neutropenic: *S aureus* (GPC), *Pseudomonas* sp. (GNR), klebsiella, enterobacter (GNR), *Bacteroides* sp. and other oral anaerobes, legionella, candida, aspergillus, mucor. Transplant recipients: CMV (60–70%), *P aeruginosa* (GNR), *S aureus* (GPC), *S pneumoniae* (GPDC), legionella (GNR), RSV, influenza virus, *P jiroveci,* aspergillus, *P boydii,* nocardia, strongyloides.	Expectorated sputum for Gram stain and bacterial culture, if purulent. Sputum induction or bronchiolar lavage for Giemsa or methenamine silver staining or DFA for *P carinii* trophozoites or cysts; for mycobacterial, fungal staining and culture, for legionella culture, and for CMV culture. Nasal washings or swab for viral respiratory direct fluorescent antibody (DFA) and viral culture. Urine for legionella and histoplasma antigen test. Blood for CMV antigenemia, human herpes virus-6 PCR or fungal galactomannan antigen test from transplant patients. Blood or bone marrow fungal culture for histoplasmosis (positive in 50%), coccidioidomycosis (positive in 30%). Blood cultures for bacteria. Blood cultures are more frequently positive in HIV-infected patients with bacterial pneumonia and often are the only source where a specific organism is identified; bacteremic patients have higher mortality rates. Histoplasma polysaccharide antigen positive in 90% of AIDS patients with disseminated histoplasmosis; antigen increases >2 RIA units with relapse. Immunodiffusion or CIE is useful for screening for, and CF for confirmation of, suspected histoplasmosis or coccidioidomycosis. Serum cryptococcal antigen when pulmonary cryptococcosis is suspected. Serum lactate dehydrogenase (LDH) levels are elevated in 63% and hypoxemia with exercise (Pao$_2$ <75 mm Hg) occurs in 57% of PCP cases.	In PCP, the sensitivities of the various diagnostic tests are: sputum induction 80% (in experienced labs), bronchoscopy with lavage 90–97%, transbronchial biopsy 94–97%. In PCP, chest x-ray may show interstitial (36%) or alveolar (25%) infiltrates or may be normal (39%), particularly if leukopenia is present. Recurrent episodes of bacterial pneumonia are common. Kaposi sarcoma of the lung is a common neoplastic process that can imitate infection in homosexual and African HIV-infected patients. Arch Intern Med 2001;161:2141. [PMID: 11570945] Crit Care Clin 2001;17:647. [PMID: 11525052] N Engl J Med 2001;344:481. [PMID: 11172189] Thorax 2001;56:379. [PMID: 11312407] Am Fam Physician 2005;72:1761. [PMID: 16300038]

	LUNG
	Mycobacterial pneumonia

Organism	Specimen/Diagnostic Tests	Comments
Mycobacterial pneumonia *M tuberculosis* (MTb, AFB, acid-fast beaded rods), *M kansasii, M avium–intracellulare* complex (MAC), other mycobacteria. (*M abscessus, M xenopi, M fortuitum, M chelonae*).	Sputum for AFB stain and culture. First morning samples are best, and at least three samples are required. Culture systems detect mycobacterial growth in as little as several days to 6 weeks. Bronchoalveolar lavage for AFB stain and culture or gastric washings for AFB culture can be used if sputum tests are negative. Sputum or bronchoalveolar lavage for PCR to MTb available for confirmation of smear positive (99%), less sensitive for smear negative (75%). Once AFB has been detected on solid media or in broth culture, nucleic acid probes or high-performance liquid chromatography can be used to identify the mycobacterial species. CT- or ultrasound-guided transthoracic fine-needle aspiration cytology can be used if clinical or radiographic features are nonspecific or if malignancy is suspected. Blood culture for MTb (15%). Pleural fluid culture for MTb (25%).	Acid-fast bacilli (AFB) found on sputum stain do not necessarily make the diagnosis of tuberculosis, because *M kansasii* and MAC look identical. Tuberculosis is very common in HIV-infected patients, in whom the chest x-ray appearance may be atypical and occasionally (4%) may mimic PCP (especially in patients with CD4 cell counts <200/mcL). Consider HIV testing if MTb is diagnosed. Delayed diagnosis of pulmonary tuberculosis is common (up to 20% of cases), especially among patients who are older or who do not have respiratory symptoms. In any patient with suspected tuberculosis, respiratory isolation is required. Am J Respir Crit Care Med 2000;161(4 part 1): 1376. [PMID: 10764337]Am J Med Sci 2001;321:49. Am J Med Sci 2001;321:49. [PMID:11202480] Lancet 2003;362:887. [PMID: 13678977]

LUNG	
Empyema	

Empyema

Neonate: *E coli* (GNR), group A or B streptococcus (GPC), *S aureus* (GPC), *Pseudomonas* sp (GNR).

Infant/child (<5 years): *S aureus* (60%) (GPC), *S pneumoniae* (27%) (GPC), *H influenzae* (GNCB), anaerobes.

Child (>5 years)/adult, acute: *S pneumoniae* (GPC), group A streptococcus (GPC), *S aureus* (GPC), *H influenzae* (GNCB), legionella, coagulase-negative staphylococci, viridans streptococci (GPC in chains).

Child (>5 years)/adult, chronic: Anaerobic streptococci, *Bacteroides* sp., *Prevotella* sp., *Porphyromonas* sp., *Fusobacterium* sp. (anaerobes 36–76%), Enterobacteriaceae, *E coli*, *Klebsiella pneumoniae*, *M tuberculosis*, *Actinomyces* sp.

Pleural fluid for cell count (WBCs 25,000–100,000/mcL, mostly PMNs), protein >50% of serum), glucose (<serum, often very low), pH (<7.20), LDH (>60% of serum). (See Pleural fluid profiles, Table 8–16))

Blood cultures for bacteria.

Sputum for Gram stain and bacterial culture. Special culture can also be performed for legionella when suspected.

Pleural fluid for Gram stain and bacterial culture (aerobic and anaerobic).

Chest tube drainage is paramount.

The clinical presentation of empyema is nonspecific.

Chest CT with contrast is helpful in demonstrating pleural fluid accumulations due to mediastinal or subdiaphragmatic processes and can identify loculated effusions, bronchopleural fistulae, and lung abscesses.

About 25% of cases result from trauma or surgery.

Bronchoscopy is indicated when the infection is unexplained. Occasionally, multiple thoracenteses may be needed to diagnose empyema.

N Engl J Med 2001;344:481. [PMID: 11172189]

Thorax 2001;56:379. [PMID: 11312407]

Pediatrics 2004;113:1735. [PMID: 15173499]

	HEART AND VESSELS
	Pericarditis

Organism	Specimen/Diagnostic Tests	Comments
Pericarditis Viruses: Enteroviruses (coxsackie, echo), influenza, Epstein-Barr, HZV, mumps, HIV, CMV, varicella, rubella, parvovirus, adenovirus, hepatitis. Bacteria: *S aureus* (GPC), *S pyogenes* (GPC), mycoplasma, *S pneumoniae* (GPC), Enterobacteriaceae (GNR), *N meningitidis* (GNDC), *N gonorrhoeae* (GDNC), *Haemophilus* sp. Fungi: *Candida* sp., histoplasma, aspergillus, coccidioides, blastomyces, nocardia, actinomyces (immunocompromised). Parasites: *Echinococcus*, amebiasis, toxoplasmosis	In acute pericarditis, specific bacterial diagnosis is made in only 19%. Pericardial fluid aspirate for Gram stain and bacterial culture (aerobic and anaerobic). In acute pericarditis, only 54% have pericardial effusions. Blood for buffy coat, stool or throat for enteroviral culture. PCR available in reference laboratories. Surgical pericardial drainage with biopsy of pericardium for culture (22%) and histologic examination. Paired sera for enterovirus (coxsackie) and mycoplasma.	Viral pericarditis is usually diagnosed clinically (precordial pain, muffled heart sounds, pericardial friction rub, cardiomegaly). The diagnosis is rarely aided by microbiologic tests. CT and MRI may demonstrate pericardial thickening. Bacterial pericarditis is usually secondary to surgery, immunosuppression (including HIV), esophageal rupture, endocarditis with ruptured ring abscess, extension from lung abscess, aspiration pneumonia or empyema, or sepsis with pericarditis. Curr Cardiol Resp 2002;4:13. [PMID: 11743917] Heart 2004;90:252. [PMID: 14966036] Lancet 2004;363:717. [PMID: 15001332] N Engl J Med 2004;351:2195. [PMID: 15548780] Postgrad Med 2004;115:67. [PMID: 15038256]

HEART AND VESSELS
Tuberculous Pericarditis

Tuberculous pericarditis

Mycobacterium tuberculosis (MTb, AFB, acid-fast beaded rods)

PPD skin testing should be performed (negative in a sizable minority).

Pericardial fluid obtained by needle aspiration can show AFB by smear (rare) or culture (low yield).

The yield is improved by obtaining three or four repeated specimens for smear and culture.

Pericardial biopsy for culture and histologic examination for granulomatous inflammation has highest diagnostic yield.

Pericardial fluid may show markedly elevated levels of adenosine deaminase.

Pericardial fluid for cell count, protein (elevated), PMN (elevated leukocytes, 700–5400/mL).

Spread from nearby caseous mediastinal lymph nodes or pleurisy is the most common route of infection. Acutely, serofibrinous pericardial effusion develops with substernal pain, fever, and friction rub. Tamponade may occur.

Tuberculosis accounts for 4% of cases of acute pericarditis, 7% of cases of cardiac tamponade, and 6% of cases of constrictive pericarditis.

One-third to one-half of patients develop constrictive pericarditis despite drug therapy. Constrictive pericarditis occurs 2–4 years after acute infection.

Clin Infect Dis 2001;33:954. [PMID: 11528565]

Chest 2002;122:900. [PMID: 12226030]

	HEART AND VESSELS
	Infectious myocarditis

Organism	Specimen/Diagnostic Tests	Comments
Infectious myocarditis Enteroviruses (especially coxsackie B), Epstein-Barr, adenovirus, influenza virus, HIV, CMV, *Borrelia burgdorferi* (Lyme disease), scrub typhus, *Rickettsia rickettsii* (Rocky Mountain spotted fever), *Coxiella burnetii* (Q fever), *Mycoplasma pneumoniae*, *Chlamydia pneumoniae*, *C diphtheriae* (GPR), *Trichinella spiralis* (trichinosis), *Trypanosoma cruzi* (Chagas disease), toxoplasma.	Endomyocardial biopsy for pathologic examination, PCR, and culture in selected cases. Indium-111 antimyosin antibody imaging is more sensitive than endomyocardial biopsy. Stool or throat swab for enterovirus culture. Blood for enterovirus PCR (reference labs) and culture of white cells. Paired sera for coxsackie B, *M pneumoniae, C pneumoniae,* scrub typhus, *R rickettsii, C burnetii,* trichinella, toxoplasma. Serum for HIV, *B burgdorferi, T cruzi.* Gallium scanning is sensitive but not specific for myocardial inflammation. Antimyosin antibody scintigraphy has a high specificity but a lower sensitivity for the detection of myocarditis.	Acute infectious myocarditis should be suspected in a patient with dynamically evolving changes in ECG, echocardiography, and serum CK levels and symptoms of an infection. The value of endomyocardial biopsy in such cases has not been established. In contrast, an endomyocardial biopsy is needed to diagnose lymphocytic inflammatory response with necrosis or giant cell myocarditis. The incidence of myocarditis in AIDS may be as high as 46%. Many patients with acute myocarditis progress to dilated cardiomyopathy. New Engl J Med 2000;343:1388. [PMID: 11070105] Circulation 2001;104:1076. [PMID: 11524405] Circulation 2002;106:1420. [PMID: 12221062]

HEART AND VESSELS
Infective endocarditis

Infective endocarditis		
S aureus (GPC), coagulase-negative staphylococci (GPC), viridans group streptococci (GPC in chains), enterococci (GPC), Abiotrophin sp., nutritionally deficient streptococci (GPC), S pneumoniae (GPC), other β-hemolytic streptococci (GPC), Erysipelothrix rhusiopathiae (GPR), brucella (GVCB), other gram-negative bacilli, yeast, Coxiella burnetii, C pneumoniae, bartonella. Slow-growing fastidious GNRs: HACEK (H parainfluenzae, H aphrophilus, Actinobacillus actinomycetemcomitans, Cardiobacterium hominis, Eikenella corrodens, Kingella kingae).	Blood cultures for bacteria are positive in 97%, if three sets are drawn at least 1 hour apart from peripheral vein and before start of antibiotic therapy. Blood cultures are frequently positive with gram-positive organisms but can be negative (5%) with gram-negative or anaerobic organisms, fungi, HACEK, and organisms that won't grow on artificial media. If the patient is not acutely ill, therapy can begin after cultures identify an organism. Transesophageal echocardiography (TEE) can help in diagnosis by demonstrating the presence of valvular vegetations (sensitivity >90%), prosthetic valve dysfunction, valvular regurgitation, secondary "jet" or "kissing" lesions, and paravalvular abscess. SPECT immunoscintigraphy with antigranulocyte antibody can be used in cases of suspected infective endocarditis if echocardiography is non-diagnostic.	Patients with congenital or valvular heart disease should receive prophylaxis before dental procedures or surgery of the upper respiratory, genitourinary, or gastrointestinal tract. In left-sided endocarditis, patients should be watched carefully for development of valvular regurgitation or ring abscess. The size and mobility of valvular vegetations on TEE can help to predict the risk of arterial embolization. Streptococci previously accounted for 60% of cases, but currently S aureus and coagulase-negative staphylococci ccount for 60% and 80–90% of tricuspid valve endocarditis. These staphylococci are methicillin-resistant strains (resistant to all β-lactam antibiotics). Arch Intern Med 2002;162:90. [PMID: 11784225] Clin Infect Dis 2003;36:615. [PMID: 12594643] Med (Baltimore) 2003;82:333. [PMID: 14530782] Circulation 2006;114:84. [PMID: 16880336] Curr Infect Dis Resp 2006;8:265. [PMID: 16822369]

HEART AND VESSELS

Prosthetic valve infective endocarditis

Organism	Specimen/Diagnostic Tests	Comments
Prosthetic valve infective endocarditis (PVE) Early (<2 months): coagulase-negative staphylococci (usually *S epidermidis* with 80%–87% methicillin-resistant) (GPC) (27%), *S aureus* (GPC) (20%), Enterobacteriaceae (GNR), enterococcus (GPC), diphtheroids (GPR), candida (yeast). Late (>2 months): viridans streptococci (GPC in chains) (42%), coagulase-negative staphylococci (22–30%), *S aureus* (11%), enterococcus (GPC), Enterobacteriaceae (GNR), HACEK group.	Blood cultures for bacteria and yeast are positive in 97%, if 3 sets are drawn at least 1 hour apart from peripheral vein and prior to start of antibiotic therapy. Although more invasive, TEE is superior in predicting which patients with infective endocarditis have perivalvular abscess or prosthetic valve dysfunction and which are most susceptible to systemic embolism.	In a large series using perioperative prophylaxis, the incidences of early and late-onset PVE were 0.78% and 1.1%, respectively. The portals of entry of early-onset PVE are intraoperative contamination and postoperative wound infections. The portals of entry of late-onset PVE appear to be the same as those of native valve endocarditis, and the microbiologic profiles are also similar. Clinically, patients with late-onset PVE resemble those with native valve disease. However, those with early-onset infection are often critically ill, more often have other complicating problems, are more likely to go into shock, and are more likely to have conduction abnormalities due to ring abscess. Arch Intern Med 2002;162:90. [PMID: 11784225] Clin Infect Dis 2003;36:615. [PMID: 12594643]. Curr Infect Dis Rep 2006;8:265. [PMID: 16822369]

HEART AND VESSELS
Infectious thrombophlebitis

Infectious thrombophlebitis

Associated with venous catheters: *S aureus* (GPC) (65–78%), coagulase-negative staphylococci (GPC), *Candida* sp. (yeast), *Pseudomonas* sp. (GNR), Enterobacteriaceae (GNR), streptococci (GPC), enterococci (GPC), CMV, anaerobes. Hyperalimentation with catheter: *Candida* sp., *Malassezia furfur* (yeast).

Indwelling venous catheter (eg, Broviac, Hickman, Gershorn): *S aureus*, coagulase-negative staphylococci, diphtheroids (GPR), *Pseudomonas* sp., Enterobacteriaceae, *Candida* sp.

Postpartum or postabortion pelvic thrombophlebitis: Bacteroides (GNR), Enterobacteriaceae, clostridium (GPR), streptococcus (GPC).

Blood cultures for bacteria are positive in 97%, if three sets are drawn at least 1 hour apart from peripheral vein and before start of antibiotic therapy. Catheter tip for bacterial culture to document etiology. More than 15 colonies (CFUs) suggests colonization or infection.

CT and MRI are the studies of choice in the evaluation of puerperal septic pelvic thrombophlebitis.

Thrombophlebitis is an inflammation of the vein wall. Infectious thrombophlebitis is associated with microbial invasion of the vessel and is associated with bacteremia and thrombosis.

Risk of infection from an indwelling peripheral venous catheter goes up significantly after 4 days.

Ann Intern Med 2001;134:409. [PMID: 11242501]

Arch Intern Med 2003;163:1657. [PMID: 12885680]

	ABDOMEN	
	Gastritis	**Infectious esophagitis**

Organism	Specimen/Diagnostic Tests	Comments
Gastritis *Helicobacter pylori*	Serum for antibody test (76–90% sensitivity but low specificity). Stool for antigen detection test (90%) and [¹³C] and [¹⁴C] urea breath test (99%) are specific noninvasive tests. Gastric mucosal biopsy for rapid urea test (90%), culture (89%), histology (92%), and PCR (99%) (reference laboratories).	Also associated with duodenal ulcer, gastric carcinoma, and gastroesophageal reflux disease. Proton pump inhibitors may cause false-negative urea breath tests and fecal antigen tests, and should be withheld for at least 7 days before testing. Aliment Pharmacol Ther 2002;16(Suppl 4)105. [PMID: 12030945] Arch Intern Med 2002;1361:1. [PMID: 11797613] Aliment Pharmacol Ther 2003;(Suppl 2):89. [PMID: 12786619] Curr Opin Infect Dis 2003;16:455. [PMID: 14501997]
Infectious esophagitis *Candida* sp. (yeast), HSV, CMV, VZV, *Helicobacter pylori* (GNR), cryptosporidium. (Rare causes: *M tuberculosis* [AFB], aspergillus, histoplasma, blastomyces, HIV).	Barium esophagram reveals abnormalities in the majority of cases of candidal esophagitis. Endoscopy with biopsy and brushings for culture and cytology has the highest diagnostic yield (57%) and should be performed if clinically indicated or if empiric antifungal therapy is unsuccessful.	Thrush (25%) and odynophagia (50%) in an immunocompromised patient warrants empiric therapy for candida. Factors predisposing to infectious esophagitis include HIV infection, exposure to radiation, cytotoxic chemotherapy, recent antibiotic therapy, corticosteroid therapy, and neutropenia. Am J Gastroenterol 2000;95(9):2171. Curr Treat Options Gastroenterol 2004;7:71. [PMID: 14723840]

ABDOMEN
Infectious colitis/dysentery

Infectious colitis/dysentery

Infant: *E coli* (enteropathogenic).

Child/adult without travel, afebrile, no gross blood or WBCs in stool: Rotavirus, caliciviruses (eg, Norwalk agent), *E coli* (GNR).

Child/adult with fever, bloody stool or history of travel to subtropics/tropics (varies with epidemiology): *Campylobacter jejuni* (GNR), *E coli* (GNR) (enterotoxigenic, enteroinvasive, enteropathogenic, enteroaggregative, diarrhea-associated hemolytic and cytolethal distending toxin-producing, enterohemorrhagic O157: H7), shigella (GNR), salmonella (GNR), *Yersinia enterocolitica* (GNR), *Clostridium difficile* (GPR), aeromonas (GNR), plesiomonas (GNR), vibrio (GNR), cryptosporidium, *Entamoeba histolytica*, *Giardia lamblia*, cyclospora, strongyloides, edwardsiella (GNR), anaerobes, histoplasma (fungi) (in HIV infection).

Child/adult with vomiting and no fever: *S aureus* (GPC), *Bacillus cereus* (GPR).

Stool for occult blood helpful in diagnosis of *E coli* /O157:H7, salmonella, shigella, campylobacter, and *E histolytica*.

Stool for culture and ova and parasites (3 specimens); the sensitivity of culture is 72%, but its specificity is 100%. Special stool culture techniques are needed for yersinia, *E coli* O157:H7, vibrio, aeromonas, plesiomonas, and *C difficile*.

Stool cultures for salmonella, shigella, and campylobacter are not helpful from patients who have been hospitalized for >3 days.

Specific examination for *C difficile* or its toxin is appropriate for patients who have been hospitalized for >3 days. *C difficile* produces two toxins: Toxin A is an enterotoxin and toxin B is a cytotoxin. Rapid EIA test for both toxin A and B has 80–90% sensitivity for 1 stool specimen, >90% sensitivity for 2 stool specimens. *C difficile* tissue culture assay has a high sensitivity (94–100%) and specificity (99%) and is the definitive test, but its turn-around time is >48 hours.

Immunodiagnosis of *G lamblia*, *E histolytica*, *Cryptosporidium parvum* cysts in stools is highly sensitive and specific.

Proctosigmoidoscopy is indicated in patients with chronic or recurrent diarrhea or in diarrhea of unknown cause for smears of aspirates and biopsy. Culture of a biopsy specimen has a slightly higher sensitivity than routine stool culture.

Obtain rectal and jejunal biopsies on HIV-infected patients; culture for bacterial pathogens and Mycobacteria (eg, MAC), and perform modified acid-fast stains for cryptosporidium, isospora, and cyclospora.

Acute dysentery is diarrhea with bloody, mucoid stools, tenesmus, and pain on defecation and implies an inflammatory invasion of the colonic mucosa. BUN and serum electrolytes may be indicated for supportive care. Severe dehydration is a medical emergency.

Necrotizing enterocolitis is a fulminant disease of premature newborns; cause is unknown, but human breast milk is protective. Air in the intestinal wall (pneumatosis intestinalis), in the portal venous system, or in the peritoneal cavity seen on plain x-ray can confirm diagnosis. 30–50% of these infants will have bacteremia or peritonitis. Risk factors for infectious colitis include poor hygiene and immune compromise (infancy, advanced age, corticosteroid or immunosuppressive therapy, HIV infection).

Gastroenterol Clin North Am 2001;96:766. [PMID: 11280548].

Gastroenterol Clin North Am 2002;97:1769. [PMID: 12135033]

N Engl J Med 2002;346:334. [PMID: 11821511]

	ABDOMEN
	Antibiotic-associated colitis

Organism	Specimen/Diagnostic Tests	Comments
Antibiotic-associated pseudomembranous colitis *Clostridium difficile* (GPR) toxin, *Clostridium perfringens* (GPR), *Staphylococcus aureus* (GPC), *Klebsiella oxytoca* (GNR), *Candida albicans* (yeast).	Send stool for *C difficile* cytotoxin B by tissue culture, but test takes >48 hours (sensitivity 90–100%, specificity 99%); or send stool for rapid EIA toxin A or toxin A and B, a less sensitive immunoassay, but test takes only 2–4 hours (sensitivity 70–90%, specificity 99%). Testing two stools on different days increases sensitivity; toxin testing for test-of-cure is not recommended. The toxin is very labile and can be present in infants with no disease. Fecal WBCs are present in 30–50% of cases. Stool culture is not recommended because nontoxigenic strains occur. Colonoscopy and visualization of characteristic 1–5 mm raised yellow plaques provides the most rapid diagnosis. However, an ultrasound appearance of grossly thickened bowel wall with luminal narrowing or CT findings of thickened bowel wall, presence of an "accordion" sign, heterogeneous contrast enhancement pattern ("target sign"), pericolonic stranding, ascites, pleural effusion, and subcutaneous edema can suggest the diagnosis of pseudomembranous colitis.	Antibiotics cause changes in normal intestinal flora, allowing overgrowth of *C difficile* and elaboration of toxin. Other risk factors for *C difficile*-induced colitis are GI manipulations, advanced age, female sex, inflammatory bowel disease, HIV, chemotherapy, and renal disease. *C difficile* nosocomial infection can be controlled by handwashing. Antibiotic-associated diarrhea may include uncomplicated diarrhea, colitis, or pseudomembranous colitis. Only 10–20% of cases are caused by infection with *C difficile*. Most clinically mild cases are due to functional disturbances of intestinal carbohydrate or bile acid metabolism, to allergic and toxic effects of antibiotics on intestinal mucosa, or to their pharmacologic effects on motility. Gastroenterol Clin North Am 2001;96:766. [PMID: 11280548] Arch Intern Med 2002;162:2177. [PMID: 12390059] Curr Gastroenterol Rep 2002;4:279. [PMID: 12149168] Gastroenterol Clin North Am 2002;97:1769. [PMID: 12135033] N Engl J Med 2002;346:334. [PMID: 11821511] Gastroenterol Clin North Am 2006;35:315. [PMID: 16680068]

ABDOMEN
Diarrhea in HIV

Diarrhea in the HIV-infected host Same as child-adult infectious colitis with addition of CMV, adenovirus, cryptosporidium, *Isospora belli*, microsporidia (*Enterocytozoon bieneusi* and *E intestinalis*), *C difficile*, *Giardia intestinalis*, MAC (AFB), HSV, *Entamoeba histolytica*, *Balantidium coli*, *Sarcocystis* sp.	Stool for stain for fecal leukocytes, culture (especially for salmonella, shigella, yersinia, and campylobacter), *C difficile* toxins (A and B by EIA), ova and parasite examination, and AFB smear. Multiple samples are often needed. Proctosigmoidoscopy with fluid aspiration and biopsy is indicated in patients with chronic or recurrent diarrhea or in diarrhea of unknown cause for smears of aspirates (may show organisms) and histologic examination and culture of tissue. Rectal and jejunal biopsies may be necessary, especially in patients with tenesmus or bloody stools. Need modified acid-fast stain for cryptosporidium, isospora, and cyclospora. Intranuclear inclusion bodies on histologic examination suggest CMV. Immunodiagnosis of giardia, cryptosporidium, and *E histolytica* cysts in stool is highly sensitive and specific.	Most patients with HIV infection will develop diarrhea at some point in their illness. Cryptosporidium causes a chronic debilitating diarrheal infection that rarely remits spontaneously and is still without effective treatment. Diarrhea seems to be the result of malabsorption and produces a cholera-like syndrome. Between 15% and 50% of HIV-infected patients with diarrhea have no identifiable pathogen. Curr Opin Infect Dis 2002;15:519. [PMID: 12686886] Curr Opin Infect Dis 2002;15:523. [PMID: 12686887] Gut 2003;52(Suppl 5):v1. [PMID: 12801941] Clin Infect Dis 2005;41:1621. [PMID: 16267735]

		ABDOMEN
		Peritonitis
Organism	**Specimen/Diagnostic Tests**	**Comments**
Peritonitis Primary or spontaneous (associated with nephrosis or cirrhosis) peritonitis (SBP): Enterobacteriaceae (GNR) (69%), enterococci (GPC), viridans streptococci (GPC in chains), *S pneumoniae* (GPC), group A streptococcus (GPC), *S aureus* (GPC), anaerobes (5%). Secondary (bowel perforation, hospital acquired, or antecedent antibiotic therapy): Enterobacteriaceae, enterococcus (GPC), *Bacteroides fragilis* group (GNR), *Pseudomonas aeruginosa* (GNR) (3–15%). Chronic ambulatory peritoneal dialysis (CAPD): Coagulase-negative staphylococci (GPC) (43%), *S aureus* (14%), *Streptococcus* sp (12%), Enterobacteriaceae (14%), *Pseudomonas aeruginosa, Corynebacterium* sp. (GPR), candida (2%), aspergillus (rare), cryptococcus (rare).	Peritoneal fluid sent for WBC >1000/mcL in SPB, >100/mcL in CAPD) with PMN (>250/mcL in SBP and secondary peritonitis, 50% PMN in CAPD); total protein (>1 g/dL); glucose (<50 mg/dL), and LDH (>225 units/mL) in secondary; pH (<7.35 in 57% of SBP). Gram stain (sensitivity 22–77% for SBP); submit large volumes of peritoneal fluid for bacterial culture. (See Ascitic fluid profiles, Table 8–5.) Blood cultures for bacteria positive in 85% of SBP cases. Catheter-related infection is associated with a WBC >500/mcL.	In nephrotic patients, Enterobacteriaceae and *S aureus* are most frequent. In cirrhotics, 69% of cases are due to Enterobacteriaceae. Cirrhotic patients (40%) with low ascitic fluid protein levels (≤1 g/dL) and high bilirubin level or low platelet count are at high risk of developing spontaneous bacterial peritonitis. "Bacterascites," a positive ascitic fluid culture without an elevated PMN count, is seen in 8% of cases of SBP and probably represents early infection. Neutrocytic ascites can have a negative culture in 10–30% of cases. In secondary peritonitis, factors influencing the incidence of postoperative complications and death include age, presence of certain concomitant diseases, site of origin of peritonitis, type of admission, and the ability of the surgeon to eliminate the source of infection (appendicitis [with or without rupture], diverticulitis, perforated ulcer, perforated gallbladder). J Hepatol 2000;32:142. [PMID: 10673079] Aliment Pharmacol Ther 2001;15:1851. Gastroenterology 2001;120:726. [PMID: 11179247] Am J Gastroenterol 2003;98:1675. [PMID: 12907318]

ABDOMEN

Tuberculous peritonitis/enterocolitis

Tuberculous peritonitis/enterocolitis

Mycobacterium tuberculosis (MTb, AFB, acid-fast beaded rods).

Ascitic fluid for appearance (clear, hemorrhagic or chylous), RBCs (can be high). WBCs (>1000/mcL, >70% lymphs), protein (>3.5 g/dL), serum/ascites albumin gradient (SAAG) (<1.1), LDH (>90 units/L). AFB culture (<50% positive). (See Ascitic fluid profiles, Table 8–5.) With coexistent chronic liver disease, protein level and SAAG are usually not helpful, but LDH >90 units/L is a useful predictor.

Culture or AFB smear from other sources (especially from respiratory tract) can help confirm diagnosis.

Abdominal ultrasound may demonstrate free or loculated intra-abdominal fluid, intra-abdominal abscess, ileocecal mass, and retroperitoneal lymphadenopathy. Ascites with fine, mobile septations shown by ultrasound and peritoneal and omental thickening detected by CT strongly suggest tuberculous peritonitis.

Marked elevations of serum CA 125 have been noted; levels decline to normal with antituberculous therapy.

Diagnosis of enterocolitis rests on biopsy of colonic lesions via endoscopy if pulmonary or other extrapulmonary infection cannot be documented.

Diagnosis is best confirmed by laparoscopy with peritoneal biopsy and culture.

Operative procedure may be needed to relieve obstruction or for diagnosis.

Infection of the intestines can occur anywhere along the GI tract but occurs most commonly in the ileocecal area or mesenteric lymph nodes. It often complicates pulmonary infection. Peritoneal infection usually is an extension of intestinal disease. Symptoms may be minimal even with extensive disease.

In the United States, 29% of patients with abdominal tuberculosis have a normal chest x-ray.

Presence of AFB in the feces does not correlate with intestinal involvement.

Clin Liver Dis 2000;4:151. [PMID: 11232182]
BMJ 2001;322:416. [PMID: 11179165]
Gastrointest Endosc Clin N Am 2001;11:79. [PMID: 11175976]
Am J Surg 2003;185:567. [PMID: 12781888]

	ABDOMEN
	Diverticulitis

Organism	Specimen/Diagnostic Tests	Comments
Diverticulitis Enterobacteriaceae (GNR), *Bacteroides* sp. (GNR), enterococcus (GPC in chains).	Identification of organism is not usually sought. Ultrasonography or flat and upright x-rays of abdomen are crucial to rule out perforation (free air under diaphragm) and to localize abscess (air-fluid collections). Barium enema can (82%) show presence of diverticula, but ultrasound (85%) and CT (79–98%) have greater accuracy in the evaluation of patients with diverticulitis.	Pain usually is localized to the left lower quadrant because the sigmoid and descending colon are the most common sites for diverticula. It is important to rule out other abdominal disease (eg, colon carcinoma, Crohn's disease, ischemic colitis, appendicitis), and gynecologic disorders (eg, ectopic pregnancy, ovarian cyst or torsion). Int Surg 2001;86:1991. Best Pract Res Clin Gastroenterol 2002;16:529. [PMID: 12406449] Br J Surg 2002;89:1137. [PMID: 12190679]

ABDOMEN
Liver abscess

Liver abscess Usually polymicrobial: Enterobacteriaceae, especially *E coli, Enterobacter* sp., *Proteus* sp., *Klebsiella* sp.(GNR), enterococcus (GPC in chains), *Bacteroides* sp. (GNR), actinomyces (GPR), *S aureus* (GPC) (MRSA), other streptococci (GPC), *Candida* sp., *Entamoeba histolytica*.	CT scan with contrast and ultrasonography are the most accurate tests for the diagnosis of liver abscess. Antibodies against *E histolytica* should be obtained on all patients (see Amebic serology, Chapter 3). Complete removal of abscess material obtained via surgery or percutaneous aspiration is recommended for culture and direct examination for *E histolytica*. *E histolytica* has a complex of two species: *E dispar* (commensal parasite) and *E histolytica* (pathogenic parasite). *E dispar* is 90% of the complex, is avirulent, and produces an asymptomatic carrier state. *E histolytica* is invasive of the intestinal wall, and it can be carried to the liver by the blood where it may develop abscesses. Stool for antigen detection has a sensitivity of 93% and specificity of 97%, and can distinguish the two species. Chest x-ray is often useful with raised hemidiaphragm, right pleural effusion, or right basilar atelectasis in 41% of patients. Elevation of serum alkaline phosphatase level in 78%.	Travel to and origin in an endemic area are important risk factors for amebic liver abscess. 60% of patients have a single lesion; 40% have multiple lesions. Biliary tract disease is the most common underlying disease, accounting for 40–60% of cases, followed by malignancy (biliary tract or pancreatic), colonic disease (diverticulitis), diabetes mellitus, liver disease, and alcoholism. *BMJ* 2001;322:537. *Clin Liver Dis* 2002;6:203. *Diagn Microbiol Infect Dis* 2003;46:245. [PMID: 12944014] *Hepatology: A Textbook of Liver Diseases,* 4th ed. Saunders 2003. *Lancet* 2003;361:1025. [PMID: 12660071] *N Engl J Med* 2003;348:1565. [PMID: 12700071]

ABDOMEN
Cholangitis/cholecystitis

Organism	Specimen/Diagnostic Tests	Comments
Cholangitis/cholecystitis Enterobacteriaceae (GNR) (68%), enterococcus (GPC in chains) (14%), *Pseudomonas aeruginosa* (GNR) (10%), bacteroides (GNR) (7%), *Clostridium* sp. (GPR) (7%), microsporidia (*Enterocytozoon bieneusi*) cryptosporidia, *Ascaris lumbricoides, Opisthorchis viverrini, O felineus, Clonorchis sinensis, Fasciola hepatica, Echinococcus granulosus, E multilocularis,* hepatitis C virus, hepatitis B virus, CMV.	Ultrasonography is the best test to quickly demonstrate gallstones or phlegmon around the gallbladder or dilation of the biliary tree. (See Abdominal Ultrasound, Chapter 6.) CT scanning is useful in cholangitis in detecting the site and cause of obstruction. (See Abdominal CT, Chapter 6.) Blood cultures for bacteria. WBC elevated (12,000–15,000 per mcL) Serum total bilirubin elevated (1–4 mg/dL). Serum for aminotransferase, alkaline phosphatase and amylase elevated.	90% of cases of acute cholecystitis are calculous, 10% are acalculous. Risk factors for acalculous disease include prolonged illness, fasting, hyperalimentation, HIV infection, and carcinoma of the gallbladder or bile ducts. Biliary obstruction and cholangitis can develop before biliary dilation is detected. Common bile duct obstruction secondary to tumor or pancreatitis seldom results in infection (0–15%). There is a high incidence of acalculous cholecystitis in AIDS patients with CD4 counts <200/mcL, due to cryptosporidium, CMV, yeast, tuberculosis, and *M avium-intracellulare.* J Clin Gastroenterol 2002;34:183. [PMID: 11782616] Am J Surg 2003;185:91. [PMID: 12559435] Gastroenterol Clin North Am 2003;32:1145. [PMID: 14696301] JAMA 2003;289:80. [PMID: 12503981] Rev Gastroenterol Disord 2003;3:187. [PMID: 14668691]

	GENITOURINARY	
	Urinary tract infection	**Prostatitis**
Urinary tract infection (UTI)/cystitis/pyuria-dysuria syndrome Enterobacteriaceae (GNR, especially *E coli* [80%]), *Chlamydia trachomatis*, *Staphylococcus saprophyticus* (GPC) (in young women), enterococci (GPC), group B streptococci (GPC), *Candida* sp. (yeast), *N gonorrhoeae* (GNCB), HSV, adenovirus, *Corynebacterium glucuronolyticum* (GPR), *Ureaplasma urealyticum* (GPR).	Urinalysis and culture reveal the two most important signs: bacteriuria and pyuria (>10 WBCs/mcL). 30% of patients have hematuria. Cystitis (95%) is diagnosed by >10² CFU/mL of bacteria; other urinary infections (90%) by >10⁵ CFU/mL. Culture is generally not necessary for uncomplicated cystitis in women. Combination of current symptoms (eg, dysuria, frequency, and hematuria) and prior history yields a >90% probability of UTI. However, pregnant women should be screened for asymptomatic bacteriuria and promptly treated. Both Gram stain for bacteria and dipstick analysis for nitrite and leukocyte esterase perform similarly in detecting UTI in children and are superior to microscopic analysis for pyuria. Nitrite or leukocyte esterase maybe negative in 19% of patients with bacteremia due to enterococci and staphylococci. DNA amplification tests for chlamydia and gonorrhea are available.	Most men with UTIs have a functional or anatomic genitourinary abnormality. In catheter-related UTI, cure is unlikely unless the catheter is removed. In asymptomatic catheter-related UTI, antibiotics should be given only if patients are at risk for sepsis (old age, underlying disease, diabetes mellitus, pregnancy). Up to one-third of cases of acute cystitis have "silent" upper tract involvement. Am J Med 2002;113(Suppl A):145. J Urol 2002;168:2351. [PMID: 12441917] BMJ 2003;327:1204. [PMID: 14630757] Dis Mon 2003;49:53. [PMID: 12601337] N Engl J Med 2003;349:259. [PMID: 12867610] Clin Infect Dis 2004;38:1150. [PMID: 15095222]
Prostatitis Acute and chronic: *E coli* (80%) (GNR), other Enterobacteriaceae (GNR), *Pseudomonas* sp. (GNR), enterococci (GPC in chains), CMV, *Staphylococcus* sp. (GPC), chlamydiae, mycoplasma, ureaplasma. HIV: *M tuberculosis*, *Candida* sp., coccidioides, cryptococcus, histoplasma.	Urinalysis shows pyuria, bacteriuria and hematuria (variable). Urine culture usually identifies causative organism. Prostatic massage is useful in chronic prostatitis to retrieve organisms but is contraindicated in acute prostatitis (it may cause bacteremia). Bacteriuria is first cleared by antibiotic treatment. Then urine cultures are obtained from first-void, bladder, and postprostatic massage urine specimens. A higher organism count in the postprostatic massage specimen localizes infection to the prostate (91%) (Meares-Stamey 3-glass test).	Acute prostatitis is a severe illness characterized by fever, dysuria, and a boggy or tender prostate. Chronic prostatitis often has no symptoms of dysuria or perineal discomfort and a normal prostate examination. Nonbacterial prostatitis (prostatodynia) represents 90% of prostatitis cases. Its etiology is unknown, although chlamydia antigen can be found in up to 25% of patients. Urology 2002;60(Suppl 6):14. [PMID: 12521581] Curr Urol Rep 2006;7:320. [PMID: 16930504] N Engl J Med 2006;355:1690. [PMID: 17050893]

	GENITOURINARY		
	Pyelonephritis		**Perinephric abscess**

Organism	Specimen/Diagnostic Tests	Comments
Pyelonephritis Acute, uncomplicated (usually young women): Enterobacteriaceae (especially *E coli*) (GNR), enterococci (GPC in chains), *S aureus* (GPC). Complicated (older women; men; postcatheterization, obstruction, post-renal transplant): Enterobacteriaceae (especially *E coli*), *Pseudomonas aeruginosa* (GNR), enterococcus (GPC), *Staphylococcus saprophyticus* (GPC), *S aureus* (GPC).	Urine culture is indicated when pyelonephritis is suspected. Urinalysis will usually show pyuria (>5 WBC/hpf) and may show WBC casts. Blood cultures for bacteria if sepsis is suspected. In uncomplicated pyelonephritis, ultrasonography is not necessary. In severe cases, however, ultrasound is the optimal procedure for ruling out urinary tract obstruction, pyonephrosis, and calculi. Doppler ultrasonography (88%) has a specificity of 100% for acute pyelonephritis.	Patients usually present with fever, chills, nausea, vomiting, and costovertebral angle tenderness. 20–30% of pregnant women with untreated bacteriuria develop pyelonephritis. Emerg Med Clin North Am 2001;19:655. [PMID: 1154280] Am J Med 2002;113(Suppl 1A):14S. [PMID: 12113867] J Clin Microbiol 2005;43:6064. [PMID: 16331100]
Perinephric abscess Associated with staphylococcal bacteremia: *S aureus* (GPC). Associated with pyelonephritis: Enterobacteriaceae (GNR), *Candida* sp. (yeast), coagulase-negative staphylococci (GPC).	CT scan with contrast is more sensitive than ultrasound in imaging abscess and confirming diagnosis. (See Abdominal CT, Chapter 6.) Urinalysis may be normal or may show pyuria. Urine culture (positive in 60–72%). Blood cultures for bacteria (positive in 20–40%). Bacterial culture of abscess fluid via needle aspiration or drainage (percutaneous or surgical).	Most perinephric abscesses are the result of extension of an ascending urinary tract infection. Often they are very difficult to diagnose. They should be considered in patients who fail to respond to antibiotic therapy, in patients with anatomic abnormalities of the urinary tract, and in patients with diabetes mellitus. J Urol 2002;168(4 Pt 1):1337. [PMID: 12352387]

GENITOURINARY		
	Urethritis	**Epididymitis/orchitis**
Urethritis (gonococcal and nongonococcal) Gonococcal (GC): *Neisseria gonorrhoeae* (GNDC). Nongonococcal (NGU): *Chlamydia trachomatis* (50%), *Ureaplasma urealyticum*, *Trichomonas vaginalis*, HSV, *Mycoplasma genitalium*, adenoviruses, *Gardnerella vaginalis*.	Urethral discharge collected with urethral swab usually shows >4 WBCs per oil-immersion field. Gram stain (identify gonococcal organisms as gram-negative intracellular diplococci), PMNs (in GC, >95% of WBCs are PMNs; in NGU usually <80% are PMNs). Urethral discharge for GC culture (80%) or ligase chain reaction (LCR) (>95%) (usually not needed for diagnosis); urine (90–95%) or urethral discharge (97%) for detection of *C trachomatis* by LCR amplification or wet mount for *T vaginalis*. Culture or nonamplified assays are considerably less sensitive for diagnosis of *C trachomatis*. VDRL should be checked in all patients because of high incidence of associated syphilis.	About 50% of patients with GC will have concomitant NGU infection. Always treat sexual partners. Recurrence may be secondary to failure to treat partners. Frequently, no pathogen can be isolated. Persistent or recurrent episodes with adequate treatment of patient and partners may warrant further evaluation for other causes (eg, prostatitis). Clin Infect Dis 2001;32:995. [PMID: 11264026] MMWR 2002;5(RR-6):1. [PMID: 12184549] Sex Transm Infect 2004;80:289. [PMID: 15295128] Am Fam Physician 2006;73:1411. [PMID: 16669564] Clin Infect Dis 2006;193:336. [PMID: 16388480]
Epididymitis/orchitis Age <35 years, homosexual men: *Chlamydia trachomatis*, *U urealyticum*, *E coli* (GNR), *Enterococcus faecalis* (GPC), *P aeruginosa* (GNR), brucella (GVCB). Age >35 years, or children: Enterobacteriaceae (especially *E coli*) (GNR), *Pseudomonas* sp. (GNR), salmonella (GNR), *Haemophilus influenzae* (GNCB), VZV, mumps. Immunosuppression: *H influenzae*, *Mycobacterium tuberculosis* (AFB), *Candida* sp. (yeast), CMV.	Urinalysis may reveal pyuria. Patients aged >35 years will often have midstream pyuria and scrotal edema. Culture urine and expressible urethral discharge when present. Prostatic secretions for Gram stain and bacterial culture are helpful in older patients. When testicular torsion is considered, Doppler ultrasound or radionuclide scan can be useful in diagnosis.	Testicular torsion is a surgical emergency that is often confused with orchitis or epididymitis. Sexual partners should be examined for signs of sexually transmitted diseases. In non–sexually transmitted disease, evaluation for underlying urinary tract infection or structural defect is recommended. BJU Int 2001;87:747. *Diseases of the Kidney*. Schrier RW ed. Lippincott Williams & Wilkins. 2001:1–17. J Androl 2002;23:453. [PMID: 12065446] Int J STD AIDS 2003;14:372. [PMID: 12816663] Rev Urol 2003;5:209. [PMID: 16985840]

	GENITOURINARY
	Vaginitis/vaginosis

Organism	Specimen/Diagnostic Tests	Comments
Vaginitis/vaginosis *Candida* sp. (yeast), *Trichomonas vaginalis*, *Gardnerella vaginalis* (GPR), bacteroides (non-*fragilis*) (GNR), mobiluncus (GPR), peptostreptococcus (GPC), *Mycoplasma hominis*, groups A and B streptococci (GPC), HSV.	Vaginal discharge for appearance (in candidiasis, area is pruritic with thick "cheesy" discharge: in trichomoniasis, copious foamy, yellow–green or discolored discharge), pH (about 4.5 for candida; 5.0–7.0 in trichomonas; 5.0–6.0 with bacterial), saline ("wet") preparation (motile organisms seen in trichomonas; cells covered with organisms—clue cells—in gardnerella; yeast and hyphae in candida, "fishy" odor on addition of KOH with gardnerella infection). Vaginal fluid pH as a screening test for bacterial vaginosis showed a sensitivity of 74.3%, but combined with clinical symptoms and signs its sensitivity increased to 81.3%. (See Vaginitis table, Table 8–27) Atrophic vaginitis is seen in postmenopausal patients, often with bleeding, scant discharge, and pH 6.0–7.0. Cultures for gardnerella are not useful and are not recommended. Culture for *T vaginalis* has greater sensitivity than wet mount. Culture for groups A and B streptococci and rare causes of bacterial vaginosis may be indicated. Gram stain of discharge is more reliable than wet mount for diagnosis of bacterial vaginosis (93% vs. 70%, respectively).	Bacterial vaginosis results from massive over-growth of anaerobic vaginal bacterial flora (especially gardnerella). Serious infectious sequelae associated with bacterial vaginosis include abscesses, endometritis and pelvic inflammatory disease. There is also a danger of miscarriage, premature rupture of the membranes, and premature labor. Am Fam Physician 2000;62:1095. [PMID: 10997533] Clin Infect Dis 2000;31:1225. [PMID: 11073756] MMWR Recomm Rep 2002;51(RR-6):1. [PMID: 12184549] Am Fam Physician 2004;70:2125. [PMID: 15606061]

GENITOURINARY

Cervicitis

Cervicitis, mucopurulent

Chlamydia trachomatis (50%), *N gonorrhoeae* (GNDC) (8%), HSV, *Mycoplasma genitalium.*

Cervical swab specimen for appearance (yellow or green purulent material), cell count (>10 WBCs per high-power oil immersion field and culture (58–80%) or nucleic acid assay (93%) for GC; urine for nucleic acid assay (93%) for GC; urine (80–92%) or cervical swab (97%) for detection of *C trachomatis* by nucleic acid amplification. Culture (52%) or nonamplified assays (50–80%) are considerably less sensitive for diagnosis of *C trachomatis.*

Because of the danger of false-positive amplified nucleic acid assays, culture is the preferred method in cases of suspected child abuse.

In one study of pregnant women, a wet mount preparation of endocervical secretions with <10 PMNs per high-power field had a negative predictive value of 99% for gonococcus-induced cervicitis and of 96% for *C trachomatis*-induced cervicitis. In family planning clinics, however, a mucopurulent discharge with >10 PMNs/hpf had a low positive predictive value of 29.2% for *C trachomatis*-related cervicitis.

Mucopurulent discharge may persist for 3 months or more even after appropriate therapy.

Am Fam Physician 2000;61:374. [PMID: 10670504]

Clin Infect Dis 2003;36:663. [PMID: 12594649]

J Infect Dis 2003;187:650. [PMID: 1599082]

Am J Obstet Gynecol 2004;190:1004.

J Infect Dis 2006;193:617.

GENITOURINARY

Salpingitis / Chorioamnionitis/endometritis

Organism	Specimen/Diagnostic Tests	Comments
Salpingitis/pelvic inflammatory disease (PID) Usually polymicrobial: *N gonorrhoeae* (GNDC), *Chlamydia trachomatis*, bacteroides, peptostreptococcus, *G vaginalis*, and other anaerobes; Enterobacteriaceae (GNR), streptococci (GPC in chains), *Mycoplasma hominis* (debatable).	Gram stain and culture or amplified nucleic acid assays of urethral or endocervical exudate. Ultrasonographic findings include thickened fluid-filled tubes, polycystic-like ovaries, and free pelvic fluid. MRI imaging findings for PID (95%) include fluid-filled tube, pyosalpinx, tubo-ovarian abscess, or polycystic-like ovaries and free fluid. Laparoscopy supplemented by microbiologic tests and fimbrial biopsy is the diagnostic standard for PID. Transvaginal ultrasonography (81%) has a lower specificity than MRI. Laparoscopy is the most specific test to confirm the diagnosis of PID. VDRL should be checked in all patients because of the high incidence of associated syphilis.	PID typically progresses from cervicitis to endometritis to salpingitis. PID is a sexually transmitted disease in some cases, not in others. All sexual partners should be examined. All IUDs should be removed. A strategy of identifying, testing, and treating women at increased risk for cervical chlamydial infection can lead to a reduced incidence of acute PID. All patients with diagnosis of acute PID should also be tested for HIV infection. Am J Obstet Gynecol 2001;184:856. Am J Obstet Gynecol 2002;186:929. [PMID: 12025517] Sex Transm Infect 2002;78:18. MMWR Recomm Rep 2005;51(RR-6):1. [PMID: 12184549] Am Fam Physician 2006;73:859. [PMID: 16629095]
Chorioamnionitis/endometritis Group B streptococcus (GPC), *E coli* (GNR), *Listeria monocytogenes* (GPR), *Mycoplasma hominis*, *M genitalium*, *Ureaplasma urealyticum*, *Gardnerella vaginalis*, enterococci (GPC), viridans streptococci (GPC in chains), *N gonorrhoeae* (GDNC) bacteroides (GNR), prevotella (GNR), and other anaerobic flora, *Chlamydia trachomatis*, group A streptococcus (GPC).	Amniotic fluid for Gram stain, leukocyte esterase, glucose levels <10–20 mg/dL, and aerobic and anaerobic culture; blood for culture (10–20%). Sonographic evaluation of fetus can be helpful, but findings are nonspecific.	Risk factors include bacterial vaginosis, preterm labor, duration of labor, parity, internal fetal monitoring. N Engl J Med 2001;345:266. [PMID: 11474666] Am J Obstet Gynecol 2002;186:690. Ann NY Acad Sci 2002;955:1. [PMID: 11949938] Clin Evid 2002;7:1654. [PMID: 12230778] Lancet 2002;359:765. Am Fam Physician 2006;73:859. [PMID: 16629095]

BONE		
Osteomyelitis		
Osteomyelitis *Staphylococcus aureus* (GPC) (60%). Infant: *S aureus*, Enterobacteriaceae (GNR), groups A and B streptococci (GPC). Child (<3 years): *H influenzae* (GNCB), *S aureus*, streptococci. Child (>3 years) to adult: *S aureus*, Group A streptococci, *Pseudomonas aeruginosa*. Postoperative: *S aureus*, Enterobacteriaceae, *Pseudomonas* sp (GNR), *Bartonella henselae* (GNR). Joint prosthesis: Coagulase-negative staphylococci, peptostreptococcus (GPC), *Propionibacterium acnes* (GPR), viridans streptococci (GPC in chains). Immunocompromised patients (eg, elderly, HIV-infected): *M tuberculosis*, *Candida* sp., cryptococcus, coccidiodes, histoplasma.	Blood cultures for bacteria are positive in about 60%. Cultures of percutaneous needle biopsy or open bone biopsy are needed if blood cultures are negative and osteomyelitis is suspected. Imaging with bone scan or gallium/indium scan (sensitivity 95%, specificity 60–97%) can localize areas of suspicion. Technetium methylene diphosphonate bone scan can suggest osteomyelitis days or weeks before plain bone films. Plain bone films are abnormal in acute cases after about 2 weeks of illness (33%). Indium-labeled WBC scan is useful in detecting abscesses. Ultrasound to detect subperiosteal abscesses and ultrasound-guided aspiration can assist in diagnosis and management of osteomyelitis. Ultrasound can differentiate acute osteomyelitis from vaso-occlusive crisis in patients with sickle cell disease. CT scan aids in detecting sequestra. When bone x-rays and scintigraphy are negative, MRI (98%) is useful for detecting early osteomyelitis (specificity 89%), in defining extent, and in distinguishing osteomyelitis from cellulitis. Myelography, CT, or MRI is indicated to rule out epidural abscess in vertebral osteomyelitis.	Hematogenous or contiguous infection (eg, infected prosthetic joint, chronic cutaneous ulcer) may lead to osteomyelitis in children (metaphyses of long bones) or adults (vertebrae, metaphyses of long bones). Hematogenous osteomyelitis in drug addicts occurs in unusual locations (vertebrae, clavicle, ribs). In infants, osteomyelitis is often associated with contiguous joint involvement. J Antimicrob Chemother 2002;50:805. [PMID: 12460997] Pediatr Infect Dis J 2002;21:432. [PMID: 12150182] Clin Infect Dis 2003;37:1481. [PMID: 14614671] JAMA 2003;290:2976. [PMID: 14665659] Rheum Dis Clin North Am 2003;29:89. [PMID: 12635502] J Pediatr Orthop 2005;14:362. [PMID: 16093948]

	JOINT	
	Bacterial/septic arthritis	
Organism	**Specimen/Diagnostic Tests**	**Comments**
Bacterial/septic arthritis Infant (<3 months); *S aureus* (GPC), Group A streptococci (GPC), Enterobacteriaceae (GNR), *Kingella kingae* (GNCB), *Haemophilus influenzae* (GNCB). Child (3 months to 6 years): *S aureus* (35%), *H influenzae*, group A streptococcus (GPC), Enterobacteriaceae (6%), *Borrelia burgdorferi* (Lyme) *S pneumoniae* (GPC), *K klingae*. Adult, STD not likely: *S aureus* (40%), group A streptococcus (27%), Enterobacteriaceae (23%), *Streptobacillus moniliformis* (GNR), brucella (GVCB), *Mycobacterium marinum* (AFB). Adult, STD likely: *N gonorrhoeae* (GNDC) (disseminated gonococcal infection [DGI]). Prosthetic joint, postoperative or following intraarticular injection: Coagulase-negative staphylococci (GPC in chains), enterococci (GPC), peptostreptococcus (GPC), *Propionibacterium acnes* (GPR), Enterobacteriaceae, *Pseudomonas* sp.	Joint aspiration (synovial) fluid for WBCs (in non-gonococcal infection, mean WBC is 100,000/mL), Gram stain (best on centrifuged concentrated specimen; positive in one-third of cases), culture (non gonococcal infection in adults [85–95%], DGI [25%]). (See Arthritis: Synovial fluid profiles, Chapter 8.) Yield of culture is greatest if 10 mL of synovial fluid is inoculated into a large volume of culture media, such as a blood culture bottle, within 1 hour after collection. Blood cultures for bacteria may be useful, especially in infants; nongonococcal infection in adults (50%); DGI (13%). *B burgdorferi* serology for Lyme disease. Genitourinary, throat, or rectal culture: DGI may be diagnosed by positive culture from a nonarticular source and by a compatible clinical picture. In difficult cases, MRI can help differentiate septic arthritis from transient synovitis.	It is important to obtain synovial fluid and blood for culture before starting antimicrobial treatment. Septic arthritis is usually hematogenously acquired. Prosthetic joint and diminished host defenses secondary to cancer, HIV, liver disease, or hypogammaglobulinemia are common predisposing factors. Nongonococcal bacterial arthritis is usually monarticular (and typically affects one knee joint). DGI is the most common cause of septic arthritis in urban centers and is usually polyarticular with associated tenosynovitis. Clin Microbiol Rev 2002;15:527. [PMID: 12364368] Med Clin North Am 2002;86:297. [PMID: 11982303] Best Pract Res Clin Rheumatol 2003;17:201. [PMID: 12787521] Curr Gastroenterol Rep 2003;5:379. [PMID: 12959718] Curr Rheumatol Rep 2003;5:205. [PMID: 12744812] Medicine (Baltimore) 2003;82:119. [PMID: 12640188] Infect Dis Clin North Am 2005;19:799. [PMID: 16297733]

MUSCLE
Gas gangrene

Gas gangrene		
Clostridium perfringens (GPR), (80–95%), other *Clostridium* sp.: *C ramosum, C bifermentans, C histolyticum, C septicum, C sordellii, C tertium.*	Diagnosis should be suspected in areas of devitalized tissue when gas is discovered by palpation (subcutaneous crepitation) or x-ray. Gram stain of foul-smelling, brown, or blood-tinged watery exudate can be diagnostic with gram-positive rods (can be gram variable) and a remarkable absence of neutrophils. Anaerobic culture of discharge is confirmatory.	Gas gangrene occurs in the setting of a contaminated wound. *C perfringens* produces potent exotoxins, including alpha toxin and theta toxin, which depresses myocardial contractility, induces shock, and causes direct vascular injury at the site of infection. Infections with enterobacteriaceae, other gram-negative rods, *S aureus*, streptococci, and mixed aerobic and anaerobic infections can also cause gas formation. These agents cause cellulitis rather than myonecrosis. Arch Intern Med 2002;162:517. [PMID: 11871919] Obstet Gynecol Surv 2002;57:53. [PMID: 11773832]

SKIN

Impetigo

Organism	Specimen/Diagnostic Tests	Comments
Impetigo Infant (impetigo neonatorum): Staphylococcus (GPC). Nonbullous or "vesicular": S pyogenes (GPC), S aureus (GPC), anaerobes. Bullous: S aureus.	Gram stain, culture, and smear for HSV and VZV antigen detection by DFA of scrapings from lesions may be useful in differentiating impetigo from other vesicular or pustular lesions (HSV, VZV, contact dermatitis). DFA smear can be performed by scraping the contents, base, and roof of vesicle and applying to glass slide. After fixing, the slide is stained with DFA for identification of HSV or VZV.	Impetigo neonatorum requires prompt treatment and protection of other infants (isolation). Polymicrobial aerobic-anaerobic infections are present in some patients. Patients with recurrent impetigo should have cultures of the anterior nares to exclude carriage of S aureus. Clin Microbiol Rev 2000;13:470. [PMID: 10885988] Pediatr Ann 2000;29:26. [PMID: 10941765] Curr Clin top Infect Dis 2002;22:42. [PMID: 12520646] Pediatr Infect Dis J 2003;22:389. [PMID: 12690285] Clin Infect Dis 2005;41:1373. [PMID: 16231249]

SKIN
Cellulitis

Cellulitis

Spontaneous, traumatic wound: Polymicrobial: *S aureus* (GPC), groups A, C, and G streptococci (GPC), enterococci (GPC), Enterobacteriaceae (GNR), *Clostridium perfringens* (GPR), *Clostridium tetani*, *Pseudomonas* sp. (GNR) (if water exposure).

Postoperative wound (not GI or GU): *S aureus*, group A streptococcus, Enterobacteriaceae, *Pseudomonas* sp.

Postoperative wound (GI or GU): Must add *Bacteroides* sp., anaerobes, enterococcus (GPC), groups B or C streptococci.

Diabetes mellitus: Polymicrobial: *S pyogenes*, enterococcus, *S aureus*, Enterobacteriaceae, anaerobes.

Bullous lesions, sea water contaminated abrasion, after raw seafood consumption: *Vibrio vulnificus* (GNR).

Vein graft donor site: Streptococcus.

Decubitus ulcers: Polymicrobial: *S aureus*, anaerobic streptococci, Enterobacteriaceae, *Pseudomonas* sp., *Bacteroides* sp.

Necrotizing fasciitis, type 1: streptococcus, anaerobes, Enterobacteriaceae; type 2: Group A streptococcus (hemolytic streptococcal gangrene).

Skin culture: In spontaneous cellulitis, isolation of the causative organism is difficult. In traumatic and postoperative wounds, Gram stain may allow rapid diagnosis of staphylococcal or clostridial infection. Culture of wound or abscess material after disinfection of the skin site will almost always yield the diagnosis.

MRI can aid in diagnosis of secondary abscess formation, necrotizing fasciitis, or pyomyositis. Frozen section of biopsy specimen may be useful.

Cellulitis has long been considered to be the result of an antecedent bacterial invasion with subsequent bacterial proliferation. However, the difficulty in isolating putative pathogens from cellulitic skin has cast doubt on this theory. Predisposing factors for cellulitis include diabetes mellitus, edema, peripheral vascular disease, venous insufficiency, leg ulcer or wound, tinea pedis, dry skin, obesity, and prior history of cellulitis.

Consider updating antitetanus prophylaxis for all wounds.

In the diabetic, and in postoperative and traumatic wounds, consider prompt surgical debridement for necrotizing fasciitis. With abscess formation, surgical drainage may be the mainstay of therapy and may be sufficient.

Hemolytic streptococcal gangrene may follow minor trauma and involves specific strains of streptococcus.

Ann Rev Med 2000;51:271 [PMID: 10774464]

Int J Antimicrob Agents [PMID: 10720800]

Am Fam Physician 2002;66:119.

J Antimicrob Chemother 2002;50:805. [PMID: 12460997]

	BLOOD
	Bacteremia of unknown source

Organism	Specimen/Diagnostic Tests	Comments
Bacteremia of unknown source Neonate (<4 days): Group B streptococcus (GPC), *E coli* (GNR), klebsiella (GNR), enterobacter (GNR), *S aureus* (GPC), coagulase-negative staphylococci (GPC), *Candida* sp. Neonate (>5 days): Add *H influenzae* (GNCB). Child (nonimmunocompromised): *H influenzae*, *S pneumoniae* (GPDC), *N meningitidis* (GNDC), *S aureus* (GPC), enterococci (GPC). Adult (IV drug use): *S aureus* or viridans streptococci (GPC in chains), enterococci (GPC). Adult (catheter-related, "line" sepsis): coagulase-negative staphylococci (30%), *S aureus* (12%), *Candida* sp. (11%), enterococci (9%), other streptococci (9%), *Klebsiella pneumoniae* (9%), *Enterobacter* sp. (4%), *Serratia* sp. (4%), *Pseudomonas* sp. (4%), *Acinetobacter baumanii* (1–4%), *Corynebacterium jelkeium* (1%), other yeast (1%). Adult (splenectomized): *S pneumoniae*, *H influenzae*, *N meningitidis*. Neutropenia (<500 PMN/mcL): Enterobacteriaceae, *Pseudomonas* sp., *S aureus*, coagulase-negative staphylococci, viridans streptococci (GPC in chains). Parasites: Babesia, ehrlichia, *Plasmodium* sp., filarial worms. Immunocompromised: *Bartonella* sp. (GNR), herpesvirus 8 (HHV8), *Mycobacterium avium-intracellulare* (AFB).	Blood cultures are mandatory for all patients with fever and no obvious source of infection. Often they are negative, especially in neonates. Cultures (3 sets) should be drawn 1 hour apart and before start of antibiotic therapy. Culture should be drawn from a peripheral vein by separate venipuncture, never from an IV line or from a femoral site. Culture and Gram stain of urine, wounds, and other potentially infected sites provide a more rapid diagnosis than blood cultures.	Occult bacteremia affects approximately 5% of febrile children ages 2–36 months. In infants, the findings of an elevated total WBC count (>15,000/mcL) and absolute neutrophil count (ANC >10,000/mcL) are equally sensitive in predicting bacteremia, but the ANC is more specific. Predisposing factors in adults include IV drug use, neutropenia, cancer, diabetes mellitus, venous catheterization, hemodialysis, and plasmapheresis. Catheter-related infection in patients with long-term venous access (Broviac, Hickman, etc) may be treated successfully without removal of the line, but recurrence of bacteremia is frequent. Switching needles during blood cultures does not decrease contamination rates and increases the risk of needle-stick injuries. N Engl J Med 2002;347:233. [PMID: 12140298] Clin Infect Dis 2003;37:557. [PMID: 12905141] Medicine (Baltimore) 2003;82:333. [PMID: 14530782] Clin Infect Dis 2004;39:309. [PMID: 15306996] N Engl J Med 2004;350:239. [PMID: 14724303] Arch Intern Med 2006;166:1289. [PMID: 16015111]

PART II. EMERGING (NEW) AND RE-EMERGING PATHOGENS/INFECTIOUS AGENTS[1]

Organism	Specimen/Diagnostic Tests	Comments
Avian Influenza A/H5N1 Influenza A virus subtype, H5N1, has greater virulence, easier (more efficient) human-to-human transmission, and resistance to antiviral drugs.	Sputum for bacterial culture. Blood and sputum for RT-PCR for influenza A/H5N1; RT-PCR testing is limted to state public health laboratories.	The first documented case of bird-to-human transmission occurred in 1997 in Hong Kong. The H5N1 virus is carried by birds that shed the virus in saliva, nasal secretions, and feces. Other birds/fowls are infected by fecal-oral transmission through contact with contaminated surface, feed, water, grout, etc. By 2006, almost every country in the world has reported at least one case of H5N1 influenza. Clinical symptoms and signs: mild-to-severe respiratory symptoms and fever. Emerg Infect Dis 2006;12:1650. [PMID: 16231249]
Human Metapneumovirus (huMPV) HuMPV is the causative agent of infant bronchiolitis in 5–15% of cases. There have been documented cases of co-infection with huMPV and RSV. From the family of Paramyxoviridae, the organism is a new metapneumovirus related to the turkey tracheitis virus. The first documented case of huMPV occurred in 2001 in the U.S.	Respiratory specimens for viral culture, and RT-PCR. Serum for antibodies is helpful, but not diagnostic.	huMPV is a respiratory pathogen that causes infections ranging from colds to severe bronchiolitis and pneumonia. Clinical symptoms and signs: 70–80% of infected individuals are asymptomatic, 20% have mild flulike symptoms, 6% have symptoms indistinguishable from RSV, bronchiolitis, croup, asthma, or pneumonia. J Infect Dis 2005;192:1061. [PMID: 16107960] J Clin Microbiol 2005;43:3443. [PMID: 16000473]

[1]Nearly 70% of emerging infectious disease outbreaks during the last 10 years have been zoonotic diseases transmitted from animals to humans. Controlling the diseases caused by new/re-emerging infectious agents is difficult owing to the diversity of geographic sources, potential for rapid global dissemination from the source, ecological and

social/economic influences.

Organism	Specimen/Diagnostic Tests	Comments
Human Monkeypox Monkeypox is in the Family of Orthopoxvirus, which is similar to smallpox (variola) virus. First documented case occurred in US in June, 2003. The infected humans had contact with prairie dogs that had been housed with infected Gambian giant rats from Ghana. This outbreak of 72 cases, involved patients in six states.	Respiratory samples submitted for viral culture. Blood and/or CSF samples for monkeypox virus DNA by PCR and for IgM antibodies by ELISA. Tissue samples for immunohistochemical testing or by demonstrating virus morphologically consistent with orthopoxvirus by electron microscopy.	History: Exposure to wild mammalian pet or exotic animal. Clinical symptoms and signs: Fever, chills or sweats, headaches, backache, sore throat, cough, shortness of breath, lymphadenopathy, rash (macular, papular, vesicular or pustular, generalized or localized, discrete or confluent), encephalitis. Mortality rate in Africa: approximately 10%, higher in immunocompromised patients. CDC Monkeypox Jan 2004:http://www.cdc.gov/ncidod/monkeypox J Infect Dis 2004;190:1833. [PMID: 15499541]
Severe Acute Respiratory Syndrome— Coronavirus A (SARS-CoA) First reported in Southern China in 2002; by mid 2003 over 8500 cases had been reported with nearly 800 deaths. Identified in 2003 as a Coronavirus; infection originates from wildlife (eg, civet cats and other mammals). Highly infectious, spread by close person-to-person contact.	Obtain CBC, activated PTT, serum liver tests, creatine phosphokinase (CPK), lactate dehydrogenase (LDH), chest radiograph, blood cultures, pleural fluid culture, sputum for bacterial culture and respiratory virus panel (influenzae A and B, and RSV). Respiratory sample, stool, plasma/serum may be sent to CDC for SAR-CoA RT-PCR assay. Blood or serum for SAR-CoA antibodies EIA assay performed by State Public Health laboratories. Lab abnormalities: normal or low WBC with decreased lymphocytes, prolonged activated PTT, increased transaminases, increased CPK, increased LDH.	Clinical symptoms and signs: Early symptoms include fever, chills, rigors, myalgia, and headaches. Respiratory symptoms appear 2–7 days after onset, with shortness of breath and/or dry cough; pneumonia in 60–100%. CDC SARS http://www.cdc.gov/ncidod/sars/ CDC: Public Health Guidance for Community-Level Preparedness and Response to SARS: May 3 2005:1. http://www.cdc.gov/ncidod/sars/guidance/

West Nile Virus (WNV) Although it first appeared in the US in 1999, within 5 years WNV had established itself as endemic in the US. Responsible agent is a single-strand RNA virus of the family Flavivirus. Its enzootic cycle involves several species of mosquitoes and birds before infecting humans; however, it is transmitted to humans from the bite of *Culex* species if mosquitoes. Incubation period of 2–14 days.	Serum, CSF, or tissue collected within 8 days of illness for IgM antibody ELISA; test performed by state public health laboratories.	Clinical symptoms and signs: 80% of infected individuals are asymptomatic, 20% have mild flulike symptoms: fever, headache, myalgias, skin rash and lymphadenopathy. In immunocompetent patients, illness is self-limited, lasting 3–6 days. Central nervous system infection (encephalitis or meningitis) develops in 1%, with change in mental status, movement disorders, and focal neurologic deficits. Gastrointestinal symptoms also occur. CDC Guidelines Aug 2003: Epidemic, epizootic West Nile Virus in USA. http://origin.cdc.gov/ncidod/dvbid/westnile/resources/wnvguidelines2003.pdf Pediatr Infect Dis J 2004;23:357. [PMID: 15071294] Curr Infect Dis Rep 2005;7:292. [PMID: 15963331] NIH: NIAID Research on West Nile Virus: April 2006. http://www.niaid.nih.gov/factsheets/westnile.htm
Mumps A virus from the family Paramyxovirus. Disease is spread by respiratory droplets; infectivity precedes the symptom by 1 day and may last a week. Incubation period is 14–21 days, average 18 days.	Buccal/oral swab for viral culture (gold standard) or mumps viral RNA by RT-PCR. Blood for serologic tests for serum mumps IgM antibody using EIA assay. Blood for serologic tests for serum mumps IgG antibodies in acute- and convalescent-phase using indirect EIA assay; fourfold rise in titer is considered diagnostic.	Clinical symptoms and signs: Acute onset of unilateral or bilateral, tender, self-limited swelling of the parotids (75%) or other salivary glands, lasting 2 or more days, without other apparent causes; fever, malaise, stiff neck, headaches. Complications include meningitis (30%), orchitis, pancreatitis, oophoritis, thyroiditis, neuritis, hepatitis, myocarditis, thrombocytopenia, arthralgias and nephritis. CDC: Laboratory Testing for Mump Infection http://www.dcd.gov/nip/diseases/mumps Am Fam Physician 2002;66:2113. [PMID: 12484693] MMWR Recomm Rep 2006;55(RR-16):1. [PMID: 17159833]

Organism	Specimen/Diagnostic Tests	Comments
Transmissible Spongiform Encephalopathy (TSE) Transmissible spongiform encephalopathy is a progressive, fatal, incurable, neurodegenerative prion disease occurring in both animals and humans. TSEs include bovine spongiform encephalopathy (BSE) in cattle; scrapie in sheep; chronic wasting disease in deer and elk; kuru in humans; Creutzfeldt-Jakob disease (CJD) in humans; and certain genetically determined or familial disorders (eg, fatal familial insomnia and Gerstmann-Straussler-Scheinker syndrome). There is the potential for BSE transmission to humans from eating infected meat or meat products. Another public health issue involves the potential transmission through blood transfusions or via corneal, dura mater, and other transplants.	Tissue from brain, spinal cord, eyes, tonsils, lymphoid tissue, spleen, pancreas, and nerves for immunohistochemical (IHC) analysis; and for conformation-dependent immunoassay (CDI), which is faster and uses specific antibodies that bind to all disease-causing prions in the brain.	Clinical symptoms and signs: rapidly progressive dementia, myoclonic fasciculations, ataxia, tremor, psychiatric symptoms. Lashley FR: *Emerging Infectious Diseases: Trends and Issues*, pp 43–71. Springer Publishing, 2002. Emerg Infect Dis 2004;10:977. [PMID: 15207045] Arch Neurol 2005;62:545. [PMID: 15824251] NIH News: Test could improve detection of prion disease in humans. Feb 2005. http://www.nih.gov/news/pr/feb2005/nia-14.htm NIH: NIAID research on prion diseases. May 2007. http://www.niaid.nih.gov/factsheets/priondis.htm

Lyme Disease	Serum for IgM antibodies by ELISA, needs confirmation by Western immunoblot (CDC recommendation).	Clinical symptoms and signs:
Causative agent is *Borrelia burgdorferi*. Found primarily in the Northeast, mid-Atlantic coastal, and north-central US. *Borrelia burgdorferi* is transmitted primarily by the deer tick (*Ixodes* species) after it has been attached to a host for more than 24 hours.		*Acute stage*: erythema migrans (expanding rash with area of central clearing) at the site of tick bite within 10 days; low-grade fever; headache; myalgia; arthralgia; and regional lymphadenopathy for 3–4 weeks. *Musculoskeletal symptoms*: asymmetric arthritis; may require 3–4 years to resolve (regardless of treatment). *Early neurologic involvement*: cranial neuritis, meningitis, and encephalitis. *Chronic neurologic disease*: subacute encephalophathy, axonal polyneuropathy, and leukoencephalopathy. NIAID: Tick-borne disease. March 2007. http://www.niaid.nih.gov/publications/tick.htm Emerg Infect Dis 2006;12:653. [PMID: 16704815]
Ehrlichiosis	Blood/serum for IgM or IgG antibodies by IFA or ELISA.	Clinical symptoms and signs: Illness is mild to fatal; most recover completely without treatment. Disease
Causative agents are *Ehrlichia chafeensis* and *E aqui*. Found primarily in North Atlantic states and South Central states of the U.S. Carried by various ticks: Dermacentor, *Ixodes* and *Amblyomma* species.	Blood/serum for ehrlichial DNA by PCR. CBC, liver tests. Blood abnormalities may include leukopenia, thrombocytopenia, and morulas (Ehrlichia bacteria in the cytoplasm of white blood cells). Increased transaminases.	can resemble Rocky Mountain spotted fever, lasting 1–2 weeks with rash (20%) (but not on palms and soles), fever, headache, chills, nausea, vomiting, anorexia, myalgias, cough, diarrhea, lymphadenopathy. Severe form includes blood and kidney abnormalities, respiratory failure, meningitis; may lead to human granulocytic ehrlichiosis (HGE) in which the organism parasitizes white blood cells, leading to toxic shock and death. NIAID: Tick-borne disease. March 2007. http://www.niaid.nih.gov/publications/tick.htm CDC: Human Ehrlichiosis in US. April 2000. http://www.cdc.gov/Ncidod/dvrd/ehrlichia/Index.htm

Organism	Specimen/Diagnostic Tests	Comments
Acinetobacter *Acinetobacter* species is a gram-negative rod, a nosocomial pathogen.	Stool or blood culture. Organism can survive for a long period of time in the environment and on the hands of health care workers.	Health care-associated infection caused by *Acinetobacter* has increased in the past decade where this strain has developed multi-drug resistance. In 2006, *Acinetobacter* was 92% susceptible to tigecycline in the U.S. Multi-drug-resistant strains are universally susceptible to the polymyxins (colestin, polymyxin B). Antimicrob Agents Chemother 2004;48:4479. [PMID: 15504889] Clin Infect Dis 2005;41:848. [PMID: 16107985] Emerg Infect Dis 2007;13:97. [PMID: 17370521]
Clostridium difficile *Clostridium difficile* is a gram-positive anaerobic rod. *C difficile* has been found in stool in 15–25% of patients with antibiotic-associated diarrhea, 10% of patients treated with antibiotics who do not have diarrhea, and in 95% of patients with diarrhea due to pseudomembranous colitis. DNA analysis yields over 100 types of *C difficile*. A new emerging type of *C difficile* is ribotype O27, also known as NAP-1, which produces 16–23 times more toxin A and B and is resistant to fluoroquinolones.	Stool for culture is the most sensitive test (89–100%), but 25% of isolates recovered are non-pathogenic and test takes 72 hours. *C difficile* produces 2 toxins: toxin A, which is an enterotoxin, and toxin B, which is a cytotoxin. Stool for cytotoxicity assay (toxin B) using cell cultures is considered the definitive test with 94–100% sensitivity and 90% specificity, but the test takes 48 hours. Stool for EIA testing for toxin A and B has 80–90% sensitivity for 1 sample, but sensitivity is >90% for multiple samples. Test takes only 2 hours. Flexible sigmoidoscopy may be performed in patients with severe symptomatology when a rapid diagnosis is needed; sensitivity is 51%.	Clinical symptoms and signs: watery diarrhea, fever, anorexia, and abdominal pain and tenderness. Diarrhea can be mild to severe. Severe diarrhea can lead to ulceration and bleeding from the colon (colitis) and to perforation of the intestine (peritonitis). N Engl J Med 2002;346:334. [PMID: 11821511] Best Pract Res Clin Gastroenterol 2003;17:775. [PMID: 14507587] CDC. July 2005: New strain of *C Difficile*. http://www.cdc.gov/ncidod/dhqp/id_CdiffFAQ_newstrain.html Cleve Clin J Med 2006;73:187 [PMID: 16478043] N Engl J Med 2005;353:2433. [PMID: 16322603] Clin Microbiol Infect 2006;12(Suppl 6):2. [PMID: 16965399]

Diarrheagenic Escherichia coli

Escherichia coli is a member of genus Escherichia within the family Enterobacteriaceae.

E coli can be characterized by shared liposaccharide (O) and flagellar (H) antigens that define serogroups (O antigen only) or serotypes (O and H antigens). More than 175 O antigens and 53 H antigens have been recognized, but only a few serotype combinations are associated with diarrheal diseases.

Stool culture, with special tests (see entries below). *E coli* has at least 6 different mechanisms by which to cause diarrhea, and each is associated with a different pathotype and different virulence determinants. The 6 pathotypes are Enteropathogenic *E coli* (**EPEC**), Enterohemorrhagic *E coli* (**EHEC**) (also known as Shiga toxin (Stx)-producing *E coli*, **STEC**), Enterotoxigenic *E coli* (**ETEC**), Enteroaggregative *E coli* (**EAEC**), Enteroinvasive *E coli* (**EIEC**), and diffusely adherent E coli (**DAEC**). Over 200 types of *E coli* are known to produce shiga toxins. Approximately 1% of stool samples tested in clinical laboratories contain (STEC) shiga toxins	The principal reservoir of EHEC/STEC is the intestinal tract of cattle and herbivorous animals (eg, sheep, deer, goats, birds). EHEC/STEC strains are most frequently identified as diarrheagenic *E coli* serotypes. Over 60 STEC serotypes are associated with human diseases. *E coli* O157:H7 is the most common STEC serotype. Clinical symptoms and signs: Diarrhea, dysentery (bloody diarrhea). CDC: *Escherichia coli* O157:H7. Dec 2006 http://www.cdc.gov/ncidod/dbmd/diseaseinfo/escherichiacoli_g.htm Donnenberg MS. Enterobacteriaceae. In: Mendel GL et al: *Principles and Practice of Infectious Diseases*, 6th ed. Elsevier Churchill Livingstone, 2005. Emerg Infect Dis 2003;9:1273. [PMID: 14609463] Emerg Infect Dis 2005;11:889. [PMID: 15963284] Proc Natl Acad Sci 2006;103:9667. [PMID: 16766659] Murray PR et al. *Manual of Clinical Microbiology*, 8th ed. ASM Press, 2003:162–181; 654–671; 286–330.

EIEC

Organism invades colonic epithelial cells, lyses the phagosome, multiplies intracellularly, and moves through the cell, exits and re-enters the basolateral plasma membrane. It is closely related to *Shigella* species genetically, biochemically and pathogenetically.

Stool for PCR or DNA probes for inv genes; test performed by state public health laboratories or research laboratories.	Clinical symptoms and signs: watery diarrhea, with a mechanism similar to shigella-related diarrhea and also related to induced apoptosis in infected macrophages; fever, abdominal cramps. Clinical symptoms and signs: mild to severe diarrhea.

Organism	Specimen/Diagnostic Tests	Comments
DAEC Organism elicits a characteristic diffuse aggregative pattern of adherence to HEP-2 cells.	Stool for tissue culture assay for diffuse adherence; test performed by state public health laboratories.	
ETEC Organism adheres to small bowel enterocytes and the enterotoxin causes mild to severe watery diarrhea. Produces two types of toxin: heat-labile (LT) or heat-stable (ST) toxins.	Stool for detection of toxin-producing *E coli*; test performed by state public health laboratories. Stool does not contain WBCs, mucus, or RBCs.	Clinical symptoms and signs: watery diarrhea, usually lasting 3–7 days, which can be prolonged or can relapse for months; abdominal cramps; occasional nausea; fever usually absent. Frequent cause of traveler's diarrhea.
EAEC Organism adheres to small and large bowel epithelial cells and expresses secretory enterotoxins and cytotoxins.	Stool for tissue culture adhesion assay; test performed by state public health laboratories. DNA and PCR tests lack sufficient sensitivity and specificity.	Clinical symptoms and signs: intestinal colic, bloody stool, and mucus. Persistent diarrhea in children. Chronic diarrhea in HIV-infected patients/immunocompromised patients. Correlated with interleukin-8 production.
EPEC Organism adheres to small bowel enterocytes and destroys the normal microvillar structure.	Stool for EPEC PCR or DNA probes and/or for tissue culture assay.	Clinical symptoms and signs: severe diarrhea, low-grade fever, vomiting. Prolonged diarrhea resulting in weight loss, malnutrition, and death. Infantile diarrhea, dehydration.

EHEC/STEC Organism colonizes enterocytes of the large bowel and causes a characteristic attaching and effacing pathology. It produces Shiga toxin (Stx) 1 or 2 which inhibits protein synthesis.	Stool for bacterial culture, special media for testing O157:H7. Stool for Shiga toxin by EIA.	Clinical symptoms and signs: frequently bloody diarrhea (although diarrhea without blood can occur), abdominal pain, vomiting, fever usually absent. Hemolytic uremic syndrome (HUS) develops in 10% and is more common in children. *E coli* O157:H7 EHEC/STEC causes 80% of cases of HUS. Among those with HUS, 30–50% have long-term kidney damage; 5–10% die.
Methicillin-resistant *Staphylococcus aureus* (MRSA) MRSA infections are divided into 3 categories by source: (1) nosocomial; (2) health care-associated (HA–MRSA) secondary to hospitalization, surgery, long-term care, dialysis, invasive device, etc; and (3) community-associated (CA-MRSA). Methicillin resistance is associated with the acquisition of the *mecA* gene.	Cultures of skin, soft tissue, blood. PCR-based specific molecular testing.	Clinical symptoms and signs: cellulitis, erysipelas, bacteremia. Clin Infect Dis 2005;40:562. [PMID: 15712079] N Engl J Med 2005;352:1485. [PMID: 15814886] Clin Infect Dis 2006;42:389. [PMID: 16392087] N Engl J Med 2006;355:666. [PMID: 16914702] Emerg Infect Dis 2007;13:236. [PMID: 16914702]

Organism	Specimen/Diagnostic Tests	Comments
Streptococcus pneumoniae, resistant	Cultures of sputum, blood, cerebrospinal fluid.	N Engl J Med 2006;354:1455. [PMID: 16598044]
Streptococcus pneumoniae is a gram-positive coccus that was generally susceptible to all classes of antimicrobial agents in the 1970's. With increased usage of antibiotics in patients with viral infections, *S pneumoniae* has acquired genetic material that encodes resistance to many commonly used antibiotics. It has developed resistance to β-lactamases (45%) at altered penicillin-binding protein sites, to macrolides (40%) at macrolide efflux pump (*mef* genes) and erythromycin-ribosomal methylases (*erm* genes) sites, to lincosamines (14%), to tetracycline, to folate-inhibitors (14–21%), and to fluoroquinolones (1–2%) with mutations in genes that code for DNA gyrase and to topoisomerase IV sites. Emergence of the multi-drug-resistant *S pneumoniae* serotype 19A is due in part to routine use of protein-conjugated pneumococcal vaccine in the US, since this serotype is not included in the vaccine.		
Vancomycin-resistant Enterococcus (VRE)	Cultures of stool, blood.	Clin Microbiol Rev 2000;13:686. [PMID: 11023964] Eur J Clin Microbiol Infect Dis 2005;24:808. [PMID: 15959813]
Emergence of VRE seen in both *E faecalis* and *E faecium* and at least 7 phenotypes (van A through van G). VRE implies intrinsic resistance to cephalosporins, aminoglycosides (ribosomally mediated), clindamycin (altered PBP5), trimethoprim-sulfamethoxazole. Enterococci that acquire the van A phenotype are highly resistant to vancomycin and to teicoplanin. Enterococci can also pass the van A gene cluster to *S aureus*.		

6

Diagnostic Imaging:
Test Selection and Interpretation

Benjamin M. Yeh, MD, and Susan D. Wall, MD

HOW TO USE THIS SECTION

Information in this chapter is arranged anatomically from superior to inferior. It would not be feasible to include all available imaging tests in one chapter in a book this size, but we have attempted to summarize the essential features of those examinations that are most frequently ordered in modern clinical practice or those that may be associated with difficulty or risk. Indications, advantages and disadvantages, contraindications, and patient preparation are presented. Costs of the studies are approximate and represent averages reported from several large medical centers.

$$\$ = <\$250$$
$$\$\$ = \$250–\$750$$
$$\$\$\$ = \$750–\$1000$$
$$\$\$\$\$ = >\$1000$$

RISKS OF CT AND ANGIOGRAPHIC INTRAVENOUS CONTRAST AGENTS

Although intravenous contrast is an important tool in radiology, it is not without substantial risks. Minor reactions (nausea, vomiting, hives) occur with an overall incidence between 1% and 12%. Major reactions (laryngeal edema, bronchospasm, cardiac arrest) occur in 0.16–1 cases per 1000 patients. Deaths have been reported in 1:40,000 to 1:170,000 cases. Patients with an allergic history (asthma, hay fever, allergy to foods or drugs) are at increased risk. A history of allergic-type reaction to contrast material is associated with an increased risk of a subsequent severe reaction. Prophylactic measures that may be required in such cases include corticosteroids and H_1 and H_2 blockers.

In addition, there is a risk of contrast-induced renal failure, which is usually mild and reversible. Persons at increased risk for potentially *irreversible* renal damage include patients with preexisting renal disease (particularly diabetics with borderline renal function), multiple myeloma, and severe hyperuricemia.

MRI INTRAVENOUS CONTRAST AGENTS

Contrast agents used in MRI are different from those used in most other radiology studies. Contrast-induced renal failure is not associated with MRI intravenous contrast and reactions are rare (minor reactions in approximately 0.066%; major reactions in 0.001%). Most MRI contrast agents are teratogenic and relatively contraindicated in pregnancy. Rarely, patients on dialysis develop fibrosing dermopathy after receiving MRI intravenous contrast.

In summary, intravenous contrast should be viewed in the same manner as other medications—that is, risks and benefits must be balanced before an examination using this pharmaceutical is ordered.

		HEAD	
		CT	**MRI**
Test	**Indications**	**Advantages**	**Disadvantages/Contraindications**	**Preparation**
HEAD **Computed tomography** (CT) $$$	Evaluation of acute craniofacial trauma, acute neurologic dysfunction (<72 hours) from suspected intracranial or subarachnoid hemorrhage. Further characterization of intracranial masses identified by MRI (presence or absence of calcium or involvement of the bony calvarium). Evaluation of sinus disease and temporal bone disease.	Rapid acquisition makes it the modality of choice for trauma. Superb spatial resolution. Superior to MRI in detection of hemorrhage within the first 24–48 hours.	Artifacts from bone may interfere with detection of disease at the skull base and in the posterior fossa. Generally limited to transaxial views. Direct coronal images of paranasal sinuses and temporal bones are routinely obtained if patient can lie prone. **Contraindications and risks:** Caution in pregnancy because of the potential harm of ionizing radiation to the fetus. See Risks of CT and Angiographic Intravenous Contrast Agents, p 295.	Normal hydration. Sedation of agitated patients. Recent serum creatinine determination if intravenous contrast is to be used.
HEAD **Magnetic resonance imaging** (MRI) $$$$	Evaluation of essentially all intracranial disease except those listed above for CT.	Provides excellent tissue contrast resolution, multiplanar capability. Can detect flowing blood and cryptic vascular malformations. Can detect demyelinating and dysmyelinating disease. No ionizing radiation.	Subject to motion artifacts. Inferior to CT in the setting of acute trauma because it is insensitive to acute hemorrhage, incompatible with traction devices, inferior in detection of bony injury and foreign bodies, and requires longer image acquisition time. Special instrumentation required for patients on life support. **Contraindications and risks:** Contraindicated in patients with cardiac pacemakers, intraocular metallic foreign bodies, intracranial aneurysm clips, cochlear implants, and some artificial heart valves.	Sedation of agitated patients. Screening CT or plain radiograph images of orbits if history suggests possible metallic foreign body in the eye.

Test	Indications	Advantages	Disadvantages/Contraindications	Preparation
BRAIN				
	MRA/MRV			**Brain scan**
BRAIN **Magnetic resonance angiography/venography (MRA/MRV)** $$$$	Evaluation of cerebral arteriovenous malformations, intracranial aneurysm, and blood supply of vascular tumors as aid to operative planning (MRA). Evaluation of dural sinus thrombosis (MRV).	No ionizing radiation. No iodinated contrast needed.	Subject to motion artifacts. Special instrumentation required for patients on life support. **Contraindications and risks:** Contraindicated in patients with cardiac pacemakers, intraocular metallic foreign bodies, intracranial aneurysm clips, cochlear implants, and some artificial heart valves.	Sedation of agitated patients. Screening CT or plain radiograph images of orbits if history suggests possible metallic foreign body in the eye.
BRAIN **Brain scan** (radionuclide) $$	Confirmation of brain death.	Confirmation of brain death not impeded by hypothermia or barbiturate coma. Can be portable.	Limited resolution. Delayed imaging required with some agents. Cannot be used alone to establish diagnosis of brain death. Must be used in combination with clinical examination or cerebral angiography to establish diagnosis. **Contraindications and risks:** Caution in pregnancy because of the potential harm of ionizing radiation to the fetus.	Premedicate with potassium perchlorate when using TcO_4 to block choroid plexus uptake.

BRAIN				
				Brain PET/SPECT / **Cisternography**
BRAIN **Positron emission tomography (PET)/single photon emission (SPECT)** brain scan $$$	Evaluation of suspected dementia. Evaluation of medically refractory seizures.	Provides functional information. Can localize seizure focus prior to surgical excision. Up to 82% positive predictive value for Alzheimer's dementia in appropriate clinical settings. Provides cross-sectional images and therefore improved lesion localization compared with planar imaging techniques.	Limited resolution compared with MRI and CT. Limited application in work-up of dementia due to low specificity of images and fact that test results do not alter clinical management. **Contraindications and risks:** Caution in pregnancy of potential harm of ionizing radiation to the fetus.	Sedation of agitated patients
BRAIN **Cisternography** (radionuclide) $$	Evaluation of hydrocephalus (particularly normal pressure), CSF rhinorrhea or otorrhea, and ventricular shunt patency.	Provides functional information. Can help distinguish normal pressure hydrocephalus from senile atrophy. Can detect CSF leaks.	Requires multiple delayed imaging sessions up to 48–72 hours after injection. **Contraindications and risks:** Caution in pregnancy because of the potential harm of ionizing radiation to the fetus.	Sedation of agitated patients. For suspected CSF leak, pack the patient's nose or ears with cotton pledgets prior to administration of dose. Must follow strict sterile precautions for intrathecal injection.

		NECK		
		MRI		**MRA**
Test	**Indications**	**Advantages**	**Disadvantages/Contraindications**	**Preparation**
NECK **Magnetic resonance imaging (MRI)** $$$$	Evaluation of the upper aerodigestive tract. Staging of neck masses. Differentiation of lymphadenopathy from blood vessels. Evaluation of head and neck malignancy, thyroid nodules, parathyroid adenoma, lymphadenopathy, retropharyngeal abscess, brachial plexopathy.	Provides excellent tissue contrast resolution. Tissue differentiation of malignancy or abscess from benign tumor often possible. Sagittal and coronal planar imaging possible. Multiplanar capability especially advantageous regarding brachial plexus. No iodinated contrast needed to distinguish lymphadenopathy from blood vessels.	Subject to motion artifacts, particularly those of carotid pulsation and swallowing. Special instrumentation required for patients on life support. **Contraindications and risks:** Contraindicated in patients with cardiac pacemakers, intracranial metallic foreign bodies, intracranial aneurysm clips, cochlear implants, and some artificial heart valves.	Sedation of agitated patients. Screening CT or plain radiograph images of orbits if history suggests possible metallic foreign body in the eye.
NECK **Magnetic resonance angiography (MRA)** $$$$	Evaluation of carotid bifurcation atherosclerosis, cervicocranial arterial dissection.	No ionizing radiation. No iodinated contrast needed. MRA of the carotid arteries can be a sufficient preoperative evaluation regarding critical stenosis when local expertise exists.	Subject to motion artifacts, particularly from carotid pulsation and swallowing. Special instrumentation required for patients on life support. **Contraindications and risks:** Contraindicated in patients with cardiac pacemakers, intracranial metallic foreign bodies, intracranial aneurysm clips, cochlear implants, and some artificial heart valves.	Sedation of agitated patients. Screening CT or plain radiograph images of orbits if history suggests possible metallic foreign body in the eye.

NECK				
NECK **Computed tomography (CT)** $$$	Evaluation of the upper aerodigestive tract. Staging of neck masses for patients who are not candidates for MRI. Evaluation of suspected abscess.	Rapid. Superb spatial resolution. Can guide percutaneous fine-needle aspiration of possible tumor or abscess.	Adequate intravenous contrast enhancement of vascular structures is mandatory for accurate interpretation. **Contraindications and risks:** See Risks of CT and Angiographic Intravenous Contrast Agents, p 295.	Normal hydration. Sedation of agitated patients. Recent serum creatinine determination.
NECK **Ultrasound (US)** $$	Patency and morphology of arteries and veins. Evaluation of thyroid and parathyroid. Guidance for percutaneous fine-needle aspiration biopsy of neck lesions.	Can detect and monitor atherosclerotic stenosis of carotid arteries non invasively and without iodinated contrast.	Technically demanding, operator-dependent. Patient must lie supine and still for 1 hour.	None.

Test	Indications	Advantages	Disadvantages/Contraindications	Preparation
THYROID			**THYROID**	
			Ultrasound	
THYROID	Determination whether a palpable nodule is a cyst or solid mass and whether multiple nodules are present. Assessment of response to suppressive therapy. Screening patients with a history of prior radiation to the head and neck. Guidance for biopsy.	Noninvasive. No ionizing radiation. Can be portable. Can image in all planes.	Cannot distinguish between benign and malignant lesions unless local invasion is demonstrated. Technique very operator-dependent. **Contraindications and risks:** None.	None.
Ultrasound (US)				
$$				

THYROID

Test	Clinical indications	Advantages	Comments (Contraindications and risks)	Preparation
THYROID — **Thyroid uptake and scan** (radionuclide) — $$	Uptake indicated for evaluation of clinical hypothyroidism, hyperthyroidism, thyroiditis, effects of thyroid-stimulating and -suppressing medications, and for calculation of therapeutic radiation dosage. Scanning indicated for above as well as evaluation of palpable nodules, mediastinal mass, and screening of patients with history of head and neck irradiation for thyroid cancer. Total body scanning used for postoperative evaluation of thyroid cancer metastases.	Demonstrates both morphology and function. Can identify ectopic thyroid tissue and "cold" nodules that have a greater risk of malignancy. Imaging of whole body with one dose (^{131}I).	Substances interfering with test include iodides in vitamins and medicines, antithyroid drugs, steroids, and intravascular contrast agents. Delayed imaging is required with iodides (^{123}I, 6 hours and 24 hours; ^{131}I total body, 72 hours). Test may not visualize thyroid gland in subacute thyroiditis. **Contraindications and risks:** Not advised in pregnancy because of the risk of ionizing radiation to the fetus (iodides cross placenta and concentrate in fetal thyroid). Significant radiation exposure occurs in total body scanning with ^{131}I; patients should be instructed about precautionary measures by nuclear medicine personnel.	Administration of dose after a 4- to 6-hour fast aids absorption. Discontinue all interfering substances prior to test, especially thyroid-suppressing medications: T_3 (1 week), T_4 (4–6 weeks), propylthiouracil (2 weeks).
THYROID — **Thyroid therapy** (radionuclide) — $$$	Hyperthyroidism and some thyroid carcinomas (papillary and follicular types are amenable to treatment, whereas medullary and anaplastic types are not).	Noninvasive alternative to surgery.	Rarely, radiation thyroiditis may occur 1–3 days after therapy. Hypothyroidism occurs commonly as a long-term complication. Higher doses that are required to treat thyroid carcinoma may result in pulmonary fibrosis. **Contraindications and risks:** Contraindicated in pregnancy and lactation. Contraindicated in patients with metastatic thyroid cancer to the brain, because treatment may result in brain edema and subsequent herniation, and in those <20 years of age with hyperthyroidism because of possible increased risk of thyroid cancer later in life. After treatment, a patient's activities are restricted to limit total exposure of any member of the general public until radiation level is ≤0.5 rem.	After treatment, patients must isolate all bodily secretions from household members. High doses for treatment of thyroid carcinoma may necessitate hospitalization.

The header labels appearing at the top: **THYROID** — **Thyroid uptake and scan** | **Radionuclide therapy**.

Test	Indications	Advantages	Disadvantages/Contraindications	Preparation
PARATHYROID				
Radionuclide scan				
PARATHYROID **Parathyroid scan** (radionuclide) $$	Evaluation of suspected parathyroid adenoma.	Identifies hyperfunctioning tissue, which is useful when planning surgery.	Small adenomas (<500 mg) may not be detected. **Contraindications and risks:** Caution in pregnancy is advised because of the risk of ionizing radiation to the fetus.	Requires strict patient immobility during scanning.

CHEST		
	Chest radiograph	**CT**
CHEST **Chest radiograph** $	Evaluation of pleural and parenchymal pulmonary disease, mediastinal disease, cardiogenic and noncardiogenic pulmonary edema, congenital and acquired cardiac disease. Screening for traumatic aortic rupture (though CT is playing an increasing role). Evaluation of possible pneumothorax (expiratory upright film) or pleural effusion	Inexpensive. Widely available.	Difficult to distinguish between causes of hilar and mediastinal enlargement (ie, vasculature versus adenopathy). **Contraindications and risks:** Caution in pregnancy because of the potential harm of ionizing radiation to the fetus.	None.
CHEST **Computed tomography (CT)** $$$	Evaluation of thoracic trauma. Evaluation of mediastinal and hilar tumor. Evaluation and staging of primary and metastatic lung neoplasm. Characterization of pulmonary nodules. Differentiation of parenchymal versus pleural process (ie, lung abscess versus empyema). Evaluation of interstitial lung disease (1-mm thin sections), aortic dissection, and aneurysm.	Rapid. Superb spatial resolution. Can guide percutaneous fine-needle aspiration of possible tumor or abscess.	Patient cooperation required for appropriate breath-holding. **Contraindications and risks:** Caution in pregnancy because of the potential harm of ionizing radiation to the fetus. See Risks of CT and Angiographic Intravenous Contrast Agents, p 295.	Preferably NPO for 2 hours before study. Normal hydration. Sedation of agitated patients. Recent serum creatinine determination.

	CHEST	
	MRI	**PET/CT**

Test	Indications	Advantages	Disadvantages/Contraindications	Preparation
CHEST **Magnetic resonance imaging (MRI)** $$$$	Evaluation of mediastinal masses. Discrimination between hilar vessels and enlarged lymph nodes. Tumor staging (especially when invasion of vessels or pericardium is suspected). Evaluation of aortic dissection, aortic aneurysm, congenital and acquired cardiac disease.	Provides excellent tissue contrast resolution and multiplanar capability. No ionizing radiation.	Subject to motion artifacts. **Contraindications and risks:** Contraindicated in patients with cardiac pacemakers, intraocular metallic foreign bodies, intracranial aneurysm clips, cochlear implants, and some artificial heart valves.	Sedation of agitated patients. Screening CT of the orbits if history suggests possible metallic foreign body in the eye.
CHEST **Positron emission tomography/Computed tomography (PET/CT)** $$$$	Evaluation for mediastinal masses and metastases. Discrimination between benign and malignant lymph nodes. Tumor staging.	Combines metabolic and anatomic information. Large area of coverage (can image whole body)	Patient cooperation required for appropriate breath-holding. **Contraindications and risks:** Contraindicated in pregnancy because of the potential harm of ionizing radiation to the fetus. See Risks of CT and Angiographic Intravenous Contrast Agents, p 295.	Preferably NPO for 2 hours prior to study. Normal hydration. Sedation of agitated patients. Recent serum creatinine determination.

LUNG				
Ventilation-perfusion scan			**CT**	

	Indications	Comments	Contraindications	Preparation
LUNG **Ventilation-perfusion scan** (radionuclide) $\dot{V} = \$\$$ $\dot{Q} = \$\$$ $\dot{V} + \dot{Q} =$ $\$\$\$-\$\$\$\$$	Evaluation of pulmonary embolism or burn inhalation injury. Preoperative evaluation of patients with chronic obstructive pulmonary disease and of those who are candidates for pneumonectomy.	Noninvasive. Provides functional information in preoperative assessment. Permits determination of differential and regional lung function in preoperative assessment. Documented pulmonary embolism is extremely rare with normal perfusion scan.	Patients must be able to cooperate for ventilation portion of the examination. There is a high proportion of intermediate probability studies in patients with underlying lung disease. The likelihood of pulmonary embolism ranges from 20%–80% in these cases. A patient who has a low probability scan still has a chance ranging from nil to 19% of having a pulmonary embolus. **Contraindications and risks:** Patients with severe pulmonary artery hypertension or significant right-to-left shunts should have fewer particles injected. Caution advised in pregnancy because of risk of ionizing radiation to the fetus.	Current chest radiograph is mandatory for interpretation.
LUNG **Computed tomography (CT)** $\$\$\$$	Evaluation of clinically suspected pulmonary embolism.	Rapid. High sensitivity and specificity for clinically relevant pulmonary emboli. Allows determination of causes other than pulmonary embolism for dyspnea. Evaluation of pulmonary vein anatomy before electrophysiology ablation.	Respiratory motion artifacts can be a problem in dyspneic patients and older CT scanners. High-quality study requires breath-holding of approximately 10–20 seconds. Specific imaging protocol utilized which limits diagnostic information for other abnormalities. **Contraindications and risks:** Caution in pregnancy because of potential harm of ionizing radiation to fetus. See Risks of CT and Angiographic Intravenous Contrast Agents, p 295.	Large gauge intravenous access (minimum 20-gauge) required. Prebreathing oxygen may help dyspneic patients perform adequate breath hold. Normal hydration. Preferably NPO for 2 hours prior to study. Recent serum creatinine determination.

Test	Indications	Advantages	Disadvantages/Contraindications	Preparation
BREAST				
Mammogram				
			BREAST	
			Mammogram	
Mammogram $	Screening for breast cancer in asymptomatic women: (1) every 1–2 years between ages 40 and 49; (2) every year after age 50. If prior history of breast cancer, mammogram should be performed yearly at any age. Indicated at any age for symptoms (palpable mass, bloody discharge) or before breast surgery.	Newer digital and film screen techniques generate lower radiation doses (0.1–0.2 rad per film, mean glandular dose). A 23% lower mortality has been demonstrated in patients screened with combined mammogram and physical examination compared with physical examination alone. In a screening population, more than 40% of cancers are detected by mammography alone and cannot be palpated on physical examination.	Detection of breast masses is more difficult in patients with radiographically dense breasts. Breast compression may cause patient discomfort. In a screening population, 9% of cancers are detected by physical examination alone and are not detectable by mammography. **Contraindications and risks:** Radiation from repeated mammograms can theoretically cause breast cancer; however, the benefits of screening mammograms greatly outweigh the risks.	None.

HEART			
Myocardial perfusion scan			
HEART **Myocardial perfusion scan** (thallium scan, technetium-99m methoxy-isobutyl isonitrile (sestamibi) scan, others) $-$$-$$$ (broad range)	Evaluation of atypical chest pain. Detection of presence, location, and extent of myocardial ischemia.	Highly sensitive for detecting physiologically significant coronary stenosis. Noninvasive. Able to stratify patients according to risk for myocardial infarction. Normal examination associated with average risk of cardiac death or nonfatal myocardial infarction of <1% per year.	The patient must be carefully monitored during treadmill or pharmacologic stress—optimally, under the supervision of a cardiologist. False-positive results may be caused by exercise-induced spasm, aortic stenosis, or left bundle branch block; false-negative results may be caused by inadequate exercise, mild or distal disease, or balanced diffuse ischemia. **Contraindications and risks:** Aminophylline (inhibitor of dipyridamole) is a contraindication to the use of dipyridamole. Treadmill or pharmacologic stress carries a risk of arrhythmia, ischemia, infarct, and, rarely, death. Caution in pregnancy because of the risk of ionizing radiation to the fetus.	In case of severe peripheral vascular disease, severe pulmonary disease, or musculoskeletal disorder, pharmacologic stress with dipyridamole or other agents may be used. Tests should be performed in the fasting state. Patient should not exercise between stress and redistribution scans.

		HEART	
		CT Coronary artery calcium scoring/angiography	**Ventriculography**
Preparation		May require medication with β-blocker to decrease heart rate.	Requires harvesting, labeling, and reinjecting the patient's red blood cells. Sterile technique required in handling of red cells.
Disadvantages/Contraindications		Gated data acquisition may be difficult in patients with severe arrhythmias or rapid heart rate. If high calcium score or coronary artery stenosis is found, patient may need to undergo coronary artery angioplasty or bypass grafting for treatment. **Contraindications and risks:** Caution in pregnancy because of potential harm of ionizing radiation to fetus. See Risks of CT and Angiographic Intravenous Contrast Agents, p 295.	Gated data acquisition may be difficult in patients with severe arrhythmias. **Contraindications and risks:** Recent infarct is a contraindication to exercise ventriculography (arrhythmia, ischemia, infarct, and rarely death may occur with exercise). Caution is advised in pregnancy because of the risk of ionizing radiation to the fetus.
Advantages		Noninvasive. Higher coronary artery calcium score correlates with high risk for significant coronary artery stenosis.	Noninvasive. Ejection fraction is a reproducible index that can be used to follow course of disease and response to therapy.
Indications		Screening evaluation for coronary artery calcification.	Evaluation of patients with ischemic heart disease and other cardiomyopathies. Evaluation of response to pharmacologic therapy and effects of cardiotoxic drugs.
Test		HEART **Computed tomography coronary artery calcium scoring/ angiography** $$-$$$	HEART **Radionuclide ventriculography** (multigated acquisition [MUGA]) $$-$$$-$$$$

ABDOMEN		
	KUB	**Ultrasound**

Imaging Study	Indications	Advantages	Comments / Contraindications	Preparation
ABDOMEN **Abdominal plain radiograph** (KUB [kidneys, ureters, bladder] x-ray) $	Assessment of bowel gas patterns (eg, to distinguish ileus from obstruction). To rule out pneumoperitoneum, order an upright abdomen and chest radiograph (acute abdominal series).	Inexpensive. Widely available.	Supine film alone is inadequate to rule out pneumoperitoneum (see Indications). Obstipation may obscure lesions. **Contraindications and risks:** Contraindicated in pregnancy because of the risk of ionizing radiation to the fetus.	None.
ABDOMEN **Ultrasound** (US) $$	Differentiation of cystic versus solid lesions of the liver and kidneys. Detection of intra- and extrahepatic biliary ductal dilation, cholelithiasis, gallbladder wall thickness, pericholecystic fluid, peripancreatic fluid and pseudocyst, hydronephrosis, abdominal aortic aneurysm, appendicitis, ascites, primary and metastatic liver carcinoma.	Noninvasive. No ionizing radiation. Can be portable. Imaging in all planes. Can guide percutaneous fine-needle aspiration of tumor or abscess.	Technique very operator-dependent. Organs (particularly pancreas and distal aorta) may be obscured by bowel gas. **Contraindications and risks:** None.	NPO for 6 hours.

	ABDOMEN
	CT

Test	Indications	Advantages	Disadvantages/Contraindications	Preparation
ABDOMEN **Computed tomography (CT)** $$$–$$$$	Morphologic evaluation of all abdominal and pelvic organs. Evaluation of abscess, trauma, mesenteric and retroperitoneal lymphadenopathy, bowel obstruction, obstructive biliary disease, pancreatitis, appendicitis, peritonitis, visceral infarction, and retroperitoneal hemorrhage. Staging and monitoring of malignancy in the liver, pancreas, kidneys, and other abdominopelvic organs and spaces. Determination of tumor resectability. Excellent screening tool for evaluation of suspected renal and ureteral stones or other cause of upper urinary tract bleeding. CT angiography evaluates the aorta and its branches. Can provide preoperative assessment of abdominal aortic aneurysm and dissection size, proximal and distal extent, relationship to renal arteries, and presence of anatomic anomalies. CT colonography useful in patients with failed colonoscopy or patients unable to undergo colonoscopy. Differentiation of benign from malignant adrenal adenoma.	Rapid. Complete coverage of abdomen and pelvis. Superb spatial resolution. Not limited by overlying bowel gas, as with ultrasound. Can guide fine-needle aspiration and percutaneous drainage. Noncontrast is the standard of reference for determining the extent and locations of urinary tract stone disease.	Barium or Hypaque, surgical clips, and metallic prostheses can cause artifacts and degrade image quality. **Contraindications and risks:** Contraindicated in pregnancy because of the potential harm of ionizing radiation to the fetus. See Risks of CT and Angiographic Intravenous Contrast Studies, p 295.	Preferably NPO for 4–6 hours. Normal hydration. Distention of gastrointestinal tract with water or oral contrast material. Sedation of agitated patients. Recent serum creatinine determination if intravenous contrast material is to be given.

ABDOMEN				
	MRI		PET/CT	

Modality	Indications	Advantages	Comments	Preparation
ABDOMEN — Magnetic resonance imaging (MRI) — $$$$	Assessment and preoperative staging of intraabdominal cancers. Differentiation of benign from malignant adrenal masses. Complementary to CT in evaluation of liver lesions (especially metastatic disease and possible tumor invasion of hepatic or portal veins). Differentiation of benign from malignant liver tumors. Differentiation of retroperitoneal lymphadenopathy from blood vessels or the diaphragmatic crus.	Provides excellent tissue contrast resolution, multiplanar capability. No ionizing radiation.	Subject to motion artifacts. Gastrointestinal opacification not yet readily available. Special instrumentation required for patients on life support. **Contraindications and risks:** Contraindicated in patients with cardiac pacemakers, intraocular metallic foreign bodies, intracranial aneurysm clips, cochlear implants, and some artificial heart valves.	NPO for 4–6 hours. Intramuscular glucagon to inhibit peristalsis. Sedation of agitated patients. Screening CT or plain radiograph images of orbits if history suggests possible metallic foreign body in the eye.
ABDOMEN/PELVIS — Positron emission tomography/computed tomography (PET/CT) — $$$$	Evaluation for abdominopelvic malignancy and metastases. Discrimination between benign and malignant lymph nodes. Tumor staging.	Combines metabolic and anatomic information. Large area of coverage (can image whole body).	Patient cooperation required for appropriate breath-holding. **Contraindications and risks:** Contraindicated in pregnancy because of the potential harm of ionizing radiation to the fetus. See Risks of CT and Angiographic Intravenous Contrast Agents, p 295.	Preferably NPO for 2 hours before study. Normal hydration. Sedation of agitated patients. Recent serum creatinine determination.

	ABDOMEN
	Mesenteric angiography

Test	Indications	Advantages	Disadvantages/Contraindications	Preparation
ABDOMEN **Mesenteric angiography** $$$$	Gastrointestinal hemorrhage that does not resolve with conservative therapy and cannot be treated endoscopically. Localization of gastrointestinal bleeding site. Acute mesenteric ischemia, intestinal angina, splenic or other splanchnic artery aneurysm. Evaluation of possible vasculitis, such as polyarteritis nodosa. Detection of islet cell tumors not identified by other studies. Abdominal trauma.	Therapeutic embolization of gastrointestinal vessels during hemorrhage is often possible.	Invasive. Patient may need to remain supine with leg extended for 6 hours following the procedure to protect the common femoral artery at the catheter entry site. **Contraindications and risks:** Allergy to iodinated contrast material may require corticosteroid and H_1 blocker or H_2 blocker premedication. Contraindicated in pregnancy because of the potential harm of ionizing radiation to the fetus. Contrast nephrotoxicity may occur, especially with preexisting impaired renal function due to diabetes mellitus or multiple myeloma; however, any creatinine elevation following the procedure is usually reversible (see p 325, 336).	NPO for 4–6 hours. Good hydration to limit possible renal insult due to iodinated contrast material. Recent serum creatinine determination, assessment of clotting parameters, reversal of anticoagulation. Performed with conscious sedation. Requires cardiac, respiratory, blood pressure, and pulse oximetry monitoring.

	GASTROINTESTINAL	
	UGI	**Enteroclysis**
GI **Upper GI study** (UGI) $$	Double-contrast barium technique demonstrates esophageal, gastric, and duodenal mucosa for evaluation of inflammatory disease and other subtle mucosal abnormalities. Single-contrast technique assesses bowel motility, peristalsis, possible outlet obstruction, gastroesophageal reflux and hiatal hernia, esophageal cancer, and varices. Water-soluble contrast (Gastrografin) is suitable for evaluation of anastomotic leak or gastrointestinal perforation.	Good evaluation of mucosa with double-contrast examination. No sedation required. Less expensive than endoscopy. Aspiration of water-soluble contrast material may occur, resulting in severe pulmonary edema. Leakage of barium from a perforation may cause granulomatous inflammatory reaction. Identification of a lesion does not prove it to be the site of blood loss in patients with gastrointestinal bleeding. Barium precludes endoscopy and body CT examination. Retained gastric secretions prevent mucosal coating with barium. **Contraindications and risks:** Caution in pregnancy because of the potential harm of ionizing radiation to the fetus.
		NPO for 8 hours.
GI **Enteroclysis** $$	Barium fluoroscopic study for location of site of intermittent partial small bowel obstruction. Evaluation of extent of Crohn disease or small bowel disease in patient with persistent gastrointestinal bleeding and normal UGI and colonic evaluations. Evaluation of metastatic disease to the small bowel.	Clarifies lesions noted on more traditional barium examination of the small bowel. Best means of establishing small bowel as normal. Requires nasogastric or orogastric tube placement and manipulation to beyond the ligament of Treitz. **Contraindications and risks:** Radiation exposure is substantial, because lengthy fluoroscopic examination is required. Therefore, the test is contraindicated in pregnant women and should be used sparingly in children and women of childbearing age.
		Clear liquid diet for 24 hours. Colonic cleansing.

	GASTROINTESTINAL		
	CT Enterography/CT Enteroclysis	**Small bowel follow-through**	**Peroral pneumocolon**
Test	GI **CT Enterography/CT Enteroclysis** $$$	GI **Small bowel follow-through** $$	GI **Peroral pneumocolon** $
Indications	Assessment for small bowel strictures before capsule endoscopy. Assess for extent of inflammatory bowel disease, postoperative adhesions, and small bowel tumors.	Barium fluoroscopic study for location of site of intermittent partial small bowel obstruction. Evaluation of extent of Crohn disease or small bowel disease in patient with normal endoscopy and colonic evaluations. Evaluation of metastatic disease to the small bowel.	Fluoroscopic evaluation of the terminal ileum by insufflating air per rectum after orally ingested barium has reached the cecum.
Advantages	Noninvasive. Complete visualiztion of the small bowel. Evaluates extraluminal disease, including extent of intraabdominal abscesses and fistulas.	Less invasive and better tolerated than enteroclysis. May be combined with UGI.	Best evaluation of the terminal ileum. Can be performed concurrently with UGI.
Disadvantages/Contraindications	Requires drinking large amounts of water or oral contrast material. CT enteroclysis requires sedation and placement of nasojejunal tube. Improved images obtained if antiperistaltic agent given at time of examination. **Contraindications and risks:** Caution in pregnancy because of the potential harm of ionizing radiation to the fetus.	Less diagnostic power than enteroclysis for mucosal detail. Requires nasogastric or orogastric tube placement and manipulation to beyond the ligament of Treitz. **Contraindications and risks:** Radiation exposure is substantial, because lengthy fluoroscopic examination is required. Therefore, the test is contraindicated in pregnant women and should be used sparingly in children and women of childbearing age.	Undigested food in the small bowel interferes with the evaluation. **Contraindications and risk:** Contraindicated in pregnancy because of the potential harm of ionizing radiation to the fetus.
Preparation	NPO for 4–6 hours. Consume 1–2 liters of water orally or contrast material 45 minutes before scan.	Clear liquid diet for 24 hours. Colonic cleansing.	Clear liquid diet for 24 hours.

	GASTROINTESTINAL		
		Barium enema	**CT colonography**
GI **Barium enema** (BE) $$	Double-contrast technique for evaluation of colonic mucosa for suspected inflammatory bowel disease or neoplasm. Single-contrast technique for investigation of possible fistulous tracts, anastomotic leak, bowel obstruction, and for examination of debilitated patients.	Good mucosal evaluation. No sedation required.	Retained fecal material limits evaluation of mucosa. Requires patient cooperation. Marked diverticulosis precludes evaluation for possible neoplasm in involved area. Evaluation of right colon occasionally incomplete or limited by reflux of barium across ileocecal valve and overlapping opacified small bowel. Use of barium delays subsequent colonoscopy and body CT. **Contraindications and risks:** Contraindicated in patients with toxic megacolon and immediately after full-thickness colonoscopic biopsy.	Colon cleansing with enemas, cathartic, and clear liquid diet (1 day in young patients, 2 days in older patients). Intravenous glucagon (which inhibits peristalsis) sometimes given to distinguish colonic spasm from a mass lesion.
GI **CT colonography** $$	Thin section CT for evaluation of possible colonic polyps and masses.	Has ability to evaluate extracolonic intrabdominal disease (AAA, renal cell cancer, kidney stones). No IV contrast. Less invasive than colonoscopy.	Retained fecal material limits study. Requires patient cooperation. If polyps or masses are found, patient will need to undergo colonoscopy or sigmoidoscopy for tissue diagnosis.	Requires colonic preparation that varies from institution to institution.

Test	Indications	Advantages	Disadvantages/Contraindications	Preparation
GASTROINTESTINAL				
	Hypaque enema			
GI **Hypaque enema** $$	Water-soluble contrast for fluoroscopic evaluation of colonic anatomy, anastomotic leak, or other perforation. Differentiation of colonic versus small bowel obstruction. Therapy for obstipation.	Water-soluble contrast medium is evacuated much faster than barium because it does not adhere to the mucosa. Therefore, Hypaque enema can be followed immediately by oral ingestion of barium for evaluation of possible distal small bowel obstruction.	Demonstrates only colonic morphologic features and not mucosal changes. **Contraindications and risks:** Contraindicated in patients with toxic megacolon. Hypertonic solution may lead to fluid imbalance in debilitated patients and children.	Colonic cleansing is desirable but not always necessary.
	Esophageal reflux study			
GI **Esophageal reflux study** (radionuclide) $$	Evaluation of heartburn, regurgitation, recurrent aspiration pneumonia.	Noninvasive and well tolerated. More sensitive for reflux than fluoroscopy, endoscopy, and manometry; sensitivity similar to that of acid reflux test. Permits quantitation of reflux. Can identify aspiration into the lung.	Incomplete emptying of esophagus may mimic reflux. Abdominal binder—used to increase pressure in the lower esophagus—may not be tolerated in patients who have undergone recent abdominal surgery. **Contraindications and risks:** Contraindicated in pregnancy because of the potential harm of ionizing radiation to the fetus.	NPO for 4–6 hours. During test, patient must be able to consume 300 mL of liquid.

GASTROINTESTINAL		
Gastric emptying study	**GI bleeding scan**	
GI **Gastric emptying study** (radionuclide) $$	Evaluation of dumping syndrome, vagotomy, gastric outlet obstruction due to inflammatory or neoplastic disease, effects of drugs, and other causes of gastroparesis (eg, diabetes mellitus).	Gives functional information not available by other means.	Reporting of meaningful data requires adherence to standard protocol and establishment of normal values. **Contraindications and risks:** Contraindicated in pregnancy because of the potential harm of ionizing radiation to the fetus.	NPO for 4–6 hours. During test, patient must be able to eat a 300-g meal consisting of both liquids and solids.
GI **GI bleeding scan** (labeled red cell scan, radionuclide) $$–$$$	Evaluation of upper or lower gastrointestinal blood loss. Distinguishing hemangioma of the liver from other mass lesions of the liver.	Noninvasive compared with angiography. Longer period of imaging possible, which aids in detection of intermittent bleeding. Labeled red cells and sulfur colloid can detect bleeding rates as low as 0.05–0.10 mL/min (angiography requires rate of about 0.5 mL/min). 90% sensitivity for blood loss >500 mL/24 h.	Bleeding must be active during time of imaging. Presence of free TcO_4 (poor labeling efficiency) can lead to gastric, kidney, and bladder activity that can be misinterpreted as sites of bleeding. Uptake in hepatic hemangioma, varices, arteriovenous malformation, abdominal aortic aneurysm, and bowel wall inflammation can also lead to false-positive examination. **Contraindications and risks:** Contraindicated in pregnancy because of the potential harm of ionizing radiation to the fetus.	Sterile technique required during in vitro labeling of red cells.

	BLOOD
	Indium scan

Test	Indications	Advantages	Disadvantages/Contraindications	Preparation
BLOOD **Leukocyte scan** (indium scan, labeled white blood cell [WBC] scan, technetium-99m hexamethylpropylene amine oxime [Tc99m-HMPAO]-labeled WBC scan, radionuclide) $$–$$$	Evaluation of fever of unknown origin, suspected abscess, pyelonephritis, osteomyelitis, inflammatory bowel disease. Examination of choice for evaluation of suspected vascular graft infection.	Highly specific (98%) for infection (in contrast to gallium). Highly sensitive in detecting abdominal source of infection. In patients with fever of unknown origin, total body imaging is advantageous compared with CT scan or ultrasound. Preliminary imaging as early as 4 hours is possible with indium but less sensitive (30–50% of abscesses are detected at 24 hours).	24-hour delayed imaging may limit the utility of indium scan in critically ill patients. False-negative scans occur with antibiotic administration or in chronic infection. Perihepatic or splenic infection can be missed because of normal leukocyte accumulation in these organs; liver and spleen scan is necessary adjunct in this situation. False-positive scans occur with swallowed leukocytes, bleeding, indwelling tubes and catheters, surgical skin wound uptake, and bowel activity due to inflammatory processes. Pulmonary uptake is nonspecific and has low predictive value for infection. Patients must be able to hold still during relatively long acquisition times (5–10 minutes). Tc99m-HMPAO WBC may be suboptimal for detecting infection involving the genitourinary and gastrointestinal tracts because of normal distribution of the agent to these organs. **Contraindications and risks:** Contraindicated in pregnancy because of the hazard of ionizing radiation to the fetus. High radiation dose to spleen.	Leukocytes from the patient are harvested, labeled in vitro, and then reinjected; process requires 12 hours. Scanning takes place 24 hours after injection of indium-labeled WBC and 1–2 hours after injection of Tc99m-HMPAO WBC. Homologous donor leukocytes should be used in neutropenic patients.

GALLBLADDER				
	Ultrasound		**HIDA scan**	

Test	Indications	Advantages	Disadvantages / Contraindications	Patient Preparation
GALLBLADDER **Ultrasound** (US) $	Demonstrates cholelithiasis (95% sensitive), sonographic Murphy sign, gallbladder wall thickening, pericholecystic fluid, intra- and extrahepatic biliary dilation.	Noninvasive. No ionizing radiation. Can be portable. Imaging in all planes. Can guide fine-needle aspiration, percutaneous transhepatic cholangiography, and biliary drainage procedures.	Technique very operator-dependent. Presence of barium obscures sound waves. Difficult in obese patients. Administration of excessive pain medication prior to exam limits accuracy of diagnosing acute cholecystitis. **Contraindications and risks:** None.	Preferably NPO for 6 hours to enhance visualization of gallbladder.
GALLBLADDER **Hepatic imi-nodiacetic acid scan** (HIDA) $$	Evaluation of suspected acute cholecystitis or common bile duct obstruction. Evaluation of bile leaks, biliary atresia, and biliary enteric bypass patency.	95 percent sensitive and 99% specific for diagnosis of acute cholecystitis. Hepatobiliary function assessed. Defines pathophysiology underlying acute cholecystitis. Rapid. Can be performed in patients with elevated serum bilirubin. No intravenous contrast used.	Does not demonstrate the cause of obstruction (eg, tumor or gallstone). Not able to evaluate biliary excretion if hepatocellular function is severely impaired. Sensitivity may be lower in acalculous cholecystitis. False-positive results can occur with hyperalimentation, prolonged fasting, and acute pancreatitis. **Contraindications and risks:** Contraindicated in pregnancy because of the potential harm of ionizing radiation to the fetus.	NPO for at least 4 hours but preferably less than 24 hours. Premedication with cholecystokinin can prevent false-positive examination in patients who are receiving hyperalimentation or who have been fasting longer than 24 hours. Avoid administration of morphine prior to examination if possible.

Test	Indications	Advantages	Disadvantages/Contraindications	Preparation
PANCREAS/BILIARY TREE				
PANCREAS/BILIARY TREE **Endoscopic retrograde cholangiopancreatography (ERCP)** $$$$	Demonstrates cause, location, and extent of extrahepatic biliary obstruction (eg, choledocholithiasis). Can diagnose chronic pancreatitis. Primary sclerosing cholangitis, AIDS-associated cholangitis, and cholangiocarcinomas.	Avoids surgery. Less invasive than percutaneous transhepatic cholangiography. Offers therapeutic potential (sphincterotomy and extraction of common bile duct stone, balloon dilatation of strictures, placement of stents). Finds gallstones in up to 14% of patients with symptoms but negative ultrasound.	Requires endoscopy. May cause pancreatitis (1%), cholangitis (<1%), peritonitis, hemorrhage (if sphincterotomy performed), and death (rare). **Contraindications and risks:** Relatively contraindicated in patients with concurrent or recent (<6 weeks) acute pancreatitis or suspected pancreatic pseudocyst. Contraindicated in pregnancy because of the potential harm of ionizing radiation to the fetus.	NPO for 6 hours. Sedation required. Vital signs should be monitored by the nursing staff. Not possible in patient who has undergone Roux-en-Y hepaticojejunostomy.
PANCREAS/BILIARY TREE **Magnetic resonance cholangiopancreatography (MRCP)** $$$$	Evaluation of intra- and extra-hepatic biliary and pancreatic duct dilatation, and the cause of obstruction.	Noninvasive. No ionizing radiation. Imaging in all planes. Can image ducts beyond the point of obstruction. Evaluates extra-luminal disease.	Special instrumentation required for patients on life support. **Contraindications and risks:** Contraindicated in patients with cardiac pacemakers, intraocular metallic foreign bodies, intracranial aneurysm clips, cochlear implants, and some artificial heart valves.	Preferably NPO for 6 hours.

LIVER

Imaging Modality	Preparation	Limitations / Contraindications	Strengths	Indications
Ultrasound (US) $	Preferably NPO for 6 hours.	Technique very operator-dependent. Presence of barium obscures sound waves. More difficult in obese patients. The presence of fatty liver or cirrhosis can limit the sensitivity of ultrasound for focal mass lesions. **Contraindications and risks:** None.	Noninvasive. No radiation. Can be portable. Imaging in all planes. Can guide fine-needle aspiration, percutaneous transhepatic cholangiography, and biliary drainage procedures.	Differentiation of cystic versus solid intrahepatic lesions. Evaluation of intra- and extrahepatic biliary dilation, primary and metastatic liver tumors, and ascites. Evaluation of patency and flow velocity of portal vein, hepatic arteries, and hepatic veins.
Computed tomography (CT) $$$–$$$$	NPO for 4–6 hours. Recent creatinine determination. Administration of oral contrast material for opacification of stomach and small bowel. Specific hepatic protocol with arterial, portal venous, and delayed images used for evaluation of neoplasm.	Requires iodinated contrast material administered intravenously. **Contraindications and risks:** Contraindicated in pregnancy because of the potential harm of ionizing radiation to the fetus. See Risks of CT and Angiographic Intravenous Contrast Agents, p 295.	Excellent spatial resolution. Can direct percutaneous fine-needle aspiration biopsy. Excellent evaluation of hepatic vasculature.	Suspected metastatic or primary tumor, gallbladder carcinoma, biliary obstruction, abscess.
Magnetic resonance imaging (MRI) $$$$	Screening CT or plain radiograph images of orbits if history suggests possible metallic foreign body in the eye. Intramuscular glucagon is used to inhibit intestinal peristalsis.	Subject to motion artifacts, particularly those of respiration. Special instrumentation required for patients on life support. **Contraindications and risks:** Contraindicated in patients with cardiac pacemakers, intraocular metallic foreign bodies, intracranial aneurysm clips, cochlear implants, some artificial heart valves.	Requires no iodinated contrast material. Provides excellent tissue contrast resolution, multiplanar capability.	Characterization of hepatic lesions, including suspected cyst, hepatocellular carcinoma, focal nodular hyperplasia, and metastasis. Suspected metastatic or primary tumor. Differentiation of benign cavernous hemangioma from malignant tumor. Evaluation of hemochromatosis, hemosiderosis, fatty liver, and suspected focal fatty infiltration.

	LIVER/BILIARY TREE			
	PTC			
Test	Indications	Advantages	Disadvantages/Contraindications	Preparation
LIVER/BILIARY TREE **Percutaneous transhepatic cholangiogram (PTC)** $$$	Evaluation of biliary obstruction in patients in whom ERCP has failed or patients with Roux-en-Y hepaticojejunostomy.	Best examination to assess site and morphology of obstruction close to the hilum (as opposed to ERCP, which is better for distal obstruction). Can characterize the nature of diffuse intrahepatic biliary disease such as primary sclerosing cholangitis. Provides guidance and access for percutaneous transhepatic biliary drainage and possible stent placement to treat obstruction.	Invasive; requires special training. Performed with conscious sedation. **Contraindications and risks:** Ascites may present a contraindication.	NPO for 4–6 hours. Sterile technique, assessment of clotting parameters, correction of coagulopathy. Performed with conscious sedation.

LIVER			
Hepatic angiography			
LIVER **Hepatic angiography** $$$$	Preoperative evaluation for liver transplantation, vascular malformations, trauma, Budd-Chiari syndrome, portal vein patency (when ultrasound equivocal) prior to transjugular intrahepatic portosystemic shunt (TIPS) procedure. In some cases, evaluation of hepatic neoplasm or transcatheter embolotherapy of hepatic malignancy.	Gold standard assessment of hepatic arterial anatomy, which is highly variable. More accurate than ultrasound with respect to portal vein patency when the latter suggests occlusion.	Invasive. Patient must remain supine with leg extended for 6 hours following the procedure to protect the common femoral artery at the catheter entry site. **Contraindications and risks:** Allergy to iodinated contrast material may require corticosteroid and H$_1$ blocker or H$_2$ blocker premedication. Contraindicated in pregnancy because of the potential harm of ionizing radiation to the fetus. Contrast nephrotoxicity may occur, especially with preexisting impaired renal function due to diabetes mellitus or multiple myeloma; however, any creatinine elevation following the procedure is usually reversible.	NPO for 4–6 hours. Good hydration to limit possible renal insult due to iodinated contrast material. Recent serum creatinine determination, assessment of clotting parameters, reversal of anticoagulation. Performed with conscious sedation. Requires cardiac, respiratory, blood pressure, and pulse oximetry monitoring.

Test	Indications	Advantages	Disadvantages/Contraindications	Preparation
LIVER/SPLEEN				
Liver, spleen scan				
LIVER-SPLEEN **Liver, spleen scan** (radionuclide) $$	Identification of functioning splenic tissue to localize an accessory spleen or evaluate suspected functional asplenia. Assessment of size, shape, and position of liver and spleen. Characterization of a focal liver mass with regard to inherent functioning reticuloendothelial cell activity (in particular focal nodular hyperplasia). Confirmation of patency and distribution of hepatic arterial perfusion catheters.	May detect isodense lesions missed by CT. Useful to detect location of active GI bleed (see GI bleeding scan, above).	Diminished sensitivity for small lesions (less than 1.5–2.0 cm) and deep lesions. SPECT increases sensitivity (can detect lesions of 1.0–1.5 cm). Nonspecific; unable to distinguish solid versus cystic or inflammatory versus neoplastic tissue. Lower sensitivity for diffuse hepatic tumors. **Contraindications and risks:** Caution in pregnancy advised because of the risk of ionizing radiation to the fetus.	None.

PANCREAS		
	CT	Ultrasound
PANCREAS **Computed tomography (CT)** $$$–$$$$	Evaluation of pancreatic and biliary obstruction and possible adenocarcinoma. Staging of pancreatic carcinoma. Evaluation of complications and causes of acute pancreatitis.	Can guide fine-needle biopsy or placement of a drainage catheter. Can identify early necrosis in pancreatitis.	Optimal imaging requires special protocol, including precontrast plus arterial and venous phase contrast-enhanced images. **Contraindications and risks:** Contraindicated in pregnancy because of the potential harm of ionizing radiation to the fetus. See Risks of CT and Angiographic Intravenous Contrast Agents, p 295.	Preferably NPO for 4–6 hours. Normal hydration. Opacification of gastrointestinal tract with oral Gastrografin. Sedation of agitated patients. Recent serum creatinine determination.
PANCREAS **Ultrasound (US)** $	Identification of peripancreatic fluid collections, pseudocysts, and pancreatic ductal dilation.	Noninvasive. No radiation. Can be portable. Imaging in all planes. Can guide fine-needle aspiration or placement of drainage catheter.	Pancreas may be obscured by overlying bowel gas. Technique very operator dependent. Presence of barium obscures sound waves. Less sensitive than CT. **Contraindications and risks:** None.	Preferably NPO for 6 hours.

	ADRENAL
	MIBG scan

Test	Indications	Advantages	Disadvantages/Contraindications	Preparation
ADRENAL **MIBG (meta-iodobenzyl-guanidine)** (radionuclide) $$$$	Suspected pheochromocytoma when CT is negative or equivocal. Also useful in evaluation of neuroblastoma, carcinoid, and medullary carcinoma of thyroid.	Test is useful for localization of pheochromocytomas (particularly extra-adrenal). 80–90% sensitive for detection of pheochromocytoma.	High radiation dose to adrenal gland. High cost and limited availability of MIBG. Delayed imaging (at 1, 2, and 3 days) necessitates return of patient. **Contraindications and risks:** Contraindicated in pregnancy because of the risk of ionizing radiation to the fetus. Because of the relatively high dose of ^{131}I, patients should be instructed about precautionary measures by nuclear medicine personnel.	Administration of Lugol's iodine solution (to block thyroid uptake) before and after administration of MIBG.

GENITOURINARY			
GENITOURINARY **Computed tomography (CT)** $$$	Evaluation for possible kidney or ureteral stones. Evaluation of staging of renal parenchymal tumors, hydronephrosis, pyelonephritis, and perinephric abscess.	Rapid. Can guide percutaneous procedures. Excellent spatial resolution.	Generally limited to transaxial views. **Contraindications and risks:** Caution in pregnancy because of the risk of ionizing radiation to the fetus. See Risks of CT and Angiographic Intravenous Contrast Agents, p 295.	Sedation of agitated patients.
GENITOURINARY **Ultrasound (US)** $$	Evaluation of renal morphology, hydronephrosis, size of prostate, and residual urine volume. Differentiation of cystic versus solid renal lesions.	Noninvasive. No radiation. Can be portable. Imaging in all planes. Can guide fine-needle aspiration or placement of drainage catheter.	Technique very operator-dependent. More difficult in obese patients. **Contraindications and risks:** None.	Preferably NPO for 6 hours. Full urinary bladder required for pelvic studies.
GENITOURINARY **Magnetic resonance imaging (MRI)** $$$$	Staging of cancers of the uterus, cervix, and prostate. Can provide information additional to what is obtained by CT in some cases of cancer of the kidney and urinary bladder.	Provides excellent tissue contrast resolution, multiplanar capability. No ionizing radiation.	Subject to motion artifacts. Gastrointestinal opacification not yet readily available. Special instrumentation required for patients on life support. **Contraindications and risks:** Contraindicated in patients with cardiac pacemakers, intraocular metallic foreign bodies, intracranial aneurysm clips, cochlear implants, and some artificial heart valves.	Sedation of agitated patients. Screening CT or plain radiograph images of orbits if history suggests possible metallic foreign body in the eye.

		GENITOURINARY	
		IVP	Radionuclide scan

Test	Indications	Advantages	Disadvantages/Contraindications	Preparation
GENITOURI-NARY **Intravenous pyelogram (IVP)** $$$	Fluoroscopic evaluation of uroepi-thelial neoplasm, calculus, papillary necrosis, and medullary sponge kidney. Screening for urinary system injury after trauma.	Permits evaluation of collecting system in less invasive manner than retrograde pyelo-gram. Can assess both renal morphology and function.	Suboptimal evaluation of the renal parenchyma. Does not adequately evaluate cause of ureteral deviation. **Contraindications and risks:** Caution in pregnancy is advised because of the risk of ionizing radiation to the fetus. See Risks of CT and Angiographic Intravenous Contrast Agents, p 295.	Adequate hydration. Colonic cleansing is pre-ferred but not essential. Recent serum creatinine determination.
GENITOURI-NARY **Renal scan** (radionuclide) $$	Determination of relative renal function. Evaluation of suspected renal vascular hypertension. Differentiation of a dilated but non-obstructed system from one that has a urodynamically significant obstruction. Evaluation of renal blood flow and function in acute or chronic renal failure. Evaluation of both medical and surgical complications of renal transplant. Estimation of glomerular filtration rate and effective renal plasma flow.	Provides functional information without risk of iodinated contrast used in IVP. Provides quantitative information not avail-able by other means.	Finding of poor renal blood flow does not pinpoint an etiologic diagnosis. Limited utility when renal function is extremely poor. Estimation of glomerular filtration rate and renal plasma flow often is inaccurate. **Contraindications and risks:** Caution in pregnancy because of the risk of ionizing radiation to the fetus.	Normal hydration needed for evaluation of suspected obstruc-tive uropathy because dehydration may result in false-positive exami-nation. Blood pressure should be monitored and an intravenous line started when an angiotensin-converting enzyme (ACE) inhibitor is used to evaluate renal vascu-lar hypertension. Patient should discon-tinue ACE inhibitor medication for at least 48 hours prior to exam-ination if possible.

PELVIS		
	Ultrasound	**MRI**
PELVIS **Ultrasound (US)** $$	Evaluation of ovarian mass, enlarged uterus, vaginal bleeding, pelvic pain, possible ectopic pregnancy, and infertility. Monitoring of follicular development. Localization of intrauterine device.	Use of a vaginal probe enables very early detection of intrauterine pregnancy and ectopic pregnancy and does not require a full bladder.	Transabdominal scan has limited sensitivity for uterine or ovarian pathology. Vaginal probe has limited field of view and therefore may miss large masses outside the pelvis. **Contraindications and risks:** None.	Distended bladder required (only in transabdominal examination).
PELVIS **Magnetic resonance imaging (MRI)** $$$$	Evaluation of gynecologic malignancies, particularly endometrial, cervical, and vaginal carcinoma. Evaluation of prostate, bladder, and rectal carcinoma. Evaluation of congenital anomalies of the genitourinary tract. Useful in distinguishing lymphadenopathy from vasculature.	Provides excellent tissue contrast resolution, multiplanar capability. No ionizing radiation. Best imaging evaluation of cancer of the uterus, cervix, prostate, and bladder. May provide metabolic and functional information on prostate cancer.	Subject to motion artifacts. Special instrumentation required for patients on life support. **Contraindications and risks:** Contraindicated in patients with cardiac pacemakers, intraocular metallic foreign bodies, intracranial aneurysm clips, cochlear implants, and some artificial heart valves.	Intramuscular glucagon is used to inhibit intestinal peristalsis. Sedation of agitated patients. Screening CT or plain radiograph images of orbits if history suggests possible metallic foreign body in the eye. An endorectal device (radiofrequency coil) is used for prostate MRI.

Test	Indications	Advantages	Disadvantages/Contraindications	Preparation
		BONE		
		Bone scan		
BONE **Bone scan, whole body (radionuclide)** $$–$$$	Evaluation of primary or metastatic neoplasm, osteomyelitis, arthritis, metabolic disorders, trauma, avascular necrosis, joint prosthesis, and reflex sympathetic dystrophy. Evaluation of clinically suspected but radiographically occult fractures. Identification of stress fractures.	Can examine entire osseous skeleton or specific area of interest. Highly sensitive compared with plain film radiography for detection of bone neoplasm. In osteomyelitis, bone scan may be positive much earlier (24 hours) than plain film (10–14 days).	Nonspecific. Correlation with plain film radiographs often necessary. Limited utility in patients with poor renal function. Poor resolution in distal extremities, head, and spine; in these instances, SPECT is often useful. Sometimes difficult to distinguish osteomyelitis from cellulitis or septic joint; dual imaging with gallium or with indium-labeled leukocytes can be helpful. False-negative results for osteomyelitis can occur following antibiotic therapy and within the first 24 hours after trauma. In avascular necrosis, bone scan may be "hot," "cold," or normal, depending on the stage. **Contraindications and risks:** Caution in pregnancy because of the risk of ionizing radiation to the fetus.	Patient should be well hydrated and void frequently after the procedure.

SPINE

Imaging Study	Indications	Strengths	Weaknesses and Comments	Preparation
SPINE **Computed tomography (CT)** $$$	Evaluation of structures that are not well visualized on MRI, including ossification of the posterior longitudinal ligament, tumoral calcification, osteophytic spurring, retropulsed bone fragments after trauma. Also used for patients in whom MRI is contraindicated.	Rapid. Superb spatial resolution. Can guide percutaneous fine-needle aspiration of possible tumor or abscess.	Generally limited to transaxial views. Coronal and sagittal reformation images can be generated. MRI unequivocally superior in evaluation of the spine nerve roots and cord, except for conditions mentioned here in Indications. **Contraindications and risks:** Contraindicated in pregnancy because of the potential harm of ionizing radiation to the fetus. See Risks of CT and Angiographic Intravenous Contrast Agents, p 295. Artifacts from metal prostheses degrade images.	Normal hydration. Sedation of agitated patients.
SPINE **Magnetic resonance imaging (MRI)** $$$$	Diseases involving the spine and cord except where CT is superior (ossification of the posterior longitudinal ligament, tumoral calcification, osteophytic spurring, retropulsed bone fragments after trauma).	Provides excellent tissue contrast resolution, multiplanar capability. No ionizing radiation.	Less useful in detection of calcification, small spinal vascular malformations, acute spinal trauma (because of longer acquisition time, incompatibility with life support devices, and inferior detection of bony injury). Subject to motion artifacts. Special instrumentation required for patients on life support. **Contraindications and risks:** Contraindicated in patients with cardiac pacemakers, intraocular metallic foreign bodies, intracranial aneurysm clips, cochlear implants, and some artificial heart valves.	Sedation of agitated patients. Screening CT or plain radiograph images of orbits if history suggests possible metallic foreign body in the eye.

	MUSCULOSKELETAL
	MRI

Test	Indications	Advantages	Disadvantages/Contraindications	Preparation
MUSCULO-SKELETAL SYSTEM **Magnetic resonance imaging (MRI)** $$$$	Evaluation of joints except where a prosthesis is in place. Extent of primary or malignant tumor (bone and soft tissue). Evaluation of aseptic necrosis, bone and soft tissue infections, marrow space disease, and traumatic derangements.	Provides excellent tissue contrast resolution, multiplanar capability. No ionizing radiation.	Subject to motion artifacts. Less able than CT to detect calcification, ossification, and periosteal reaction. Special instrumentation required for patients on life support. **Contraindications and risks:** Contraindicated in patients with cardiac pacemakers, intraocular metallic foreign bodies, intracranial aneurysm clips, cochlear implants, and some artificial heart valves.	Sedation of agitated patients. Screening CT or plain radiograph images of orbits if history suggests possible metallic foreign body in the eye.

VASCULATURE			
Ultrasound			
VASCULATURE **Ultrasound (US)** $$	Evaluation of deep venous thrombosis, extremity grafts, patency of inferior vena cava, portal vein, and hepatic veins. Carotid Doppler indicated for symptomatic carotid bruit, atypical transient ischemic attack, monitoring after endarterectomy, and baseline prior to major vascular surgery. Surveillance of TIPS patency and flow.	Noninvasive. No radiation. Can be portable. Imaging in all planes.	Technique operator-dependent. Ultrasound not sensitive to detection of ulcerated plaque. May be difficult to diagnose tight stenosis versus occlusion (catheter angiography may be necessary). May be difficult to distinguish acute from chronic deep venous thrombosis. **Contraindications and risks:** None.	None

	AORTA			
	Angiography			
Test	Indications	Advantages	Disadvantages/Contraindications	Preparation
AORTA AND ITS BRANCHES **Angiography** $$$	Peripheral vascular disease, abdominal aortic aneurysm, renal artery stenosis (atherosclerotic and fibromuscular disease), visceral ischemia, thoracic aortic dissection, gastrointestinal hemorrhage, vasculitis, abdominal tumors, arteriovenous malformations, abdominopelvic trauma. Preoperative evaluation for aortofemoral bypass reconstructive surgery. Postoperative assessment of possible graft stenosis, especially femoral to popliteal or femoral to distal (foot or ankle).	Can localize atherosclerotic stenosis and assess the severity by morphology, flow, and pressure gradient. Provides assessment of stenotic lesions and access for percutaneous transluminal balloon dilation as well as stent treatment of iliac stenoses. Provides access for thrombolytic therapy of acute or subacute occlusion of native artery or bypass graft.	Invasive. Patient must remain supine with leg extended for 6 hours following the procedure to protect the common femoral artery at the catheter entry site. **Contraindications and risks:** Allergy to iodinated contrast material may require corticosteroid and H$_1$ blocker or H$_2$ blocker premedication. Contraindicated in pregnancy because of the potential harm of ionizing radiation to the fetus. Contrast nephrotoxicity may occur, especially with preexisting impaired renal function due to diabetes mellitus or multiple myeloma; however, any creatinine elevation that occurs after the procedure is usually reversible.	NPO for 4–6 hours. Good hydration to limit possible renal insult due to iodinated contrast material. Recent serum creatinine determination, assessment of clotting parameters, reversal of anticoagulation. Performed with conscious sedation. Requires cardiac, respiratory, blood pressure, and pulse oximetry monitoring as well as noninvasive studies of peripheral vascular disease to verify indication for angiography and to guide the examination.

AORTA				
CTA				
AORTA AND ITS BRANCHES **Computed tomography angiography (CTA)** $$$	Preoperative assessment of aortic aneurysm. Evaluation of abdominal trauma. Evaluation of possible aortic injury.	Rapid. Excellent spatial resolution. Evaluates calcified vascular plaques.	Limited functional and hemodynamic evaluation. **Contraindications and risks:** Contraindicated in pregnancy because of potential harm of ionizing radiation to the fetus. See Risks of CT and Angiographic Intravenous Contrast Agents, p 295.	Sedation of agitated patients. Hydration.
MRA				
AORTA AND ITS BRANCHES **Magnetic resonance angiography (MRA)** $$$$	Can provide preoperative assessment of abdominal aortic aneurysm to determine aneurysm size, proximal and distal extent, relationship to renal arteries, and presence of anatomic anomalies. Permits evaluation of the hemodynamic and functional significance of renal artery stenosis.	No ionizing radiation. No iodinated contrast needed.	Subject to motion artifacts. Special instrumentation required for patients on life support. **Contraindications and risks:** Contraindicated in patients with cardiac pacemakers, intraocular metallic foreign bodies, intracranial aneurysm clips, cochlear implants, and some artificial heart valves.	Sedation of agitated patients. Screening CT or plain radiograph images of orbits if history suggests possible metallic foreign body in the eye.

7

Basic Electrocardiography

Fred M. Kusumoto, MD

HOW TO USE THIS SECTION

This chapter includes criteria for the diagnosis of basic electrocardiographic waveforms and cardiac arrhythmias. It is intended for use as a reference and assumes a basic understanding of the electrocardiogram (ECG).

Electrocardiographic interpretation is a "stepwise" procedure, and the first steps are to study and characterize the cardiac rhythm.

Step One (Rhythm)

Categorize what you see in the 12-lead ECG or rhythm strip, using the three major parameters that allow for systematic analysis and subsequent diagnosis of the rhythm:

1. Mean rate of the QRS complexes (slow, normal, or fast).
2. Width of the QRS complexes (wide or narrow).
3. Rhythmicity of the QRS complexes (characterization of spaces between QRS complexes) (regular or irregular).

Step Two (Morphology)

Step 2 consists of examining and characterizing the morphology of the cardiac waveforms.

1. Examine for atrial abnormalities and bundle branch blocks (BBBs) (pp 358–361).
2. Assess the QRS axis and the causes of axis deviations (pp 361–366).
3. Examine for signs of left ventricular hypertrophy (pp 364–365).

Adapted, with permission, from Evans GT Jr.: *ECG Interpretation Cribsheets,* 4th ed. Ring Mountain Press, 1999.

4. Examine for signs of right ventricular hypertrophy (p 366).
5. Examine for signs of myocardial infarction, if present (pp 368–387).
6. Bear in mind conditions that may alter the ability of the ECG to diagnose a myocardial infarction (p 377).
7. Examine for abnormalities of the ST segment or T wave (pp 370–384).
8. Assess the QT interval (pp 382–384).
9. Examine for miscellaneous conditions (pp 384–385).

STEP ONE: DIAGNOSIS OF THE CARDIAC RHYTHM

A. APPROACH TO DIAGNOSIS OF THE CARDIAC RHYTHM

Most electrocardiograph machines display 10 seconds of data in a standard tracing. A rhythm is defined as three or more successive P waves or QRS complexes.

Categorize the patterns seen in the tracing according to a systematic method. This method proceeds in three steps that lead to a diagnosis based upon the most likely rhythm producing a particular pattern:

1. What is the mean rate of the QRS complexes?
   Slow (<60 bpm): The easiest way to determine this is to count the total number of QRS complexes in a 10-second period. If there are no more than 9, the rate is slow.
   Another method for determining the rate is to count the number of large boxes (0.20 s) between QRS complexes and use the following formula:

   Rate = 300 ÷ (number of large boxes between QRS complexes)

   A slow heart rate (<60 bpm) has more than five large boxes between QRS complexes.
   Normal (60–100 bpm): If there are 10–16 complexes in a 10-second period, the rate is normal.
   In normal heart rates, the QRS complexes are separated by three–five large boxes.
   Fast (>100 bpm): If there are ≥17 complexes in a 10-second period, the rate is fast.
   Fast heart rates have fewer than three large boxes between QRS complexes.
2. Is the duration of the dominant QRS morphology narrow (<0.12 s) or wide (≥0.12 s)? (Refer to the section below on the QRS duration.)
3. What is the "rhythmicity" of the QRS complexes (defined as the spacing between QRS complexes)? Regular or irregular? (Any change in the spacing of the R-R intervals defines an irregular rhythm.)

TABLE 7–1. SUSTAINED REGULAR RHYTHMS.

Rate	Fast	Normal	Slow

Narrow QRS duration	Sinus tachycardia
	Atrial tachycardia
	Atrial flutter
	  (2 : 1 AV conduction)
	Junctional tachycardia
	Orthodromic AVRT
		Sinus rhythm
		Ectopic atrial rhythm
		Atrial flutter
		  (4 : 1 conduction)
		Accelerated junctional
		  rhythm
			Sinus bradycardia
			Ectopic atrial bradycardia
			
			Junctional rhythm

Wide QRS duration	All rhythms listed above under narrow QRS duration, but with BBB or IVCD patterns		
	Ventricular tachycardia Antidromic AVRT	Accelerated ventricular rhythm	Ventricular escape rhythm

AV = atrioventricular; **BBB** = bundle branch blocks; **IVCD** = intraventricular conduction delay.

Using the categorization above, refer to Tables 7–1 and 7–2 to select a specific diagnosis for the cardiac rhythm.

B. NORMAL HEART RATE

Sinus Rhythm

The sinus node is the primary pacemaker for the heart. Because the sinus node is located at the junction of the superior vena cava and the right atrium,

TABLE 7–2. SUSTAINED IRREGULAR RHYTHMS.

Rate	Fast	Normal	Slow

Narrow QRS duration	Atrial fibrillation
	Atrial flutter (variable
	  AV conduction)
	Multifocal atrial tachycardia
	Atrial tachycardia with
	  AV block (rare)
		Atrial fibrillation
		Atrial flutter (variable
		  AV conduction)
		Multiform atrial rhythm
		Atrial tachycardia with
		  AV block (rare)
			Atrial fibrillation
			Atrial flutter (variable
			  AV conduction)
			Multiform atrial rhythm
			Sinus rhythm with 2°
			  AV block

Wide QRS duration	All rhythms listed above under narrow QRS duration, but with BBB or IVCD patterns		

	Torsade de pointes
	Rarely, anterograde conduc-
	  tion of atrial fibrillation
	  over an accessory
	  pathway in patients with
	  WPW syndrome		

AV = atrioventricular; **BBB** = bundle branch blocks; **IVCD** = intraventricular conduction delay; **WPW** = Wolff-Parkinson-White syndrome.

in **sinus rhythm** the atria are activated from "right to left" and "high to low." The P wave in sinus rhythm is upright in lead II and inverted in lead aVR. In lead V_I, the P wave is usually biphasic with a small initial positive deflection due to right atrial activation and a terminal negative deflection due to left atrial activation.

The normal sinus rate is usually between 60 and 100 bpm but can vary significantly. During sleep, when parasympathetic tone is high, **sinus bradycardia** (sinus rates <60 bpm) is a normal finding, and during conditions associated with increased sympathetic tone (exercise, stress), **sinus tachycardia** (sinus rate >100 bpm) is common. In children and young adults, **sinus arrhythmia** (sinus rates that vary by more than 10% during 10 seconds) due to respiration is frequently observed.

Ectopic Atrial Rhythm

In some situations, the atria are activated by an ectopic atrial focus rather than the sinus node. In this case, the P wave will have an abnormal shape depending on where the ectopic focus is located. For example, if the focus arises from the left atrium, the P wave is inverted in leads I and aVL. If the depolarization rate of the ectopic focus is between 60 and 100 bpm, the patient has an **ectopic atrial rhythm.** If the rate is <60 bpm, the rhythm is defined as an ectopic atrial bradycardia.

Atrial Flutter With 4:1 Atrioventricular Conduction

In **atrial flutter**, the atria are activated rapidly (usually 300 bpm) due to a stable reentrant circuit. Most commonly, the reentrant circuit rotates counterclockwise around the tricuspid valve. Because the left atrium and interatrial septum are activated low-to-high, "sawtooth" flutter waves that are inverted in the inferior leads (II, III, and aVF) are usually observed. If every fourth atrial beat is conducted to the ventricles (due to slow conduction in the atrioventricular [AV] node), a relatively normal ventricular rate of 75 bpm is observed.

Accelerated Junctional Rhythm (p 341)

Premature QRS Activity

It is common to have isolated premature QRS activity that leads to mild irregularity of the heart rhythm. A premature narrow QRS complex is most often due to a normally conducted **premature atrial complex (PAC)** or more rarely a **premature junctional complex (PJC)**. A premature wide QRS complex is usually due to a **premature ventricular complex (PVC)** or to a premature supraventricular complex (PAC or PJC) that conducts to the ventricle with aberrant conduction due to block in one of the bundle branches (pp 342–350). Premature supraventricular complexes (with or without aberrant conduction) are commonly observed phenomena that are not associated with cardiac disease. Although PVCs are observed in normal individuals, they are usually associated with higher risk in patients with cardiac disease.

C. TACHYCARDIA

Tachycardias are normally classified by whether the QRS complex is narrow or wide, and whether the rhythm is regular or irregular. A narrow QRS tachycardia indicates normal activation of the ventricular tissue regardless of the tachycardia mechanism. Narrow QRS tachycardias are frequently grouped together as supraventricular tachycardia (SVT) and can be due to a number of mechanisms described below. This grouping also has clinical utility because SVTs are not usually life-threatening. In addition to QRS width, it is useful to consider the anatomic site from which the tachycardia arises: atrium, atrioventricular junction, ventricle, or utilization of an accessory pathway (Figure 7–1).

Narrow QRS Tachycardia with a Regular Rhythm: Regular SVT (Figure 7–2)

A. **Sinus Tachycardia:** Under many physiologic conditions, the sinus node discharges at a rate >100 bpm. In **sinus tachycardia,** an upright P wave can be observed in II and aVF and an inverted P wave is observed in aVR. The PR interval is usually relatively normal, because conditions associated with sinus tachycardia (most commonly sympathetic activation) also cause more rapid AV conduction.

B. **Atrial Tachycardia:** Rarely, a single atrial site other than the sinus node fires rapidly. This leads to an abnormally shaped P wave. The specific shape of the P wave depends on the specific site of **atrial tachycardia.** The PR interval depends on how quickly atrioventricular conduction occurs. As the atrial tachycardia rate increases, the AV node conduction slows (decremental conduction) and the PR interval increases; decremental conduction properties of the AV node prevent rapid ventricular rates in the presence of rapid atrial rates.

C. **Atrial Flutter:** The mechanism for **atrial flutter** is described above. Most commonly atrioventricular conduction occurs with every other flutter wave (2:1 conduction), leading to a heart rate of approximately 150 bpm. In some situations, very rapid ventricular rates can be observed due to 1:1 conduction, or slower rates observed due to 3:1 conduction.

Atrial tachycardias

   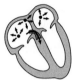

Atrial flutter   Atrial fibrillation   Atrial tachycardia   Atrial tachycardia
(MAT)

Junctional tachycardias

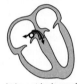

Atrioventricular node   Atrioventricular node
reentrant tachycardia   automatic tachycardia

Ventricular tachycardias

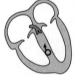 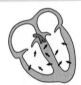

Ventricular tachycardia   Ventricular fibrillation

Accessory pathway-mediated tachycardias

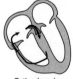

Orthodromic   Antidromic   Atrial fibrillation
atrioventricular   atrioventricular   with activation of
reentrant tachycardia   reentrant tachycardia   the ventricles via
                                            an accessory pathway
                                            and the AV node

Figure 7–1. Anatomic classification of tachycardias. (*Adapted from Kusumoto FM: Arrhythmias. In:* Cardiovascular Pathophysiology, *FM Kusumoto (editor), Hayes Barton Press, 2004.*)

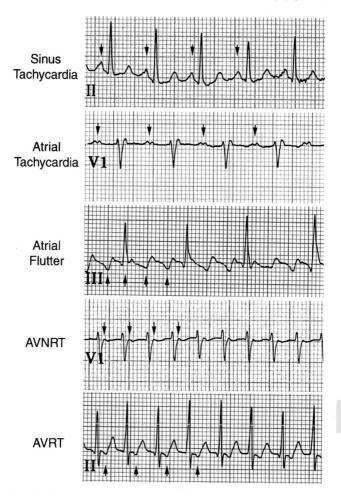

Figure 7–2. ECG appearance of different forms of regular SVTs. The arrows show the first four atrial deflections in each SVT. In *sinus tachycardia,* the P wave has a normal morphology and the PR interval is normal. In *atrial tachycardia,* the P wave is abnormal (positive in V_1 and the PR interval is prolonged because of decremental conduction in the AV node. In *atrial flutter,* inverted "saw-tooth" waves are observed in lead III. In *AVNRT,* a pseudo-R wave due to retrograde atrial activation is observed in lead V_1. In *AVRT,* a retrograde P wave is observed in the ST segment because the atria and ventricles are activated sequentially. The P wave is usually located relatively close to the preceding QRS complex because the accessory pathway conducts rapidly.

D. Junctional Tachycardia: The most common type of tachycardia to arise from tissue near the atrioventricular junction is **AV nodal reentrant tachycardia (AVNRT)**. In AVNRT, two separate parallel pathways of conduction are present within junctional and perijunctional tissue. Usually, one of the pathways has relatively rapid conduction properties but a long refractory period ("fast pathway") and the other has slow conduction and a short refractory period ("slow pathway"). In some cases, a premature atrial contraction can block one of the pathways (usually the fast pathway), conduct down the slow pathway, and activate the fast pathway retrogradely, initiating a reentrant circuit. In rare circumstances, a site within the AV node fires rapidly due to increased automaticity.

Regardless of the mechanism, because the tachycardia originates within the AV junction, the atria and ventricles are activated simultaneously. Most commonly (in approximately 50% of cases), the P wave is buried in the QRS complex and is not seen. In approximately 40% of cases, the retrograde P wave is observed in the terminal portion of the QRS complex. The easiest place to see the retrograde P wave is in lead V_1, where a low-amplitude terminal positive deflection (pseudo-R′ wave) is seen (Figure 7–2). In addition, a terminal negative deflection (pseudo-S wave) is seen in the inferior leads (II, III, and aVF). Finally, in about 10% of cases, the P wave is observed in the initial portion of the QRS complex. The location of the P wave depends on the relative speeds of retrograde activation of the atria and anterograde activation of the ventricles via the His-Purkinje system.

E. Accessory Pathway–Mediated Tachycardia: Usually, the AV node and His bundle provide the only path for AV conduction. In approximately 1 in 1000 individuals, an additional AV connection called an **accessory pathway** is present. The presence of two parallel pathways (the accessory pathway and the AV node-His bundle) for AV conduction increases the likelihood that reentrant tachycardia will occur. The most common tachycardia is a reentrant narrow QRS tachycardia in which the ventricles are activated via the His-Purkinje system and the atria are activated via retrograde activation from the accessory pathway (Figure 7–3). This type of tachycardia is frequently called **orthodromic atrioventricular reentrant tachycardia (AVRT)** because conduction through the AV node and His-Purkinje fibers occurs normally (*ortho* is Greek for straight or normal). Orthodromic AVRT is one cause of SVT; the QRS complexes are narrow and normal-appearing because the ventricles are activated via the AV node and His-Purkinje system, ventricular tissue, an accessory pathway, and atrial tissue. Because the ventricles and atria are activated sequentially, the P wave is most often observed within the ST segment (Figure 7–2). As discussed later, accessory pathways can also be associated with regular and irregular wide complex tachycardias.

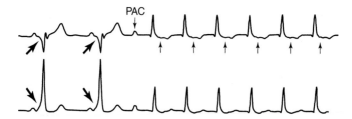

Figure 7–3. Initiation of SVT in a patient with an accessory pathway. During sinus rhythm, the ventricles are activated via the accessory pathway and the AV node-His bundle. Because the accessory pathway conducts rapidly and inserts into regular ventricular myocardium, the PR interval is short and a delta wave is observed (*large arrows*). A PAC blocks in the accessory pathway and travels only down the AV node-His bundle, leading to a narrow QRS complex. The atria are activated retrogradely by the accessory pathway (*small arrows*) and orthodromic AVRT is initiated. *(From Kusumoto FM: Cardiovascular disorders: Heart disease. In: Pathophysiology of Disease: An Introduction to Clinical Medicine, 5th ed. SJ McPhee, WF Ganong (editors), McGraw-Hill, 2006.)*

Narrow QRS Tachycardias with an Irregular Rhythm: Irregular SVT (Figure 7–4)

A. Atrial Fibrillation: Atrial fibrillation is the most common abnormal fast heart rhythm observed. Atrial fibrillation is most commonly due to multiple chaotic wandering wavelets of reentry that cause irregular activation of the atria. Because the AV node is also activated irregularly, AV conduction is variable and an irregular ventricular rhythm is observed. In atrial fibrillation, the rhythm is often called "irregularly irregular" because there is no organized atrial activity. On the ECG, continuous fibrillatory low-amplitude waves with varying morphology are observed with no easily identifiable isoelectric period. The fibrillatory waves are usually best seen in leads V_1, V_2, II, III, and aVF.

B. Multifocal Atrial Tachycardia: In **multifocal atrial tachycardia** (often called **MAT**), several atrial sites beat due to abnormal automaticity. This leads to P waves of three or more different morphologies. The rhythm is usually irregular; the different sites fire at different rates. MAT can be distinguished from atrial fibrillation by discrete P waves and isoelectric periods between the T wave and the P wave. The most common cause of MAT is chronic obstructive pulmonary disease (approximately 60% of cases).

C. Atrial Flutter With Variable Block: Atrial flutter can sometimes present as an irregular rhythm because of variable AV block. In this case, although the ventricular rhythm is irregular, there are often relatively constant intervals between the QRS complexes. For example,

Atrial fibrillation

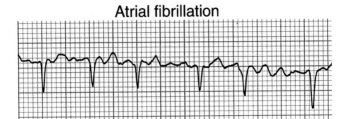

Multifocal atrial tachycardia

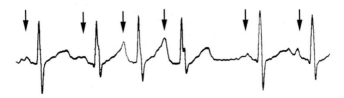

Figure 7–4. ECG appearance of atrial fibrillation and MAT. In atrial fibrillation, continuous chaotic activation of the atria results in continuous low-amplitude fibrillatory waves. In MAT, discrete P waves (*arrows*) and an isoelectric T–P segment are observed.

if the atrial flutter rate is 300 bpm, the possible ventricular rates will be 300 bpm, 150 bpm, 100 bpm, or 75 bpm for 1:1, 2:1, 3:1, and 4:1 AV conduction, respectively.

Wide QRS Complex Tachycardia With a Regular Rhythm

The most common cause of **wide QRS complex tachycardia with a regular rhythm (WCT-RR)** is sinus tachycardia with either right bundle branch block (RBBB) or left bundle branch block (LBBB). However, if a patient with structural heart disease presents with WCT-RR, one assumes a worst-case scenario and the presumptive diagnosis becomes **ventricular tachycardia (VT).** Most commonly, VT originates from a rapid reentrant circuit located at the border of infarcted and normal myocardium. Because the ventricles are not activated via the bundle branches or the Purkinje system, an abnormally wide QRS complex is observed. Any atrial or junctional tachycardias associated with aberrant conduction can also cause a WCT-RR. Finally, in very rare circumstances, patients with accessory pathways will present with **antidromic AVRT** in which the ventricles are activated via the accessory pathway (leading to a wide and bizarre QRS complex) and the atria are activated retrogradely via the His bundle-AV node (*anti* is Greek for against).

The ECG differentiation between regular SVTs with aberrant conduction (sinus tachycardia, atrial tachycardia, atrial flutter, junctional tachycardia, orthodromic AVRT) and VT can sometimes be difficult. Accurate diagnosis of VT is critical because this rhythm is frequently life-threatening. The two principal techniques for identifying VT are the presence of AV dissociation and abnormal QRS morphology.

A. **Atrioventricular Dissociation:** In **AV dissociation,** the atria and ventricles are not related in one-to-one fashion. AV dissociation can be due to several conditions:

1. Atrioventricular conduction block (p 357).
2. Slowing of the primary pacemaker, most commonly due to sinus bradycardia or sinus pauses with junctional escape rhythm (p 342).
3. Acceleration of a subsidiary pacemaker, most commonly due to VT or much less commonly due to junctional tachycardia.

The most important reason to identify AV dissociation is in wide complex tachycardia for the differentiation of SVT with aberrancy from VT. In VT, the rapid ventricular rate is often associated with retrograde block within the His-Purkinje system (ventriculoatrial block). This leads to P waves (from sinus node depolarization) that are not associated in 1:1 fashion with the QRS complexes (Figure 7–5). The presence of AV dissociation makes VT the most likely diagnosis in a patient with a regular wide complex tachycardia. In some circumstances, AV dissociation can be identified by the presence of **capture beats** or **fusion beats**. Occasionally, a properly timed P wave will conduct to the ventricles and a portion (fusion beat) or all (capture beat) of ventricular tissue will be activated by the His-Purkinje tissue for one QRS complex. It is always easier to identify AV dissociation rather than AV association; T waves can often be confused with P waves. Always examine the entire ECG for unexpected deflections in the QRS complex, ST segment and T waves that are dissociated P waves. The P waves are usually most obvious in the inferior leads (II, III, and aVF) or V_1.

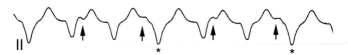

Figure 7–5. Lead II from a wide complex tachycardia. The arrows mark P waves that are not associated with every QRS complex (AV dissociation). The QRS complexes marked with an * are slightly narrower due to partial activation from the preceding P wave (fusion complex).

MORPHOLOGY ALGORITHMS FOR IDENTIFYING VT

1. METHOD ONE: QUICK METHOD FOR DIAGNOSIS OF VT (REQUIRES LEADS I, V_1, AND V_2)

This method derives from an analysis of typical waveforms of RBBB or LBBB as seen in leads I, V_1, and V_2. If the waveforms do not conform to either the common or uncommon typical morphologic patterns, the diagnosis defaults to VT.

Step One

Determine the morphologic classification of the wide QRS complexes (RB type or LB type), using the criteria below.

- **A. Determination of the Morphologic Type of Wide QRS Complexes:** Use lead V_1 only to determine the type of bundle branch block morphology of abnormally wide QRS complexes.
  - **1. RBBB- and RBB-type QRS complexes as seen in lead V_1:** A wide QRS complex with a net positive area under the QRS curve is called the right bundle branch "type" of QRS. This does not mean that the QRS conforms exactly to the morphologic criteria for RBBB. Typical morphologies seen in RBBB are shown in the box at left below. Atypical morphologies at the right are most commonly seen in PVCs or during VT.

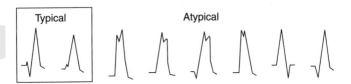

Typical   Atypical

  - **2. LBBB- and LBB-type QRS complexes as seen in lead V_1:** A wide QRS complex with a net negative area under the QRS curve is called a left bundle branch "type" of QRS. This does not mean that the QRS conforms exactly to the morphologic criteria for LBBB. Typical morphologies of LBBB are shown in the box at left below. Atypical morphologies at the right are most commonly seen in PVCs or during VT.

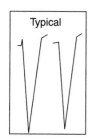 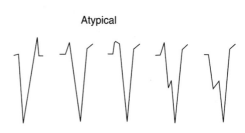

Step Two

Apply criteria for common and uncommon normal forms of either RBBB or LBBB, as described below. The waveforms may not be identical, but the morphologic descriptions must match. If the QRS complexes do not match, the rhythm is probably VT.

A. RBBB: Lead I must have a terminal broad S wave, but the R/S ratio may be <1.

In lead V_1, the QRS complex is usually triphasic but sometimes is notched and monophasic. The latter must have notching on the ascending limb of the R wave, usually at the lower left.

B. LBBB: Lead I must have a monophasic, usually notched R wave and may not have Q waves or S waves.

Both lead V_1 and lead V_2 must have a dominant S wave, usually with a small, narrow R wave. S descent must be rapid and smooth, without notching.

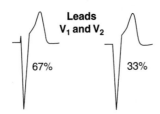

2. METHOD TWO: THE BRUGADA ALGORITHM FOR DIAGNOSIS OF VT

(Requires all six precordial leads)

Brugada and coworkers reported on a total of 554 patients with WCT-RR whose mechanism was diagnosed in the electrophysiology laboratory. Patients included 384 (69%) with VT and 170 (31%) with SVT with aberrant ventricular conduction.

1. **Is there absence of an RS complex in ALL precordial leads?**

   If Yes ($n = 83$), VT is established diagnosis (sensitivity 21%, specificity 100%). *Note:* Only QR, Qr, qR, QS, QRS, monophasic R, or rSR′ are present. qRs complexes were not mentioned in the Brugada study.

   If No ($n = 471$), proceed to next step.

2. **Is the RS interval >100 ms in ANY ONE precordial lead?**

   If Yes ($n = 175$), VT is established diagnosis (sensitivity 66%, specificity 98%). *Note:* The onset of R to the nadir of S is >100 ms (>2.5 small boxes) in a lead with an RS complex.

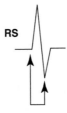

   If No ($n = 296$), proceed to next step.

3. **Is there AV dissociation?**

   If Yes ($n = 59$), VT is established diagnosis (sensitivity 82%, specificity 98%). *Note:* AV block also implies the same diagnosis.

If No (*n* = 237), proceed to next step. *Note:* Antiarrhythmic drugs were withheld from patients in this study. Clinically, drugs that prolong the QRS duration may give a false-positive sign of VT using this criterion.

4. Are morphologic criteria for VT present?

If Yes (*n* = 59), VT is established diagnosis (sensitivity 99%, specificity 97%). *Note:* RBBB type QRS in V₁ versus LBBB type QRS in V₁ should be assessed as shown in the boxes below.

If No (*n* = 169)—and if there are no matches for VT in the boxes below—the diagnosis is SVT with aberration (sensitivity 97%, specificity 99%).

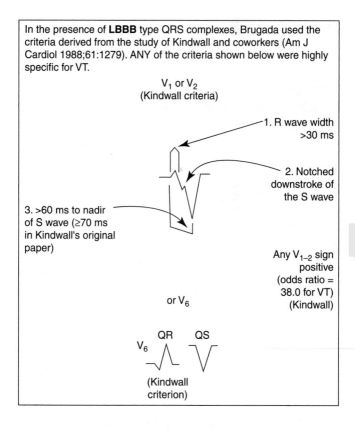

In the presence of **LBBB** type QRS complexes, Brugada used the criteria derived from the study of Kindwall and coworkers (Am J Cardiol 1988;61:1279). ANY of the criteria shown below were highly specific for VT.

V₁ or V₂
(Kindwall criteria)

1. R wave width >30 ms

2. Notched downstroke of the S wave

3. >60 ms to nadir of S wave (≥70 ms in Kindwall's original paper)

Any V₁₋₂ sign positive (odds ratio = 38.0 for VT) (Kindwall)

or V₆

QR   QS

V₆

(Kindwall criterion)

In the presence of **RBBB** type QRS complexes (dominant positive in V_1), a diagnosis of VT can be made by examination of both V_1 and V_6.

V_1 only	V_6
Monophasic R wave	QS or QR
QR or RS	R/S < 1 (seen with LAD)

3. METHOD THREE: THE GRIFFITH METHOD FOR DIAGNOSIS OF VT (REQUIRES LEADS V_1 AND V_6)

This method derives from an analysis of typical waveforms of RBBB or LBBB as seen in both leads V_1 and V_6. If the waveforms do not conform to the typical morphologic patterns, the diagnosis defaults to VT.

Step One

Determine the morphologic classification of the wide QRS complexes (RB type or LB type), using the criteria above.

Step Two

Apply criteria for normal forms of either RBBB or LBBB, as described below. A negative answer to any of the three questions is inconsistent with either RBBB or LBBB, and the diagnosis defaults to VT.

A. For QRS Complexes With RBBB Categorization:
1. Is there an rSR′ morphology in lead V_1?

2. Is there an RS complex in V_6 (may have a small septal Q wave)?

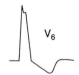

3. Is the R/S ratio in lead $V_6 > 1$?

B. For QRS Complexes With LBBB Categorization:
   1. Is there an rS or QS complex in leads V_1 and V_2?

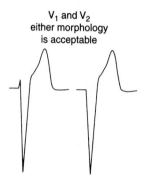

2. Is the onset of the QRS to the nadir of the S wave in lead $V_1 < 70$ ms?
3. Is there an R wave in lead V_6, without a Q wave?

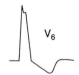

Wide QRS Tachycardia with an Irregular Rhythm

A. Polymorphic Ventricular Tachycardia and Ventricular Fibrillation
In **polymorphic ventricular tachycardia** and **ventricular fibrillation**, the ventricles are often activated continuously in chaotic fashion by disorganized wavelets of activation that produce irregular QRS complexes with no isoelectric periods. Both ventricular fibrillation and polymorphic ventricular tachycardia are life-threatening conditions that require prompt defibrillation. The distinction between ventricular fibrillation and polymorphic ventricular tachycardia is simply based on the amplitude of the QRS complexes and has very little clinical utility.

The most common cause of polymorphic ventricular tachycardia and ventricular fibrillation is myocardial ischemia due to coronary artery occlusion.

B. Torsade de Pointes

Torsade de pointes ("twisting of the points") is a specific form of polymorphic VT that is often pause dependent, has a characteristic shifting morphology of the QRS complex, and occurs in the setting of a prolonged QT interval. Torsade de pointes is associated with drug-induced states, congenital long QT syndrome, and hypokalemia (p 382).

C. Atrial Fibrillation with Anterograde Accessory Pathway Activation

If a patient with an accessory pathway develops atrial fibrillation, the ventricles are activated by both the normal AV node-His bundle axis and the accessory pathway. Because the accessory pathway does not have decremental conduction properties, it allows very rapid activation of the ventricles. The combination of an irregular wide complex rhythm with very rapid rates (250–300 bpm) should arouse suspicion of this scenario, particularly in a young, otherwise healthy patient.

D. Bradycardia

Slow heart rates can be due to failure of impulse formation (sinus node dysfunction) or blocked AV conduction.

Sinus Node Dysfunction

Sinus node dysfunction is manifested in a number of ECG findings. Most commonly, there is a sinus pause with a junctional escape beat. Alternatively, sinus bradycardia can be associated with sinus node dysfunction.

A. Sinus Bradycardia: The normal range of sinus rates changes with age. In infants less than 12 months old, the mean heart rate is 140 bpm with a range of 100–190 bpm. In contrast, the normal range for adults is probably 50–90 bpm. Sinus rates less than 60 bpm are classified as **sinus bradycardia,** but it must be remembered that sinus rates of less than 60 bpm are commonly observed (sleep, athletes). Treatment of sinus bradycardia (usually with a pacemaker) is indicated only when it is associated with symptoms, not because of a specific heart rate.

B. Sinus Pauses: In some individuals, the sinus node abruptly stops firing, leading to **sinus pauses.** Usually an escape rhythm from an ectopic atrial focus or the junction prevents asystole. Sinus pauses of up to 2 seconds are seen in normal adults. Patients with sinus pauses >3 seconds should be evaluated for the presence of sinus node dysfunction.

C. Junctional Rhythm: If the sinus node rate is very low, **sustained junctional rhythm** can sometimes be observed. In junctional rhythm, the QRS is not preceded by a P wave. A retrograde P wave can sometimes be seen in the initial portion or terminal portion of the QRS complex, but most commonly it is "buried" in the QRS complex. Normally, junctional rhythms are <60 bpm. Transient junctional rhythm can be observed in normal individuals during sleep, but sinus node dysfunction should be suspected if junctional rhythm is observed when a patient is awake.

In rare circumstances, accelerated junctional rhythms between 60 and 100 bpm are observed due to more rapid depolarization of AV nodal cells. If the junctional rate is faster than the sinus rate, the sinus node will be suppressed by retrograde atrial activation because of repetitive depolarization from the junction. Accelerated junctional rhythms can be present in digitalis toxicity, rheumatic fever, and after cardiac surgery.

AV Block

Because AV conduction normally occurs along a single axis, the AV node and His bundle, **atrioventricular (AV) block** most commonly is due to block at one of these two sites. Block within the His bundle is associated with a worse prognosis, and should be suspected in any form of AV block associated with a wide QRS complex. Electrocardiographically, AV block is usually described as first-degree, second-degree, or third-degree AV block. In **first-degree (1°) AV block,** every P wave is conducted to the ventricles, but there is an abnormal delay between atrial activation and ventricular activation (PR interval >0.2 second. In 1° AV block, the ventricular rate is not slow unless sinus bradycardia is also present.

In **second-degree (2°) AV block,** some but not all P waves are conducted to the ventricles. This leads to an irregular ventricular rhythm. Second-degree AV block is usually subclassified as **Mobitz type I** block, **Wenckebach block** or **Mobitz type II block.** In type I 2° AV block, progressive prolongation of the PR interval is observed; in type II 2° AV block, the PR interval remains relatively constant before the blocked P wave. The importance of this distinction is this: type I 2° AV block usually indicates that conduction is blocked within the AV node, whereas type II AV block suggests that conduction is blocked within the His bundle (regardless of the width of the QRS complex). The simplest way to differentiate between type I and type II 2° AV block is to compare the PR intervals before and after the block P wave. In type I 2° AV block, the PR interval after the blocked P wave is shorter than the PR interval before the blocked P wave; in type II 2° AV block, the PR intervals are the same.

In **third-degree (3°) or complete AV block,** no P waves are conducted to the ventricles. The P-to-P and QRS-to-QRS intervals are constant and unrelated (AV dissociation). The QRS rate and morphology depend on the site of the subsidiary intrinsic pacemaker. If the block is within the AV node, a lower AV nodal pacemaker often takes over and the rate is

40–50 bpm with a normal-appearing QRS complex (junctional rhythm). If the block is within the His bundle, a ventricular pacemaker with a rate of 20–40 bpm and a wide QRS will be noted (**ventricular escape rhythm**).

STEP TWO: MORPHOLOGIC DIAGNOSIS OF THE CARDIAC WAVEFORMS

A. THE NORMAL ECG: TWO BASIC QRST PATTERNS

The most common pattern is illustrated below and is usually seen in leads I or II and V_{-6}. There is a small "septal" Q wave <30 ms in duration. The T wave is upright. The normal ST segment, which is never normally iso-electric except sometimes at slow rates (<60 bpm), slopes upward into an upright T wave, whose proximal angle is more obtuse than the distal angle. The normal T wave is never symmetric.

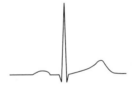

The pattern seen in the right precordial leads, usually V_{1-3}, is shown below. There is a dominant S wave. The J point—the junction between the end of the QRS complex and the ST segment—is usually slightly elevated, and the T wave is upright. The T wave in V_1 may occasionally be inverted as a normal finding in up to 50% of young women and 25% of young men, but this finding is usually abnormal in adult males. V_2 usually has the largest absolute QRS and T-wave magnitude of any of the 12 electrocardiographic leads.

B. ATRIAL ABNORMALITIES

Right Atrial Enlargement (RAE)

Diagnostic criteria include a positive component of the P wave in lead V_1 or $V_2 \geq 1.5$ mm. Another criterion is a P-wave amplitude in lead II >2.5 mm.

Note: A tall, peaked P in lead II may represent RAE but is more commonly due to either chronic obstructive pulmonary disease (COPD) or increased sympathetic tone.

Clinical correlation: RAE is seen with right ventricular hypertrophy (RVH).

Left Atrial Enlargement (LAE)

The most sensitive lead for the diagnosis of LAE is lead V_1, but the criteria for lead II are more specific. Criteria include a terminal negative wave ≥1 mm deep and ≥40 ms wide (one small box by one small box in area) for lead V_1 and >40 ms between the first (right) and second (left) atrial components of the P wave in lead II, or a P-wave duration >110 ms in lead II.

Clinical correlations: left ventricular hypertrophy (LVH), coronary artery disease, mitral valve disease, or cardiomyopathy.

C. BUNDLE BRANCH BLOCK

The normal QRS duration in adults ranges from 67–114 ms (Glasgow cohort). If the QRS duration is ≥120 ms (three small boxes or more on the electrocardiographic paper), there is usually an abnormality of conduction of the ventricular impulse. The most common causes are either RBBB or LBBB (see p 348). However, other conditions may also prolong the QRS duration.

RBBB is defined by delayed terminal QRS forces that are directed to the right and anteriorly, producing broad terminal positive waves in leads V_1 and aVR and a broad terminal negative wave in lead I.

LBBB is defined by delayed terminal QRS forces that are directed to the left and posteriorly, producing wide R waves in leads that face the left ventricular free wall and wide S waves in the right precordial leads.

RIGHT BUNDLE BRANCH BLOCK

Diagnostic Criteria

The diagnosis of uncomplicated complete RBBB is made when the following criteria are met:

1. Prolongation of the QRS duration to 120 ms or more.
2. An rsr′, rsR′, or rSR′ pattern in lead V_1 or V_2. The R′ is usually greater than the initial R wave. In a minority of cases, a wide and notched R pattern may be seen.
3. Leads V_6 and I show a QRS complex with a wide S wave (S duration is longer than the R duration or >40 ms in adults).

(See common and uncommon waveforms for RBBB under Step Two, p 351).

ST–T changes in RBBB

In uncomplicated RBBB, the ST–T segment is depressed and the T wave inverted in the right precordial leads with an R′ (usually only in lead V_1 but occasionally in V_2). The T wave is upright in leads I, V_5, and V_6.

LEFT BUNDLE BRANCH BLOCK

Diagnostic Criteria

The diagnosis of uncomplicated complete LBBB is made when the following criteria are met:

1. Prolongation of the QRS duration to 120 ms or more.
2. There are broad and notched or slurred R waves in left-sided precordial leads V_5 and V_6, as well as in leads I and aVL. Occasionally, an RS pattern may occur in leads V_5 and V_6 in uncomplicated LBBB associated with posterior displacement of the left ventricle.
3. With the possible exception of lead aVL, Q waves are absent in the left-sided leads, specifically in leads V_5, V_6, and I.
4. The R peak time is prolonged to >60 ms in lead V_5 or V_6 but is normal in leads V_1 and V_2 when it can be determined.
5. In the right precordial leads V_1 and V_3, there are small initial r waves in the majority of cases, followed by wide and deep S waves. The transition zone in the precordial leads is displaced to the left. Wide QS complexes may be present in leads V_1 and V_2 and rarely in lead V_3.

(See common and uncommon waveforms for LBBB under Step Two, p 351).

ST–T Changes in LBBB

In uncomplicated LBBB, the ST segments are usually depressed and the T waves inverted in left precordial leads V_5 and V_6 as well as in leads I and aVL. Conversely, ST-segment elevations and positive T waves are recorded in leads V_1 and V_2. Only rarely is the T wave upright in the left precordial leads. As a general rule, ST–T changes in LBBB are usually in the direction opposite the direction of the QRS complex (inverted T waves and ST-segment depression if the QRS is upright).

D. INCOMPLETE BUNDLE BRANCH BLOCKS

Incomplete LBBB

The waveforms are similar to those in complete LBBB, but the QRS duration is <120 ms. Septal Q waves are absent in I and V_6. Incomplete LBBB is synonymous with LVH and commonly mimics a delta wave in leads V_5 and V_6.

Incomplete RBBB

The waveforms are similar to those in complete RBBB, but the QRS duration is <120 ms. This diagnosis suggests RVH. Occasionally, in a normal variant pattern, there is an rSr′ waveform in lead V_1. In this case, the r′ is usually smaller than the initial r wave; this pattern is not indicative of incomplete RBBB.

Intraventricular Conduction Delay or Defect

If the QRS duration is ≥120 ms but typical waveforms of either RBBB or LBBB are not present, there is an intraventricular conduction delay or defect (IVCD). This pattern is common in dilated cardiomyopathy. An IVCD with a QRS duration of ≥170 ms is highly predictive of dilated cardiomyopathy.

E. FASCICULAR BLOCKS (HEMIBLOCKS)

1. LEFT ANTERIOR FASCICULAR BLOCK (LAFB)

Diagnostic Criteria

1. Mean QRS axis from –45 degrees to –90 degrees (possibly –31 to –44 degrees).
2. A qR pattern in lead aVL, with the R peak time, that is, the onset of the Q wave to the peak of the R wave ≥45 ms (slightly more than one small box wide), as shown below.

Clinical correlations: hypertensive heart disease, coronary artery disease, or idiopathic conducting system disease.

2. LEFT POSTERIOR FASCICULAR BLOCK (LPFB)

Diagnostic Criteria

1. Mean QRS axis from +90 degrees to +180 degrees.
2. A qR complex in leads III and aVF, an rS complex in leads aVL and I, with a Q wave ≥40 ms in the inferior leads.

Clinical correlations: LPFB is a diagnosis of exclusion. It may be seen in the acute phase of inferior myocardial injury or infarction or may result from idiopathic conducting system disease.

F. DETERMINATION OF THE MEAN QRS AXIS

The mean electrical axis is the average direction of the activation or repolarization process during the cardiac cycle. Instantaneous and mean electrical axes may be determined for any deflection (P, QRS, ST–T) in the three planes (frontal, transverse, and sagittal). The determination of the electrical axis of a QRS complex is useful for the diagnosis of certain pathologic cardiac conditions.

The Mean QRS Axis in the Frontal Plane (Limb Leads)

Arzbaecher developed the **hexaxial reference system** that allowed for the display of the relationships among the six frontal plane (limb) leads. A diagram of this system is shown below.

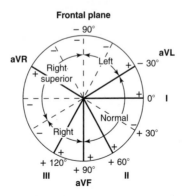

The normal range of the QRS axis in adults is –30 degrees to +90 degrees.
It is rarely important to precisely determine the degrees of the mean QRS. However, the recognition of abnormal axis deviations is critical

because it leads to a presumption of disease. The mean QRS axis is derived from the net area under the QRS curves. The most efficient method of determining the mean QRS axis uses the method of Grant, which requires only leads I and II (see below). If the net area under the QRS curves in these leads is positive, the axis falls between –30 degrees and +90 degrees, which is the normal range of axis in adults. (The only exception to this rule is in RBBB, in which the first 60 ms of the QRS is used. Alternatively, one may use the maximal amplitude of the R and S waves in leads I and II to assess the axis in RBBB.) Abnormal axes are shown below.

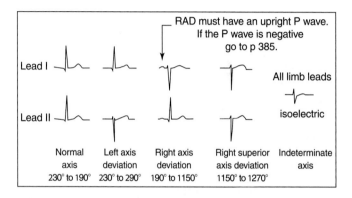

Left Axis Deviation (LAD)

The four main causes of left axis deviation are as follows:

A. Left Anterior Fascicular Block (LAFB): See criteria above.

B. Inferior Myocardial Infarction: There is a pathologic Q wave ≥30 ms either in lead aVF or lead II in the absence of ventricular preexcitation.

C. Ventricular Preexcitation (WPW Pattern): LAD is seen with inferior paraseptal accessory pathway locations. This can mimic inferoposterior myocardial infarction. The classic definition of the Wolff-Parkinson-White (WPW) pattern includes a short PR interval (<120 ms); an initial slurring of the QRS complex, called a delta wave; and prolongation of the QRS complex to >120 ms. However, because this pattern may not always be present despite the presence of ventricular preexcitation, a more practical definition is an absent PR segment and an initial slurring of the QRS complex in any lead. The diagnosis of the WPW pattern usually requires sinus rhythm.

D. COPD: LAD is seen in 10% of patients with COPD.

Right Axis Deviation (RAD)

The four main causes of right axis deviation (RAD) are as follows:

   A. **Right Ventricular Hypertrophy:** This is the most common cause (refer to diagnostic criteria, below). However, one must first exclude acute occlusion of the posterior descending coronary artery, causing LPFB, and exclude also items B and C below.

   B. **Extensive Lateral and Apical Myocardial Infarction:** Criteria include QS or Qr patterns in leads I and aVL and in leads V_{4-6}.

   C. **Ventricular Preexcitation (WPW Pattern):** RAD seen with left lateral accessory pathway locations. This can mimic lateral myocardial infarction.

   D. **Left Posterior Fascicular Block (LPFB):** This is a diagnosis of exclusion (see criteria above).

Right Superior Axis Deviation

This category is rare. Causes include RVH, apical myocardial infarction, VT, and hyperkalemia. Right superior axis deviation may rarely be seen as an atypical form of LAFB.

G. VENTRICULAR HYPERTROPHY

1. LEFT VENTRICULAR HYPERTROPHY

The ECG is very insensitive as a screening tool for LVH, but electrocardiographic criteria are usually specific. Echocardiography is the major resource for this diagnosis.

   The best electrocardiographic criterion for the diagnosis of LVH is the Cornell voltage, the sum of the R-wave amplitude in lead aVL and the S-wave depth in lead V_3, adjusted for sex:

   1. RaVL + SV_3 >20 mm (females), >25 mm (males). The R-wave height in aVL alone is a good place to start.
   2. RaVL >9 mm (females), >11 mm (males).

Alternatively, application of the following criteria will diagnose most cases of LVH.

   3. Sokolow-Lyon criteria: SV_1 + RV_5 or RV_6 (whichever R wave is taller) >35 mm (in patients age >35).
   4. Romhilt-Estes criteria: Points are scored for QRS voltage (1 point), the presence of LAE (1 point), typical repolarization abnormalities

in the absence of digitalis (1 point), and a few other findings. The combination of LAE (see above) and typical repolarization abnormalities (see below) (score ≥5 points) will suffice for the diagnosis of LVH even when voltage criteria are not met.

5. $RV_6 > RV_5$ (usually occurs with dilated LV). First exclude anterior myocardial infarction and establish that the R waves in V_5 are >7 mm tall and that in V_6 they are >6 mm tall before using this criterion.

Repolarization Abnormalities

Typical repolarization abnormalities in the presence of LVH are an ominous sign of end-organ damage. In repolarization abnormalities in LVH, the ST segment and T wave are directed opposite to the dominant QRS waveform in all leads. However, this directional rule does not apply either in the transitional lead (defined as a lead having an R-wave height equal to the S wave depth) or in the transitional zone (defined as leads adjacent to the transitional lead) or one lead to the left in the precordial leads.

Spectrum of Repolarization Abnormalities

The waveforms below, usually seen in leads I, aVL, V_5, and V_6 but more specifically in leads with dominant R waves, represent hypothetical stages in the progression of LVH.

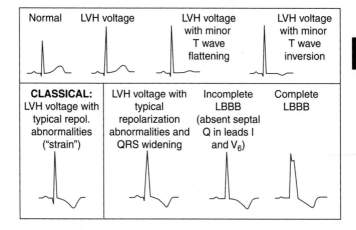

2. RIGHT VENTRICULAR HYPERTROPHY (RVH)

The ECG is insensitive for the diagnosis of RVH. In 100 cases of RVH from one echocardiography laboratory, only 33% had RAD because of the confounding effects of LV disease. Published electrocardiographic criteria for RVH are listed below, all of which have ≥97% specificity.

   With rare exceptions, right atrial enlargement is synonymous with RVH.

Diagnostic Criteria

Recommended criteria for the electrocardiographic diagnosis of RVH are as follows:

   1. Right axis deviation (>90 degrees), or
   2. An R/S ratio ≥1 in lead V_1 (absent posterior MI or RBBB), or
   3. An R wave >7 mm tall in V_1 (not the R′ of RBBB), or
   4. An rsR′ complex in V_1 (R′ ≥10 mm), with a QRS duration of <0.12 s (incomplete RBBB), or
   5. An S wave >7 mm deep in leads V_5 or V_6 (in the absence of a QRS axis more negative than +30 degrees), or
   6. RBBB with RAD (axis derived from first 60 ms of the QRS). (Consider RVH in RBBB if the R/S ratio in lead I is <0.5.)
   A variant of RVH (type C loop) may produce a false-positive sign of an anterior myocardial infarction.

Repolarization Abnormalities

The morphology of repolarization abnormalities in RVH is identical to those in LVH, when a particular lead contains tall R waves reflecting the hypertrophied RV or LV. In RVH, these typically occur in leads V_{1-2} or V_3 and in leads aVF and III. This morphology of repolarization abnormalities due to ventricular hypertrophy is illustrated above. In cases of RVH with massive dilation, all precordial leads may overlie the diseased RV and may exhibit repolarization abnormalities.

H. LOW VOLTAGE OF THE QRS COMPLEX

Low-Voltage Limb Leads Only

Defined as peak-to-peak QRS voltage <5 mm in all limb leads.

Low-Voltage Limb and Precordial Leads

Defined as peak-to-peak QRS voltage <5 mm in all limb leads and <10 mm in all precordial leads. Primary myocardial causes include multiple or massive infarctions; infiltrative diseases such as amyloidosis, sarcoidosis, or hemochromatosis; and myxedema. Extracardiac causes include pericardial effusion, COPD, pleural effusion, obesity, anasarca, and subcutaneous emphysema. When there is COPD, expect to see low voltage in the limb leads as well as in leads V_5 and V_6.

I. PROGRESSION OF THE R WAVE IN THE PRECORDIAL LEADS

The normal R-wave height increases from V_1 to V_5. The normal R-wave height in V_5 is always taller than that in V_6 because of the attenuating effect of the lungs. The normal R-wave height in lead V_3 is usually >2 mm.

"Poor R-Wave Progression"

The term "poor R-wave progression" (PRWP) is a nonpreferred term because most physicians use this term to imply the presence of an anterior myocardial infarction, although it may not be present. Other causes of small R waves in the right precordial leads include LVH, LAFB, LBBB, cor pulmonale (with the type C loop of RVH), and COPD.

Reversed R-Wave Progression (RRWP)

Reversed R-wave progression is defined as a loss of R-wave height between leads V_1 and V_2 or between leads V_2 and V_3 or between leads V_3 and V_4. In the absence of LVH, this finding suggests anterior myocardial infarction or precordial lead reversal.

J. TALL R WAVES IN THE RIGHT PRECORDIAL LEADS

Etiology

Causes of tall R waves in the right precordial leads include the following:

A. **Right Ventricular Hypertrophy:** This is the most common cause. There is an R/S ratio ≥ 1 or an R-wave height >7 mm in lead V_1.

B. **Posterior Myocardial Infarction:** There is an R wave ≥ 6 mm in lead V_1 or ≥ 15 mm in lead V_2. One should distinguish the tall R wave of RVH from the tall R wave of posterior myocardial infarction in lead V_1. In RVH, there is a downsloping ST segment and an inverted T wave, usually with right axis deviation. In contrast, in posterior myocardial infarction, there is usually an upright, commonly tall T wave and, because posterior myocardial infarction is usually associated with concomitant inferior myocardial infarction, a left axis deviation.

C. **Right Bundle Branch Block:** The QRS duration is prolonged, and typical waveforms are present (see above).

D. **The WPW Pattern:** Left-sided accessory pathway locations produce prominent R waves with an R/S ratio ≥ 1 in V_1, with an absent PR segment and initial slurring of the QRS complex, usually best seen in lead V_4.

E. **Rare or Uncommon Causes:** The normal variant pattern of early precordial QRS transition (not uncommon); the reciprocal effect of a deep Q wave in leads V_{5-6} (very rare); Duchenne muscular dystrophy; dextrocardia (very rare); chronic constrictive pericarditis (very rare); and reversal of the right precordial leads.

K. MYOCARDIAL INJURY, ISCHEMIA, AND INFARCTION

Definitions

A. **Myocardial Infarction:** Pathologic changes in the QRS complex reflect ventricular activation away from the area of infarction.

B. **Myocardial Injury:** Injury always points *outward* from the surface that is injured.
   1. **Epicardial injury:** ST elevation in the distribution of an acutely occluded artery.
   2. **Endocardial injury:** Diffuse ST-segment depression, which is really reciprocal to the primary event, reflected as ST elevation in aVR.

C. **Myocardial Ischemia:** Diffuse ST-segment depression, usually with associated T-wave inversion. It usually reflects subendocardial injury, reciprocal to ST elevation in lead aVR. In ischemia, there may only be inverted T waves with a symmetric, sharp nadir.

D. **Reciprocal Changes:** Passive electrical reflections of a primary event viewed from either the other side of the heart, as in epicardial injury, or the other side of the ventricular wall, as in subendocardial injury.

Steps in the Diagnosis of Myocardial Infarction

The following pages contain a systematic method for the electrocardiographic diagnosis of myocardial injury or infarction, arranged in seven steps. Following the steps will achieve the diagnosis in most cases.

Step 1: Identify the presence of myocardial injury by ST-segment deviations.

Step 2: Identify areas of myocardial injury by assessing lead groupings.

Step 3: Define the primary area of involvement and identify the culprit artery producing the injury.

TABLE 7–3. GUSTO STUDY DEFINITIONS.

Area of ST–Segment Elevation	Leads Defining This Area
Anterior (Ant)	V_{1-4}
Apical (Ap)	V_{5-6}
Lateral (Lat)	I, aVL
Inferior (Inf)	II, aVF, III

Step 4: Identify the location of the lesion in the artery to risk stratify the patient.

Step 5: Identify any electrocardiographic signs of infarction found in the QRS complexes.

Step 6: Determine the age of the infarction by assessing the location of the ST segment in leads with pathologic QRS abnormalities.

Step 7: Combine all observations into a final diagnosis.

STEPS ONE AND TWO

Identify presence of and areas of myocardial injury.

The GUSTO study of patients with ST-segment elevation in two contiguous leads defined four affected areas as set out in Table 7–3.

Two other major areas of possible injury or infarction were not included in the GUSTO categorization because they do not produce ST elevation in two contiguous standard leads. These are:

1. **Posterior Injury:** The most commonly used sign of posterior injury is ST depression in leads V_{1-3}, but posterior injury may best be diagnosed by obtaining posterior leads V_7, V_8, and V_9.

2. **Right Ventricular Injury:** The most sensitive sign of right ventricular injury, ST-segment elevation ≥ 1 mm, is found in lead V_4R. A very specific—but insensitive—sign of right ventricular injury or infarction is ST elevation in V_1, with concomitant ST-segment depression in V_2 in the setting of ST elevation in the inferior leads.

STEP THREE

Identify the primary area of involvement and the culprit artery.

Primary Anterior Area

ST elevation in two contiguous V_{1-4} leads defines a primary anterior area of involvement. The left anterior descending coronary artery (LAD) is the culprit artery. Lateral (I and aVL) and apical (V_5 and V_6) areas are contiguous to anterior (V_{1-4}), so ST elevation in these leads signifies more myocardium at risk and more adverse outcomes.

Primary Inferior Area

ST-segment elevation in two contiguous leads (II, aVF, or III) defines a primary inferior area of involvement. The right coronary artery (RCA) is usually the culprit artery. Apical (V_5 and V_6), posterior (V_{1-3} or V_{7-9}), and right ventricular ($V_4 R$) areas are contiguous to the inferior (II, aVF, and III) area, so ST elevation in these contiguous leads signifies more myocardium at risk and more adverse outcomes.

The Culprit Artery

In the GUSTO trial, 98% of patients with ST-segment elevation in any two contiguous V_{1-4} leads, either alone or with associated changes in leads V_{5-6} or I and aVL, had LAD obstruction. In patients with ST-segment elevation only in leads II, aVF, and III, there was RCA obstruction in 86%.

PRIMARY ANTERIOR PROCESS

Acute occlusion of the LAD produces a sequence of changes in the anterior leads (V_{1-4}).

Earliest Findings

A. **"Hyperacute" Changes:** ST elevation with loss of normal ST-segment concavity, commonly with tall, peaked T waves.

rS complex — V_2

B. **Acute Injury:** ST elevation, with the ST segment commonly appearing as if a thumb has been pushed up into it.

rS complex — V_2

Evolutionary Changes

A patient who presents to the emergency department with chest pain and T-wave inversion in leads with pathologic Q waves is most likely to be in the evolutionary or completed phase of infarction. Successful revascularization usually causes prompt resolution of the acute signs of injury or infarction and results in the electrocardiographic signs of a fully evolved infarction. The tracing below shows QS complexes in lead V_2.

  A. **Development of Pathologic Q Waves (Infarction):** Pathologic Q waves develop within the first hour after onset of symptoms in at least 30% of patients.

QS complexes
V_2 shown

day 1

  B. **ST-Segment Elevation Decreases:** T-wave inversion usually occurs in the second 24-hour period after infarction.

day 2

  C. **Fully Evolved Pattern:** Pathologic Q waves, ST segment rounded upward, T waves inverted.

chronic

PRIMARY INFERIOR PROCESS

A primary inferior process usually develops after acute occlusion of the RCA, producing changes in the inferior leads (II, III, and aVF).

Earliest Findings

The earliest findings are of acute injury (ST-segment elevation). The J point may "climb up the back" of the R wave (a), or the ST segment may rise up into the T wave (b).

Evolutionary Changes

ST-segment elevation decreases and pathologic Q waves develop. T-wave inversion may occur in the first 12 hours of an inferior myocardial infarction—in contrast to that in anterior myocardial infarction.

Right Ventricular Injury or Infarction

With right ventricular injury, there is ST-segment elevation, best seen in lead V_4R. With right ventricular infarction, there is a QS complex.

For comparison, the normal morphology of the QRS complex in lead V_4R is shown below. The normal J point averages +0.2 mm.

POSTERIOR INJURY OR INFARCTION

Posterior injury or infarction is commonly due to acute occlusion of the left circumflex coronary artery, producing changes in the posterior leads (V_7, V_8, V_9) or reciprocal ST-segment depression in leads V_{1-3}.

Acute Pattern

Acute posterior injury or infarction is shown by ST-segment depression in V_{1-3} and perhaps also V_4, usually with upright (often prominent) T waves.

V_2 or V_3 V_2

Chronic Pattern

Chronic posterior injury or infarction is shown by pathologic R waves with prominent tall T waves in leads V_{1-3}.

V_2

STEP FOUR

Identify the location of the lesion within the artery to risk stratify the patient.

Primary Anterior Process

Aside from an acute occlusion of the left main coronary artery, occlusion of the proximal LAD conveys the most adverse outcomes. Four electrocardiographic signs indicate proximal LAD occlusion:

1. ST elevation >1 mm in lead I, in lead aVL, or in both
2. New RBBB
3. New LAFB
4. New first-degree AV block

If the occlusion occurs in a more distal portion of the LAD (after the first diagonal branch and after the first septal perforator), ST-segment elevation is observed in the anterior leads but the four criteria described above are not seen. In patients with occlusion of the left main coronary artery, diffuse endocardial injury leads to ST-segment elevation in aVR, because this is the only lead that "looks" directly at the ventricular endocardium, and diffuse ST-segment depression is observed in the anterior and inferior leads.

Primary Inferior Process

Nearly 50% of patients with inferior myocardial infarction have distinguishing features that may produce complications or adverse outcomes unless successfully managed:

1. Precordial ST-segment depression in V_{1-3} (suggests concomitant posterior wall involvement);
2. Right ventricular injury or infarction (identifies a proximal RCA lesion);
3. AV block (implies a greater amount of involved myocardium);
4. The sum of ST-segment depressions in leads V_{4-6} exceeds the sum of ST-segment depressions in leads V_{1-3} (suggests multivessel disease).

Reciprocal Changes in the Setting of Acute Myocardial Infarction

ST depressions in leads remote from the primary site of injury are felt to be a purely reciprocal change. With successful reperfusion, the ST depressions usually resolve. If they persist, patients more likely have significant three-vessel disease and so-called ischemia at a distance. Mortality rates are higher in such patients.

STEP FIVE

Identify Electrocardiographic Signs of Infarction in the QRS Complexes

The 12-lead ECG shown below contains numbers corresponding to pathologic widths for Q waves and R waves for selected leads (see Table 7–4 for more complete criteria).

One can memorize the above criteria by mastering a simple scheme of numbers that represent the durations of pathological Q waves or R waves. Begin with lead V_1 and repeat the numbers in the box below in the following order. The numbers increase from "any" to 50.

TABLE 7–4. DIAGNOSIS OF MYOCARDIAL INFARCTION.

Infarct Location	ECG Lead	Criterion	Sensitivity	Specificity	Likelihood Ratio (+)	Likelihood Ratio (−)
Inferior	II	Q ≥ 30 ms	45	98	22.5	0.6
	aVF	Q ≥ 30 ms	70	94	11.7	0.3
		Q ≥ 40 ms	40	98	20.0	0.6
		R/Q ≤ 1	50	98	25.0	0.5
Anterior	V_1	Any Q	50	97	16.7	0.5
	V_2	Any Q, or R ≤ 0.1 mV and R ≤ 10 ms, or RV_2 ≤ RV_1	80	94	13.3	0.2
	V_3	Any Q, or R ≤ 0.2 mV, or R ≤ 20 ms	70	93	10.0	0.3
	V_4	Q ≥ 20 ms	40	92	5.0	0.9
		R/Q ≤ 0.5, or R/S ≤ 0.5	40	97	13.3	0.6
Anterolateral (lateral)						
	I	Q ≥ 30 ms	10	98	5.0	0.9
		R/Q ≤ 1, or R ≤ 2 mm	10	97	3.3	0.9
	aVL	Q ≥ 30 ms	7	97	0.7	1.0
		R/Q ≤ 1	2			
Apical	V_5	Q ≥ 30	5	99	5.0	1.0
		R/Q ≤ 2, or R ≤ 7 mm, or R/S ≤ 2, or notched R	60	91	6.7	0.4
		R/Q ≤ 1, or R/S ≤ 1	25	98	12.5	0.8
	V_6	Q ≤ 30	3	98	1.5	1.0
		R/Q ≤ 3, or R ≤ 6 mm, or R/S ≤ 3, or notched R	40	92	25.0	0.7
		R/Q ≤ 1, or R/S ≤ 1	10	99	10.0	0.9

(continued)

TABLE 7–4. DIAGNOSIS OF MYOCARDIAL INFARCTION. (*CONTINUED*)

Infarct Location	ECG Lead	Criterion	Sensitivity	Specificity	Likelihood Ratio (+)	Likelihood Ratio (−)
Posterolateral						
	V_1	R/S ≤ 1	15	97	5.0	0.9
		R ≥ 6 mm, or R ≥ 40 ms	20	93	2.9	0.9
		S ≤ 3 mm	8	97	2.7	0.9
	V_2	R ≥ 15 mm, or R ≥ 50 ms	15	95	3.0	0.9
		R/S ≥ 1.5	10	96	2.5	0.9
		S ≤ 4 mm	2	97	0.7	1.0

Notched R = a notch that begins within the first 40 ms of the R wave; **Q** = Q wave; **R/Q** = ratio of R-wave height to Q-wave depth; **R** = R wave; **R/S ratio** = ratio of R-wave height to S-wave depth; **RV_2 ≤ RV_1** = R-wave height in V_2 less than or equal to that in V_1; **S** = S wave.
Reproduced, with permission, from Haisty WK Jr et al: Performance of the automated complete Selvester QRS scoring system in normal subjects and patients with single and multiple myocardial infarctions. J Am Coll Cardiol 1992;19:341.

Any   Q wave in lead V_1, for anterior MI
Any   Q wave in lead V_2, for anterior MI
Any   Q wave in lead V_3, for anterior MI

20   Q wave ≥ 20 ms in lead V_4, for anterior MI
30   Q wave ≥ 30 ms in lead V_5, for apical MI
30   Q wave ≥ 30 ms in lead V_6, for apical MI

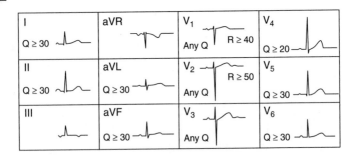

30   Q wave ≥ 30 ms in lead I, for lateral MI
30   Q wave ≥ 30 ms in lead aVL, for lateral MI
30   Q wave ≥ 30 ms in lead II, for inferior MI
30   Q wave ≥ 30 ms in lead aVF, for inferior MI

R40   R wave ≥ 40 ms in lead V_1, for posterior MI
R50   R wave ≥ 50 ms in lead V_2, for posterior MI

Test Performance Characteristics for Electrocardiographic Criteria in the Diagnosis of Myocardial Infarction

Haisty and coworkers studied 1344 patients with normal hearts documented by coronary arteriography and 837 patients with documented myocardial infarction (366 inferior, 277 anterior, 63 posterior, and 131 inferior and anterior) (Table 7–4). (Patients with LVH, LAFB, LPFB, RVH, LBBB, RBBB, COPD, or WPW patterns were excluded from analysis because these conditions can give false-positive results for myocardial infarction.) Shown above are the sensitivity, specificity, and likelihood ratios for the best-performing infarct criteria. Notice that leads III and aVR are not listed: lead III may normally have a Q wave that is both wide and deep, and lead aVR commonly has a wide Q wave.

Mimics of Myocardial Infarction

Conditions that can produce pathologic Q waves, ST-segment elevation, or loss of R-wave height in the absence of infarction are set out in Table 7–5.

TABLE 7–5. MIMICS OF MYOCARDIAL INFARCTION.

Condition	Pseudoinfarct Location
WPW pattern	Any, most commonly inferoposterior or lateral
Hypertrophic cardiomyopathy	Lateral apical (18%), inferior (11%)
LBBB	Anteroseptal, anterolateral, inferior
RBBB	Inferior, posterior (using criteria from leads V_1 and V_2), anterior
LVH	Anterior, inferior
LAFB	Anterior (may cause a tiny Q in V_2)
COPD	Inferior, posterior, anterior
RVH	Inferior, posterior (using criteria from leads V_1 and V_2), anterior, or apical (using criteria for R/S ratios from leads V_{4-6})
Acute cor pulmonale	Inferior, possibly anterior
Cardiomyopathy (nonischemic)	Any, most commonly inferior (with IVCD pattern), less commonly anterior
Chest deformity	Any
Left pneumothorax	Anterior, anterolateral
Hyperkalemia	Any
Normal hearts	Posterior, anterior

STEP SIX

Determine the Age of the Infarction

An **acute infarction** manifests ST-segment elevation in a lead with a pathologic Q wave. The T waves may be either upright or inverted.

An **old** or **age-indeterminate infarction** manifests a pathologic Q wave, with or without slight ST-segment elevation or T-wave abnormalities.

Persistent ST-segment elevation ≥1 mm after a myocardial infarction is a sign of dyskinetic wall motion in the area of infarct. Half of these patients have ventricular aneurysms.

STEP SEVEN

Combine Observations into a Final Diagnosis

There are two possibilities for the major electrocardiographic diagnosis: myocardial infarction or acute injury. If there are pathologic changes in the QRS complex, one should make a diagnosis of myocardial infarction—beginning with the primary area, followed by any contiguous areas—and state the age of the infarction. If there are no pathologic changes in the QRS complex, one should make a diagnosis of acute injury of the affected segments—beginning with the primary area and followed by any contiguous areas.

L. ST SEGMENTS

Table 7–6 summarizes major causes of ST-segment elevations. Table 7–7 summarizes major causes of ST-segment depressions or T-wave inversions. The various classes and morphologies of ST–T waves as seen in lead V_2 are shown in Table 7–8.

M. U WAVES

Normal U Waves

In many normal hearts, low-amplitude positive U waves <1.5 mm tall that range from 160–200 ms in duration are seen in leads V_2 or V_3. Leads V_2 and V_3 are close to the ventricular mass and small-amplitude signals may be best seen in these leads.

Cause: Bradycardias.

Abnormal U Waves

Abnormal U waves have increased amplitude or merge with abnormal T waves and produce T–U fusion. Criteria include an amplitude

TABLE 7–6. MAJOR CAUSES OF ST-SEGMENT ELEVATION.

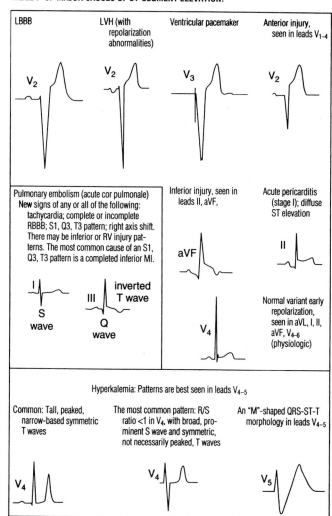

LBBB

LVH (with repolarization abnormalities)

Ventricular pacemaker

Anterior injury, seen in leads V₁₋₄

Pulmonary embolism (acute cor pulmonale) New signs of any or all of the following: tachycardia; complete or incomplete RBBB; S1, Q3, T3 pattern; right axis shift. There may be inferior or RV injury patterns. The most common cause of an S1, Q3, T3 pattern is a completed inferior MI.

S wave

inverted T wave

Q wave

Inferior injury, seen in leads II, aVF,

Acute pericarditis (stage I); diffuse ST elevation

Normal variant early repolarization, seen in aVL, I, II, aVF, V₄₋₆ (physiologic)

Hyperkalemia: Patterns are best seen in leads V₄₋₅

Common: Tall, peaked, narrow-based symmetric T waves

The most common pattern: R/S ratio <1 in V₄, with broad, prominent S wave and symmetric, not necessarily peaked, T waves

An "M"-shaped QRS-ST-T morphology in leads V₄₋₅

TABLE 7–7. MAJOR CAUSES OF ST-SEGMENT DEPRESSION OR T-WAVE INVERSION.

Whenever the ST segment or the T wave is directed counter to an expected repolarization abnormality, consider ischemia, healed MI, or drug or electrolyte effect.	In RBBB, there is an obligatory inverted T wave in right precordial leads with an R' (usually only in V_1) or its equivalent (a qR complex in septal MI). An upright T in these leads suggests completed posterior MI.	Altered depolarization RBBB V_1

LBBB	LVH (with repolarization abnormality)	Subarachnoid hemorrhage	RVH
V_5	V_6	V_4	RVH V_{1-3}

Inferior subendocardial injury	Posterior subepicardial injury	Anterior subendocardial injury or non-Q wave MI	
II	V_2	V_5	V_4

Hypokalemia	Digitalis	Antiarrhythmics	J point depression secondary to catecholamines
V_4	V_4	V_4	II
When $K^+ \leq 2.8$, 80% have ECG changes			PR interval and ST segment occupy the same curve

TABLE 7–8. VARIOUS CLASSES AND MORPHOLOGIES OF ST-T WAVES AS SEEN IN LEAD V₂.

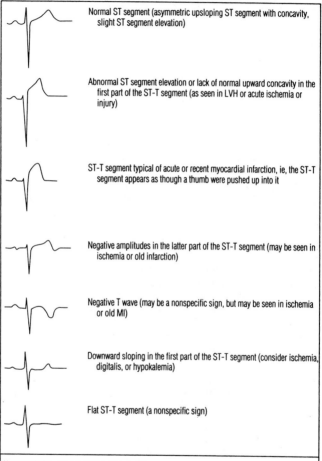

Normal ST segment (asymmetric upsloping ST segment with concavity, slight ST segment elevation)

Abnormal ST segment elevation or lack of normal upward concavity in the first part of the ST-T segment (as seen in LVH or acute ischemia or injury)

ST-T segment typical of acute or recent myocardial infarction, ie, the ST-T segment appears as though a thumb were pushed up into it

Negative amplitudes in the latter part of the ST-T segment (may be seen in ischemia or old infarction)

Negative T wave (may be a nonspecific sign, but may be seen in ischemia or old MI)

Downward sloping in the first part of the ST-T segment (consider ischemia, digitalis, or hypokalemia)

Flat ST-T segment (a nonspecific sign)

Nonspecific ST segment or T wave abnormalities
  By definition, nonspecific abnormalities of either the ST segment (ones that are only slightly depressed or abnormal in contour) or T wave (ones that are either 10% the height of the R wave that produced it, or are either flat or slightly inverted) do not conform to the characteristic waveforms found above or elsewhere.

≥1.5 mm or a U wave that is as tall as the T wave that immediately precedes it.

Causes: Hypokalemia, digitalis, antiarrhythmic drugs.

Inverted U Waves

These are best seen in leads V_{4-6}.

Causes: LVH, acute ischemia.

Table 7–9 summarizes various classes and morphologies of ST–T–U abnormalities as seen in lead V_4.

N. QT INTERVAL

A prolonged QT interval conveys adverse outcomes. The QT interval is inversely related to the heart rate. QT interval corrections for heart rate often use Bazett's formula, defined as the observed QT interval divided by the square root of the R–R interval in seconds. A corrected QT interval of ≥440 ms is abnormal.

Use of the QT Nomogram (Hodges Correction)

Measure the QT interval in either lead V_2 or V_3, where the end of the T wave can usually be clearly distinguished from the beginning of the U wave. If the rate is regular, use the mean rate of the QRS complexes. If the rate is irregular, calculate the rate from the immediately prior R-R cycle, because this cycle determines the subsequent QT interval. Use the numbers you have obtained to classify the QT interval using the nomogram on p 340. Or remember that at heart rates of ≥40 bpm, an observed QT interval ≥480 ms is abnormal.

Prolonged QT Interval

The four major causes of a prolonged QT interval are as follows:

A. Electrolyte Abnormalities: Hypokalemia, hypocalcemia

B. Drugs: Also associated with torsade de pointes.
Class Ia antiarrhythmic agents: Quinidine, procainamide, disopyramide
Class Ic agents: Propafenone
Class III agents: Amiodarone, bretylium, N-acetylprocainamide, sotalol
Antibiotics: Erythromycin, trimethoprim-sulfamethoxazole
Antifungals: Ketoconazole, itraconazole
Chemotherapeutics: Pentamidine, perhaps anthracyclines

TABLE 7–9. VARIOUS CLASSES AND MORPHOLOGIES OF ST-T-U ABNORMALITIES AS SEEN IN LEAD V₄.

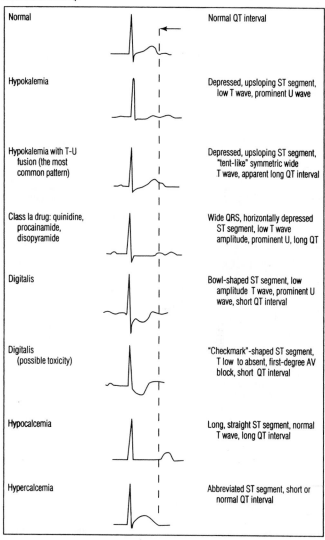

Normal	Normal QT interval
Hypokalemia	Depressed, upsloping ST segment, low T wave, prominent U wave
Hypokalemia with T-U fusion (the most common pattern)	Depressed, upsloping ST segment, "tent-like" symmetric wide T wave, apparent long QT interval
Class Ia drug: quinidine, procainamide, disopyramide	Wide QRS, horizontally depressed ST segment, low T wave amplitude, prominent U, long QT
Digitalis	Bowl-shaped ST segment, low amplitude T wave, prominent U wave, short QT interval
Digitalis (possible toxicity)	"Checkmark"-shaped ST segment, T low to absent, first-degree AV block, short QT interval
Hypocalcemia	Long, straight ST segment, normal T wave, long QT interval
Hypercalcemia	Abbreviated ST segment, short or normal QT interval

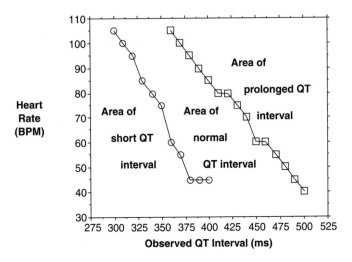

Psychotropic agents: Tricyclic and heterocyclic antidepressants, phenothiazines, haloperidol

Toxins and poisons: Organophosphate insecticides

Miscellaneous: Cisapride, prednisone, probucol, chloral hydrate

C. Congenital Long QT Syndromes: Though rare, a congenital long QT syndrome should be considered in any young patient who presents with syncope or presyncope.

D. Miscellaneous Causes:

Third-degree and sometimes second-degree AV block

At the cessation of ventricular pacing

LVH (usually minor degrees of lengthening)

Myocardial infarction (in the evolutionary stages where there are marked repolarization abnormalities)

Significant active myocardial ischemia

Cerebrovascular accident (subarachnoid hemorrhage)

Hypothermia

Short QT Interval

The five causes of a short QT interval are hypercalcemia, digitalis, thyrotoxicosis, increased sympathetic tone, and genetic abnormality.

O. MISCELLANEOUS ABNORMALITIES

Right-Left Arm Cable Reversal versus Mirror Image Dextrocardia

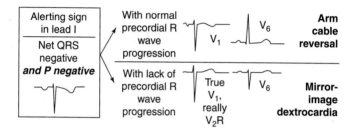

Misplacement of the Right Leg Cable

This error should not occur but it does occur nevertheless. It produces a "far field" signal when one of the bipolar leads (I, II, or III) records the signal between the left and right legs. The lead appears to have no signal except for a tiny deflection representing the QRS complex. There are usually no discernible P waves or T waves. RL–RA cable reversal is shown here.

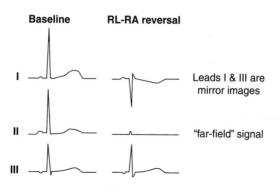

Early Repolarization Normal Variant ST–T Abnormality

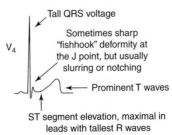

Early repolarization normal variant ST-T abnormality

V_4

Tall QRS voltage

Sometimes sharp "fishhook" deformity at the J point, but usually slurring or notching

Prominent T waves

ST segment elevation, maximal in leads with tallest R waves

Hypothermia

Hypothermia is usually characterized on the ECG by a slow rate, a long QT, and muscle tremor artifact. An Osborn wave is typically present.

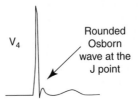

V_4

Rounded Osborn wave at the J point

Acute Pericarditis: Stage I (With PR-Segment Abnormalities)

There is usually widespread ST-segment elevation with concomitant PR-segment depression in the same leads. The PR segment in aVR protrudes above the baseline like a knuckle, reflecting atrial injury.

II

aVR

Differentiating Pericarditis From Early Repolarization

Only lead V_6 is used. If the indicated amplitude ratio A/B is ≥25%, suspect pericarditis (shown on left side). If A/B <25%, suspect early repolarization (shown on right side).

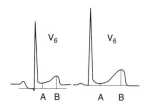

Wolff-Parkinson-White Pattern

The WPW pattern is most commonly manifest as an absent PR segment and initial slurring of the QRS complex in any lead. The lead with the best sensitivity is V_4.

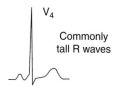

A. **Left Lateral Accessory Pathway:** This typical WPW pattern mimics lateral or posterior myocardial infarction.

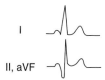

B. **Posteroseptal Accessory Pathway:** This typical WPW pattern mimics inferoposterior myocardial infarction.

COPD Pattern, Lead II

The P-wave amplitude in the inferior leads is equal to that of the QRS complexes.

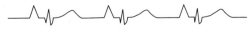

Prominent P waves with low QRS voltage

REFERENCES

Al-Khatib SM: What clinicians should know about the QT interval. JAMA 2003;289:2120. [PMID: 12709470]

Channer K et al: ABC of clinical electrocardiography: Myocardial ischemia. BMJ 2002;324:1023. [PMID: 11976247]

Chauhan VS et al: Supraventricular tachycardia. Med Clin North Am 2001;85:193. [PMID: 11233946]

Delacretaz E: Clinical practice. Supraventricular tachycardia. N Engl J Med 2006;354:1039. [PMID: 16525141]

Edhouse J, Morris F: Broad complex tachycardia—Part 1. BMJ 2002;324:719. [PMID: 11909791]

Evans GT Jr: ECG *Interpretation Cribsheets*, 4th ed. Ring Mountain Press, 1999.

Herring N et al: ECG diagnosis of acute ischemia and infarction: Past, present, and future. QJM 2006;99:219. [PMID: 16495300]

Kusumoto FM: Arrhythmias. In *Cardiovascular Pathophysiology*, FM Kusumoto (editor): Hayes Barton Press, 2004.

Stahmer SA et al: Tachydysrhythmias. Emerg Med Clin North Am 2006;24:11. [PMID: 16308111]

8

Diagnostic Tests in Differential Diagnosis and Diagnostic Algorithms

Chuanyi Mark Lu, MD, Stephen J. McPhee, MD,
Diana Nicoll, MD, PhD, MPA, and Michael Pignone, MD, MPH

HOW TO USE THIS SECTION

This section shows how diagnostic tests can be used in differential diagnosis and difficult diagnostic challenges. Material is presented in algorithmic and/or tabular forms, and contents are listed in alphabetical order by subject.

Abbreviations used throughout this section include the following:

$$
\begin{array}{rcl}
\text{N} & = & \text{Normal} \\
\text{Abn} & = & \text{Abnormal} \\
\text{Pos} & = & \text{Positive} \\
\text{Neg} & = & \text{Negative} \\
\uparrow & = & \text{Increased or high} \\
\downarrow & = & \text{Decreased or low} \\
\text{Occ} & = & \text{Occasional}
\end{array}
$$

Contents

TABLE 8–1. ACID–BASE DISTURBANCE: LABORATORY CHARACTERISTICS OF PRIMARY OR SINGLE ACID–BASE DISTURBANCE.

Disturbance	Acute Primary Change	Partial Compensatory Response	Arterial pH	Serum [K⁺] (meq/L)	Unmeasured Anions (Anion Gap¹)	Clinical Features
Normal	None	None	7.35–7.45	3.5–5.0	12–18	None
Respiratory acidosis	Pco_2 ↑ (CO_2 retention)	↑ HCO_3^-	↓	↑	N	Dyspnea, polypnea, respiratory outflow obstruction, ↑ anterior-posterior chest diameter, rales, wheezes. In severe cases, stupor, disorientation, coma.
Respiratory alkalosis	Pco_2 ↓ (CO_2 depletion)	↓ HCO_3^-	↑	↓	N or ↓	Anxiety, occasional complaint of breathlessness, frequent sighing, lungs usually clear to examination, positive Chvostek and Trousseau signs.
Metabolic acidosis	HCO_3^- depletion	↓ Pco_2	↓	↑ or ↓	N or ↑	Weakness, air hunger, Kussmaul respiration, dry skin and mucous membranes, poor skin turgor. In severe cases, poor coma, hypotension, death.
Metabolic alkalosis	HCO_3^- retention	↑ Pco_2	↑	↓	N	Weakness, positive Chvostek and Trousseau signs, hyporeflexia.

¹Anion gap = $([Na^+]+[K^+])-([HCO_3^-]+[Cl^-])$ = 12–18 meq/L normally.
Reproduced, with permission, from Stobo JD et al (editors): The Principles and Practice of Medicine, 23rd ed. Originally published by Appleton & Lange. Copyright © 1996 by Appleton & Lange.

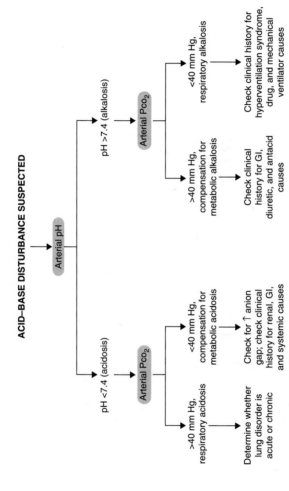

Figure 8–1. ACID–BASE DISTURBANCE: Diagnostic approach. *Reproduced, with permission, from Stobo JD et al (editors): The Principles and Practice of Medicine, 23rd ed. Originally published by Appleton & Lange. Copyright ©1996 by Appleton & Lange.*

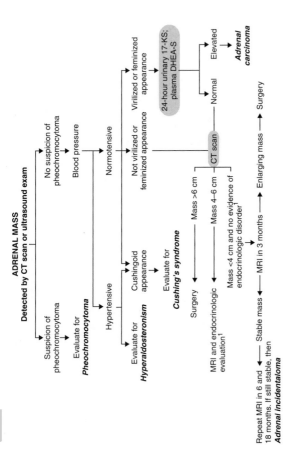

Figure 8–2. ADRENAL MASS: Diagnostic evaluation. **DHEA-S** = dehydroepiandrosterone sulfate; **17-KS** = 17-ketosteroids; **MRI** = magnetic resonance imaging.

[1] Evaluate and exclude Cushing's syndrome, pheochromocytoma, and hyperaldosteronism.

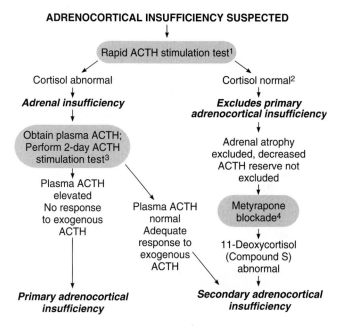

ADRENOCORTICAL INSUFFICIENCY SUSPECTED

Rapid ACTH stimulation test[1]

Cortisol abnormal

Adrenal insufficiency

Obtain plasma ACTH;
Perform 2-day ACTH
stimulation test[3]

Plasma ACTH
elevated
No response
to exogenous
ACTH

Plasma ACTH
normal
Adequate
response to
exogenous
ACTH

*Primary adrenocortical
insufficiency*

Cortisol normal[2]

*Excludes primary
adrenocortical insufficiency*

Adrenal atrophy
excluded, decreased
ACTH reserve not
excluded

Metyrapone
blockade[4]

11-Deoxycortisol
(Compound S)
abnormal

*Secondary adrenocortical
insufficiency*

[1]In the rapid ACTH stimulation test, a baseline cortisol sample is obtained; Cosyntropin, 10–25 mcg, is given IM or IV; and plasma cortisol samples are obtained 30 or 60 minutes later.
[2]The normal response is a cortisol increment >7 mcg/dL. If a cortisol level of >18 mcg/dL is obtained, the response is normal regardless of the increment.
[3]Administer ACTH, 250 mcg IV every 8 hours, as a continuous infusion for 48 hours, and measure daily urinary 17-hydroxycorticosteroids (17-OHCS) or free cortisol excretion and plasma cortisol. Urinary 17-OHCS excretion of >27 mg during the first 24 hours and >47 mg during the second 24 hours is normal. Plasma cortisol >20 mcg/dL at 30 or 60 minutes after infusion is begun and >25 mcg/dL 6–8 hours later is normal.
[4]Metyrapone blockade is performed by giving 2–2.5 g metyrapone orally at 12 midnight. Draw cortisol and 11-deoxycortisol levels at 8 AM. 11-Deoxycortisol level <7 mcg/dL indicates secondary adrenal insufficiency (as long as there is adequate blockade of cortisol synthesis [cortisol level <10 mcg/dL]).

Figure 8–3. ADRENOCORTICAL INSUFFICIENCY: Laboratory evaluation. **ACTH** = adreno-corticotropic hormone.(*Modified, with permission, from Baxter JD, Tyrrell JB: The adrenal cortex. In:* Endocrinology and Metabolism, *3rd ed. Felig P, Baxter JD, Frohman LA [editors].* McGraw-Hill, *1995; and from Harvey AM et al:* The Principles and Practice of Medicine, *22nd ed. Originally published by Appleton & Lange. Copyright © 1988 by The McGraw-Hill Companies, Inc.)*

AMENORRHEA, SECONDARY

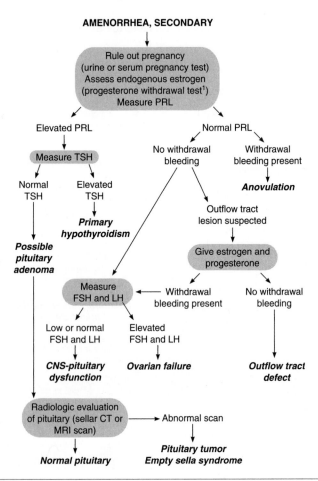

¹Give medroxyprogesterone 5–10 mg orally once daily for 5 days. If withdrawal bleeding ensues thereafter, endogenous estrogen is adequate.

Figure 8–4. AMENORRHEA. Diagnostic evaluation of secondary amenorrhea. **PRL** = prolactin; **TSH** = thyroid-stimulating hormone; **FSH** = follicle-stimulating hormone; **LH** = luteinizing hormone; **CT** = computed tomography; **MRI** = magnetic resonance imaging. (*Modified, with permission, from Greenspan FS, Baxter JD [editors]:* Basic & Clinical Endocrinology, *4th ed. Originally published by Appleton & Lange. Copyright © 1994 by The McGraw-Hill Companies, Inc.*)

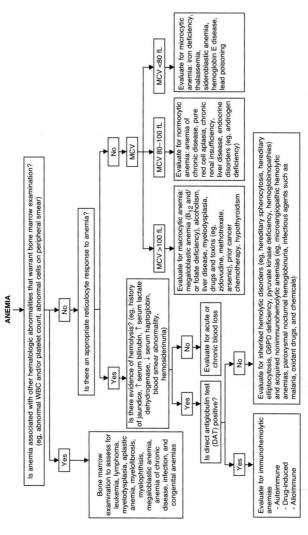

Figure 8–5. ANEMIA: General considerations and initial evaluation. The initial evaluation of anemia should include complete blood cell count, reticulocyte count, and review of peripheral blood smear. **G6PD** = glucose-6-phosphate dehydrogenase; **MCV** = mean corpuscular volume.

TABLE 8–2. ANEMIA: DIAGNOSIS OF COMMON ANEMIAS BASED ON RED CELL INDICES.

Type of Anemia	MCV (fL)	Common Causes	Common Laboratory Abnormalities	Other Clinical Findings
Microcytic, hypochromic	<80	Iron deficiency	Low reticulocyte count, low serum and bone marrow iron, high TIBC, high serum/plasma soluble transferrin receptor (sTfR).	Mucositis, blood loss.
		Thalassemias	Abnormal red cell morphology, normal serum iron levels, abnormal hemoglobin electrophoresis, high hemoglobin A_2 in β-thalassemia minor.	Asian, African, or Mediterranean descent.
		Chronic lead poisoning	Basophilic stippling of RBCs, elevated lead, and free erythrocyte protoporphyrin levels.	Peripheral neuropathy, history of exposure to lead.
		Sideroblastic anemia	High serum iron, ringed sideroblasts in bone marrow.	Dimorphic red cell population with hypochromic red cells on smear.
Normocytic, normochromic	81–100	Acute blood loss	Fecal occult blood test positive if GI bleeding is the underlying cause.	Recent blood loss.
		Hemolysis	Haptoglobin low or absent, reticulocytosis, hyperbilirubinemia, high serum LDH, spherocytes or schistocytes on smear.	Hemoglobinuria, splenomegaly.
		Chronic disease[1]	Low serum iron, TIBC low or low normal, normal sTfR, normal or high bone marrow iron stores with rare or no sideroblasts.	Depends on cause, typically chronic inflammation.

Macrocytic, normochromic	>10[1][2]	Vitamin B_{12} deficiency	Hypersegmented PMNs, macro-ovalocytes, low serum vitamin B_{12} levels, high serum/urine MMA, achlorhydria.	Peripheral neuropathy, glossitis.
		Folate deficiency	Hypersegmented PMNs, macro-ovalocytes, low serum and red cell folate levels.	Alcoholism, malnutrition.
		Liver disease	MCV usually <120 fL; normal serum vitamin B_{12} and folate levels.	Signs of liver disease.
		Reticulocytosis	Marked (>15%) reticulocytosis.	Variable, including acute hemorrhage or hemolysis.

[1]May be microcytic, hypochromic.
[2]If MCV >120–130, vitamin B_{12} or folate deficiency is likely.
MCV = mean corpuscular volume; **MMA** = methylmalonic acid; **TIBC** = total iron-binding capacity, serum; **PMN** = polymorphonuclear cell.

Modified, with permission, from Saunders CE, Ho MT (editors): Current Emergency Diagnosis & Treatment, 4th ed. Originally published by Appleton & Lange. Copyright © 1992 by The McGraw-Hill Companies, Inc.

TABLE 8–3. MICROCYTIC ANEMIA: LABORATORY EVALUATION OF MICROCYTIC, HYPOCHROMIC ANEMIAS.

Diagnosis	MCV (fL)	Serum Iron (mcg/dL)	Iron-binding Capacity (mcg/dL)	Transferrin Saturation (%)	Serum Ferritin (mcg/L)	Free Erythrocyte Protoporphyrin (mcg/dL)	Basophilic Stippling	Bone Marrow Iron Stores
Normal	80–100	50–175	250–460	16–60	16–300	<35	Absent	Present
Iron deficiency anemia	↓	<30	↑	<16	<12	↑	Absent	Absent
Anemia of chronic disease	N or ↓	<30	N or ↓	N or ↓	N or ↑	↑	Absent	Present
Thalassemia minor	↓	N	N	N	N	N	Usually present	Present

Modified, with permission, from Stobo JD et al (editors): The Principles and Practice of Medicine, 23rd ed. Originally published by Appleton & Lange. Copyright © 1996 by Appleton & Lange.

TABLE 8–4. ARTHRITIS: EXAMINATION AND CLASSIFICATION OF SYNOVIAL (JOINT) FLUID.

Type of Joint Fluid	Volume (mL)	Appearance	WBC (per mcL)	PMNs	Gram Stain & Culture	Fluid Glucose (mg/dL)	Comments
Normal	<3.5	Clear, light yellow	<200	<25%	Neg	Equal to serum	Protein 2.0–3.5 g/dL.
Non-inflammatory (Group I)	Often >3.5	Clear, light yellow	<3000	<25%	Neg	Equal to serum	Degenerative joint disease, trauma, avascular necrosis, osteochondritis dissecans, osteo-chondromatosis, neuropathic arthropathy, subsiding or early inflammation, hyper-trophic osteoarthropathy, pigmented villonodular synovitis.
Inflammatory (Group II)	Often >3.5	Cloudy to opaque, dark yellow	3000–100,000	≥50%	Neg	>25, but lower than serum	Protein >3 g/dL. Rheumatoid arthritis, acute crystal-induced synovitis (gout, pseudogout). Reiter syndrome, ankylosing spondylitis, psoriatic arthritis, sarcoidosis, arthritis accompanying ulcerative colitis and Crohn disease, rheumatic fever, SLE, scleroderma; tuberculous, viral, or mycotic infections. Phagocytic inclusions in PMNs suggest rheumatoid arthritis (RA cells). Phagocytosis of leukocytes by macrophages seen in Reiter syndrome.

(continued)

TABLE 8-4. ARTHRITIS: EXAMINATION AND CLASSIFICATION OF SYNOVIAL (JOINT) FLUID. (*CONTINUED*)

Type of Joint Fluid	Volume (mL)	Appearance	WBC (per mcL)	PMNs	Gram Stain & Culture	Fluid Glucose (mg/dL)	Comments
Infectious/ purulent (Group III)	Often >3.5	Cloudy to opaque, dark yellow to green	Usually >40,000, often >100,000	≥90%	Usually positive	<25, much lower than serum	Pyogenic bacterial infection (eg, *Neisseria gonorrhoeae, Staphylococcus aureus*). Bacteria on culture or Gram-stained smear. Most common exception: gonococci seen in only about 25% of cases. WBC count and % PMN lower with infections caused by organisms of low virulence or if antibiotic therapy already started.
Crystal-induced (Group IV)	Often >3.5	Cloudy, turbid, or white-opaque	500–200,000	<90%	Neg	>25, but lower than serum	Crystals present. Crystals diagnostic of gout or pseudogout: gout crystals (urate) show negative birefringence; pseudogout crystals (calcium pyrophosphate) show positive birefringence when red compensator filter is used with polarized light microscopy.
Hemorrhagic (Group V)	Often >3.5	Cloudy, pink to red	Usually >2000	<30%	Neg	Equal to serum	Trauma with or without fracture, hemophilia or other hemorrhagic diathesis, neuropathic arthropathy, pigmented villonodular synovitis, synovioma, hemangioma, and other benign neoplasms. Many RBCs found also. Fat globules strongly suggest intra-articular fracture.

Modified, with permission, from Rodnan GP: Primer on the rheumatic diseases: Appendix III. JAMA 1973;224(5):802. Copyright © 1973 by American Medical Association.

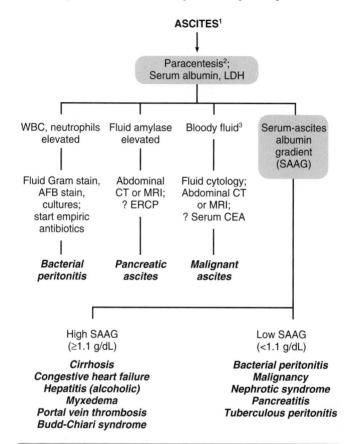

Figure 8–6. ASCITES: Diagnostic evaluation. **CEA** = carcinoembryonic antigen, serum; **CT** = computed tomography; **ERCP** = endoscopic retrograde cholangiopancreatography; **LDH** = lactate dehydrogenase; **MRI** = magnetic resonance imaging; **SAAG** = serum-ascites albumin gradient; ? = consider. (*Modified with permission, from Ferri FF: Clinical Advisor: Instant Diagnosis and Treatment, 4th ed. Mosby, 2002.*)

TABLE 8–5. ASCITES: ASCITIC FLUID PROFILES IN VARIOUS DISEASE STATES.

Diagnosis	Appearance	Fluid Protein (g/dL)	Serum-Ascites Albumin Gradient (SAAG)	Fluid Glucose (mg/dL)	WBC and Differential (per mcL)	RBC (per mcL)	Gram Stain and Culture	Cytology	Comments
Normal	Clear	<3.0		Equal to plasma glucose	<250	Few or none	Neg	Neg	
TRANSUDATES[1]									
Cirrhosis	Clear	<3.0	High[2]	N	<250, MN	Few	Neg	Neg	Occasionally turbid, rarely bloody. Fluid LDH/serum LDH ratio <0.6.
Congestive heart failure	Clear	<2.5	High[2]	N	<250, MN	Few	Neg	Neg	
Nephrotic syndrome	Clear	<2.5	Low[3]	N	<250, MN	Few	Neg	Neg	
Pseudomyxoma peritonei	Gelatinous	<2.5		N	<250	Few	Neg	Occ Pos	
EXUDATES[4]									
Bacterial peritonitis	Cloudy	>3.0	Low[3]	<50 with perforation	>500, PMN	Few	Pos	Neg	Blood cultures frequently positive.
Tuberculous peritonitis	Clear	>3.0	Low[3]	<60	>500, MN	Few, occasionally many	Stain Pos in 25%; culture Pos in 65%	Neg	Occasionally chylous. Peritoneal biopsy positive in 65%.

Malignancy	Clear or bloody	>3.0	Low[3]	<60	>500, MN, PMN	Many	Neg	Pos in 60–90%	Occasionally chylous. Fluid LDH/serum LDH ratio >0.6. Peritoneal biopsy diagnostic.
Pancreatitis	Clear or bloody	>2.5	Low[3]	N	>500, MN, PMN	Many	Neg	Neg	Occasionally chylous. Fluid amylase > 1000 IU/L, sometimes >10,000 IU/L. Fluid amylase > serum amylase.
Chylous ascites	Turbid	Varies, often >2.5		N	Few	Few	Neg	Neg	Fluid TG > 400 mg/dL (turbid). Fluid TG > serum TG.

[1] Transudates have protein concentration <2.5–3.0 g/dL; fluid LDH/serum LDH ratio <0.6 (may be useful in difficult cases).
[2] High = ≥1.1 g/dL.
[3] Low = <1.1 g/dL.
[4] Exudates have fluid protein concentration >2.5–3.0 g/dL; fluid LDH/serum LDH ratio >0.6 (may be useful in difficult cases).
MN = mononuclear cells; **PMN** = polymorphonuclear cells; **TG** = triglycerides.

TABLE 8-6. AUTOANTIBODIES: ASSOCIATIONS WITH CONNECTIVE TISSUE DISEASES.

Suspected Disease State	Test	Primary Disease Association (Sensitivity, Specificity)	Other Disease Associations (Sensitivity)	Comments
CREST syndrome	Anticentromere antibody	CREST (70–90%, high)	Scleroderma (10–15%), Raynaud disease (10–30%).	Predictive value of a positive test is >95% for scleroderma or related disease (CREST, Raynaud). Diagnosis of CREST is made clinically.
Systemic lupus erythematosus (SLE)	Antinuclear antibody (ANA)	SLE (>95%, low)	RA (30–50%), discoid lupus, scleroderma (60%), drug-induced lupus (100%), Sjögren syndrome (80%), miscellaneous inflammatory disorders.	Often used as a screening test; a negative test virtually excludes SLE; a positive test, while nonspecific, increases posttest probability. Titer does not correlate with disease activity.
	Anti-double-stranded DNA antibody (anti-ds-DNA)	SLE (60–70%, high)	Lupus nephritis, rarely RA, CTD, usually in low titer.	Predictive value of a positive test is >90% for SLE if present in high titer; a decreasing titer may correlate with worsening renal disease. Titer generally correlates with disease activity.
	Anti-Smith antibody (anti-Sm)	SLE (30–40%, high)		SLE specific. A positive test substantially increases posttest probability of SLE. Test rarely indicated.
Mixed connective tissue disease (MCTD)	Anti-ribonucleoprotein antibody (RNP)	MCTD (95–100%, low) Scleroderma (20–30%, low)	SLE (30%), Sjögren syndrome, RA (10%), discoid lupus (20–30%).	A negative test essentially excludes MCTD; a positive test in high titer, though nonspecific, increases posttest probability of MCTD.

Disease	Test	Associated disease	Other associated conditions	Comments
Rheumatoid arthritis (RA)	Rheumatoid factor (RF)	Rheumatoid arthritis (50–90%)	Other rheumatic diseases, chronic infections, some malignancies, some healthy individuals, elderly patients.	Titer does not correlate with disease activity.
	Anti-cyclic citrullinated peptide (CCP) IgG	Rheumatoid arthritis (70%)		Approximately 70% of patients with RA are positive for CCP IgG, whereas only 2% of random blood donors and disease controls are positive. The diagnostic value of antibodies to CCP in juvenile rheumatoid arthritis patients has not been determined.
Scleroderma	Anti-Scl-70 antibody	Scleroderma (15–20%, high)		Predictive value of a positive test is >95% for scleroderma.
Sjögren syndrome	Anti-SSA/Ro	Sjögren syndrome (60–70%, low)	SLE (30–40%), RA (10%), subacute cutaneous lupus, vasculitis.	Useful in counseling women of childbearing age with known CTD, because a positive test is associated with a small but real risk of neonatal SLE and congenital heart block.
Wegener granulomatosis	Antineutrophil cytoplasmic	Wegener granulomatosis (systemic necrotizing vasculitis) (56–96%, high)	Crescentic glomerulonephritis or other systemic vasculitis (eg, polyarteritis nodosa).	Ability of this assay to reflect disease activity remains unclear.

CTD = connective tissue disease; **SSA** = Sjögren syndrome A antibody; **CREST** = calcinosis, Raynaud phenomenon, esophageal dysmotility, sclerodactyly and telangiectasia.
Modified, with permission, from Stobo JD et al (editors): The Principles and Practice of Medicine, 23rd ed. Originally published by Appleton & Lange, 1996. Copyright 1996 by Appleton & Lange; from White RH, Robbins DL: Clinical significance and interpretation of antinuclear antibodies. West J Med 1987;147:210; and from Tan EM: Autoantibodies to nuclear antigens (ANA): Their immunobiology and medicine. Adv Immunol 1982;33:173.

TABLE 8–7. BLEEDING DISORDERS: LABORATORY EVALUATION.

Suspected Diagnosis	Platelet Count	PT	PTT	TT	Further Diagnostic Tests
Idiopathic thrombocytopenic purpura, drug effect, bone marrow suppression	↓	N	N	N	Platelet antibody, bone marrow examination.
Disseminated intravascular coagulation	↓	↑	↑	↑	Fibrinogen assay, D-dimers.
Platelet function defect, salicylates, or uremia	N	N	N	N	PFA-100 CT, platelet aggregation, blood urea nitrogen, creatinine.
von Willebrand disease	N	N	↑ or N	N	PFA-100 CT, factor VIII assay, vWF antigen & activity, vWF multimer analysis.
Factor VII deficiency or inhibitor	N	↑	N	N	Factor VII assay (normal plasma should correct PT if no inhibitor is present).
Factor V, X, II, I deficiencies as in liver disease or with anticoagulants	N	↑	↑	N or ↑	Liver function tests.
Factor VIII (hemophilia), IX, XI, or XII deficiencies or inhibitor	N	N	↑	N	Inhibitor screen, individual factor assays, Bethesda assay.
Factor XIII deficiency	N	N	N	N	5M urea solubility test (screen test); factor XIII assay.
Increase in fibrinolytic activity	N	N	N	N	Euglobulin clot lysis time (screening test), α₂-antiplasmin, plasminogen activator inhibitor-1 (PAI-1)

Note: In approaching patients with bleeding disorders, try to distinguish clinically between platelet disorders (eg, patient has petechiae, mucosal bleeding) and factor deficiency states (eg, patient has hemarthrosis).

PFA-100CT = platelet function analyzer-100CT; **PT** = prothrombin time; **PTT** = activated partial thromboplastin time; **TT** = thrombin time.

Modified, with permission, from Tierney LM Jr, McPhee SJ, Papadakis MA (editors): Current Medical Diagnosis & Treatment 2005. Originally published by Appleton & Lange. Copyright © 2005 by The McGraw-Hill Companies, Inc.; and from Stobo JD et al (editors): The Principles and Practice of Medicine, 23rd ed. Originally published by Appleton & Lange. Copyright © 1996 by Appleton & Lange.

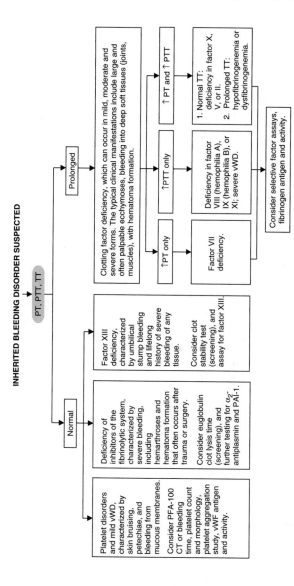

Figure 8–7. BLEEDING DISORDERS: Evaluation of suspected inherited bleeding disorders. **PAI-1** = plasminogen activator inhibitor 1; **PFA-100 CT** = platelet function analyzer-100 closure time; **PT** = prothrombin time; **PTT** = activated partial thromboplastin time; **TT** = thrombin time; **vWD** = von Willebrand disease; **vWF** = von Willebrand factor.

TABLE 8–8. CEREBROSPINAL FLUID (CSF): CSF PROFILES IN CENTRAL NERVOUS SYSTEM DISEASES.

Diagnosis	Appearance	Opening Pressure (mm H_2O)	RBC (per mcL)	WBC & Diff (per mcL)	CSF Glucose (mg/dL)	CSF Protein (mg/dL)	Smears	Culture	Comments
Normal	Clear, colorless	70–200	0	≤5 MN, 0 PMN	45–85	15–45	Neg	Neg	
Bacterial meningitis	Cloudy	↑↑↑	0	200–20,000, mostly PMN	<45	>50	Gram stain Pos	Pos	PMN predominance may be seen early in course.
Tuberculous meningitis	N or cloudy	↑↑	0	100–1000, mostly MN	<45	>50	AFB stain Pos	±	Counterimmunoelectrophoresis or latex agglutination may be diagnostic. CSF and serum cryptococcal antigen positive in cryptococcal meningitis.
Fungal meningitis	N or cloudy	N or ↑	0	100–1000, mostly MN	<45	>50		±	
Viral (aseptic) meningitis	N	N or ↑	0	100–1000, mostly MN	45–85	N or ↑	Neg	Neg	RBC count may be elevated in herpes simplex encephalitis. Glucose may be decreased in herpes simplex or mumps infections. Viral cultures may be helpful.

	Appearance			Cells	Glucose	Protein	Cytology	Serology	Comments
Parasitic meningitis	N or cloudy	N or ↑	0	100–1000, mostly MN, E	<45	N or ↑	Amebae may be seen on wet smear	±	
Carcinomatous meningitis	N or cloudy	N or ↑	0	N or 100–1000, mostly MN	<45	N or ↑	Cytology Pos	Neg	
Cerebral lupus erythematosus	N	N or ↑	0	N or ↑, mostly MN	N	N or ↑	Neg	Neg	
Subarachnoid hemorrhage	Pink-red, supernatant yellow	↑	↑ crenated or fresh	N or 100–1000, mostly PMN	N or ↓	N or ↑	Neg	Neg	Blood in all tubes equally. Pleocytosis and low glucose sometimes seen several days after subarachnoid hemorrhage, reflecting chemical meningitis caused by subarachnoid blood.
"Traumatic" tap	Bloody, supernatant clear	N	↑↑↑ fresh	↑	N	↑	Neg	Neg	Most blood in tube #1, least blood in tube #4.

(continued)

TABLE 8–8. CEREBROSPINAL FLUID (CSF): CSF PROFILES IN CENTRAL NERVOUS SYSTEM DISEASES. (CONTINUED)

Diagnosis	Appearance	Opening Pressure (mm H$_2$O)	RBC (per mcL)	WBC & Diff (per mcL)	CSF Glucose (mg/dL)	CSF Protein (mg/dL)	Smears	Culture	Comments
Spirochetal, early, acute syphilitic meningitis	Clear to turbid	↑	0	25–2000, mostly MN	15–75	>50	Neg	Neg	PMN may predominate early. Positive serum RPR or VDRL. CSF VDRL insensitive. If clinical suspicion is high, institute treatment despite negative CSF VDRL.
Late CNS syphilis	Clear	Usually N	0	N or ↑	N	N or ↑	Neg	Neg	CSF VDRL insensitive.
"Neighborhood" meningeal reaction	Clear or turbid, often xantho-chromic	Variable, usually N	Variable	↑	N	N or ↑	Neg	Usually Neg	May occur in mastoiditis, brain abscess, sinusitis, septic thrombophlebitis, brain tumor, intrathecal drug therapy.
Hepatic encephalopathy	N	N	0	≤5	N	N	Neg	Neg	CSF glutamine >15 mg/dL.
Uremia	N	Usually ↑	0	N or ↑	N or ↑	N or ↑	Neg	Neg	
Diabetic coma	N	Low	0	N or ↑	↑	N	Neg	Neg	

MN = mononuclear cells (lymphocytes or monocytes); **PMN** = polymorphonuclear cells; **E** = eosinophils; **CNS** = central nervous system; **WBC** = white blood cells.

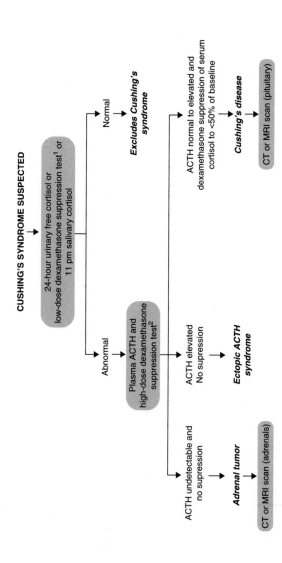

Figure 8–8. CUSHING SYNDROME: Diagnostic evaluation. **ACTH** = adrenocorticotropic hormone; **CT** = computed tomography; **MRI** = magnetic resonance imaging.

[1]Low dose: Give 1 mg dexamethasone orally at 11 PM; draw serum cortisol at 8 AM the next morning. Normally, AM cortisol is <5 mcg/dL.
[2]High dose: Give 4mg or 8 mg dexamethasone orally at 11 PM; draw serum cortisol at 8 AM the next morning, and the result is reported in % of baseline.

TABLE 8–9. GENETIC DISEASES: MOLECULAR DIAGNOSTIC TESTING.

Test/Range/Collection	Physiologic Basis	Interpretation	Comments
Breast cancer *BRCA1* and *BRCA2* mutations Blood Lavender $$$$	Mutations in two genes, *BRCA1* and *BRCA2*, are the major cause of familial early-onset breast cancer. A mutation in either gene confers an 80–90% lifetime risk of breast cancer. Although many mutations have been reported in *BRCA1* and *BRCA2*, three mutations found in Ashkenazi Jews have carrier frequencies high enough to warrant a preliminary screen before comprehensive and expensive testing such as DNA sequencing.	This assay will detect the 185 del AG and 5382 ins C mutations in *BRCA1* and the 6174 del T mutation in *BRCA2*. These three mutations have a combined carrier frequency of approximately 1.7% in the Ashkenazi Jewish population.	Oncogene 2000;19:6159. [PMID: 11156530] Semin Cancer Biol 2001;11:375. [PMID: 11562180]
Cystic fibrosis mutation PCR + reverse dot blot Blood Lavender $$$$	Cystic fibrosis is caused by a mutation in the cystic fibrosis transmembrane regulator gene (*CFTR*). Over 800 mutations have been found, with the most common being ΔF508, present in 68% of cases.	Test specificity approaches 100%, so a positive result should be considered diagnostic of a cystic fibrosis mutation. Because of the wide range of mutations, an assay for the F508 mutation alone is 68% sensitive. Screening for 64 mutations provides a sensitivity of 70–95% in all U.S. ethnic groups except Asians; and >81% when the U.S. population is considered as a whole. The test can distinguish between heterozygous carriers and homozygous patients.	Cystic fibrosis is the most common inherited disease in North American Caucasians, affecting 1 in 2500 births. Caucasians have a carrier frequency of 1 in 25. The disease is autosomal recessive. Carrier screening might be offered to individuals and couples in high-risk groups (eg, Ashkenazi Jews, central or northern Europeans), one partner with cystic fibrosis, and individuals with a family history of cystic fibrosis) who seek preconception counseling, infertility care, or prenatal care. Clin Perinatol 2001;28:383. [PMID: 11499059]

Deafness nonsyndromic recessive connexin 26 mutations Blood Lavender or blue $$$$	The connexins are a family of proteins present in gap junctions of adherent cells. A common frameshift-mutation (35 del G) in connexin 26, found to occur at a carrier frequency of 1 in 35 to 1 in 79 in Europe, segregates worldwide in families with nonsyndromic recessive deafness. Another frameshift mutation (167 del T) is present at a carrier frequency of 1 in 25 among Ashkenazi-Jewish individuals.	This test detects both mutations. Both are deleterious when they occur either in homozygous or compound heterozygous forms.	Genet Med 2001;3:168. [PMID: 11388756] Pediatrics 2001;107:280. [PMID: 11158459] Clin Chem 2002;48:1121. [PMID: 12089190]
Dementia, frontotemporal (FTD) tau gene mutations Blood Lavender $$$$	The microtubule-associated protein, tau, located on chromosome 17q21, coassembles with tubulin to form microtubules. Tau is mostly found in axons and when hyperphosphorylated appears to form tangles of paired helical filaments, which can damage the neuronal cytoskeleton and lead to neurodegeneration. Mutations in the gene encoding tau are found in individuals with frontotemporal dementia and pallidopontonigral degeneration.	This test detects three mutations, two missense mutations commonly found in the *tau* gene (P301L, A279L), and a splice isoform mutant (IVS 10, 14C to T).	Brain Res Rev 2000;32:181. [PMID: 10751668] J R Soc Med 2002;95:171. [PMID: 11934905] Annu Rev Neurosci 2001;24:1121. [PMID: 11520930] Med Clin North Am 2002;86:501. [PMID: 12168557]

(continued)

TABLE 8–9. GENETIC DISEASES: MOLECULAR DIAGNOSTIC TESTING. (CONTINUED)

Test/Range/Collection	Physiologic Basis	Interpretation	Comments
Factor II (prothrombin) G20210A mutation Blood Lavender $$$$	The factor II (prothrombin) 20210A mutation is a common genetic risk factor for thrombosis and is associated with elevated prothrombin levels. Higher concentrations of prothrombin lead to increased rates of thrombin generation, resulting in excessive growth of fibrin clots. It is an autosomal dominant disorder, with heterozygotes being at a 3- to 11-fold greater risk for thrombosis. Although homozygosity is rare, inheritance of two G20210A mutations would further increase the risk for developing thrombosis. The estimated frequency of FII G20210A in white populations is between 1% and 6%.	Positive in: Hypercoagulability secondary to FII (prothrombin) G20210A mutation (sensitivity and specificity approach 100%).	If a patient is heterozygous for both the prothrombin G20210A and the factor V Leiden mutation, the combined heterozygosity leads to an earlier onset of thrombosis and tends to be more severe than single-gene heterozygosity. Polymerase chain reaction (PCR) is the most commonly used method for the detection of FII G20210A mutation. Arch Intern Med 2006;166:729. [PMID: 16606808] Mol Genet Metab 2005;86:91. [PMID: 16185908] Br J Haematol 2001;113:630. [PMID: 11380448]
Factor V (Leiden) mutation Blood Lavender $$$$	The Leiden mutation is a single-base mutation (G1691A) in the Factor V gene, leading to an amino acid substitution (Arg506Glu) at one of the sites where coagulation Factor V is cleaved by activated protein C (APC). This mutation results in a substantially reduced anticoagulant response to APC, because FVa$_{Leiden}$ is inactivated about 10 times more slowly than normal FVa. The frequency of FV$_{Leiden}$ in white populations is between 2–15%. Factor V mutations may be present in up to half of the cases of unexplained venous thrombosis and are seen in more than 90% of patients with APC resistance.	Positive in: Hypercoagulability secondary to Factor V$_{Leiden}$ mutation (sensitivity and specificity approach 100%).	The Factor V Leiden mutation is the most common genetic risk factor for thrombosis and accounts for >90% of cases with APC resistance. The presence of the mutation is only a risk factor for thrombosis, not an absolute marker for disease. Homozygotes have a 50- to 100-fold increase in risk of thrombosis (relative to the general population), and heterozygotes have a 7-fold increase in risk. Polymerase chain reaction (PCR) is the most commonly used method for the detection of gene mutation. Arch Intern Med 2006;166:729. [PMID: 16606808] Mol Genet Metab 2005;86:91. [PMID: 16185908] Lancet 1994;343:1361;1535. [PMID: 7910348;7911872]

| **Familial adenomatous polyposis (FAP)**

PCR, Sequencing

Lavender
$$$$ | Familial adenomatous polyposis is an autosomal dominant condition, which predisposes the mutation carrier to colorectal cancer in early adulthood. The condition is characterized by hundreds to thousands of adenomatous polyps in the colon that usually develop in the second to third decade of life. A milder condition, termed Attenuated FAP (AFAP), with patients having fewer polyps and an older age of onset. FAP has been linked to germline mutations of the APC gene that encodes a protein with 2,843 amino acids that has important functions in the regulation of cell growth. | A PCR-based assay is used to amplify all exons of the APC gene, and direct sequence analysis of PCR products corresponding to the entire APC coding region is performed.
The testing is used only to confirm clinical diagnosis of FAP and AFAP and to identify affected but asymptomatic family members in FAP/AFAP families in which a familial mutation has been identified. | Numerous germline mutations have been located between codons 156 and 2011 of the APC gene. Mutations spanning the region between codons 543 and 1309 are strongly associated with congenital hypertrophy of retinal pigment epithelium. Mutations between codons 1310 and 2011 are associated with increased risk of desmoid tumors. Mutations at codon 1309 are associated with early development of colorectal cancer. Mutations between codons 976 and 1067 are associated with increased risk of duodenal adenomas. The cumulative frequency of extracolonic manifestations is highest for mutations between codons 976 and 1067.
J Clin Oncol 2003;21:1698. [PMID: 12721244] |
| **Fragile X syndrome**

PCR, Southern blot

Blood, cultured amniocytes

Lavender
$$$$ | Fragile X syndrome results from a mutation in the familial mental retardation–1 gene (FMRI), located at Xq27.3. Fully symptomatic patients have abnormal methylation of the gene (which blocks transcription) during oogenesis. The gene contains a variable number of repeating CGG sequences and, as the number of sequences increases, the probability of abnormal methylation increases. The number of copies increases with subsequent generations so that women who are unaffected carriers may have offspring who are affected. | Normal patients have 6–52 CGG repeat sequences. Patients with 52–230 repeat sequences are asymptomatic carriers. Patients with more than 230 repeat sequences are very likely to have abnormal methylation and to be symptomatic. | Fragile X syndrome is the most common cause of inherited mental retardation, occurring in 1 in 1000–1500 men and 1 in 2000–2500 women. Full mutations can show variable penetration in females, but most such women will be at least mildly retarded.
Genet Test 2000;4:289. [PMID:11142761]
Diagn Mol Pathol 2001;10:34. [PMID: 11277393]
Expert Rev Mol Diagn 2001;1:226. [PMID: 11901818]
Health Technol Assess 2001;5:1. [PMID: 11262423] |

(continued)

TABLE 8–9. GENETIC DISEASES: MOLECULAR DIAGNOSTIC TESTING. (CONTINUED)

Test/Range/Collection	Physiologic Basis	Interpretation	Comments
Hemochromatosis, hereditary Blood Lavender $$$	Hereditary hemochromatosis is an autosomal recessive disorder of iron metabolism that varies in clinical severity. Three *HFE* gene mutations (C282Y, H63D, and S65C) have been described in the majority of patients with hemochromatosis.	Homozygosity for the C282Y mutation is responsible for up to 90% of hemochromatosis patients. The estimated penetrance is 80% for men and 35% for women over 40. Compound heterozygosity (C282Y/H63D or C282Y/S65C) may cause hemochromatosis, but the penetrance is very low. Homozygous H63D genotypes (H63D/H63D) rarely show symptoms of hemochromatosis. Heterozygotes for C282Y (C282Y/WT), H63D (H63D/WT), or S65C (S65C/WT) are not significantly associated with hemochromatosis.	Annu Rev Med 2006;57:331. [PMID 16409153] Clin Gastroenterol Hepatol 2005; 3:945. [PMID 16234038]
Hemophilia A Southern blot Blood, cultured amniocytes Lavender $$$	Approximately half of severe hemophilia A cases are caused by an inversion mutation within the factor VIII gene. The resulting rearrangement of BCL1 sites can be detected by Southern blot hybridization assays.	Test specificity approaches 100%, so a positive result should be considered diagnostic of a hemophilia A inversion mutation. Because of a variety of mutations, however, test sensitivity is only about 50%.	Hemophilia A is one of the most common X-linked diseases in humans, affecting 1 in 5000 men. Haemophilia 2001;7:20. [PMID: 11136376] J Biochem Biophys Meth 2001: 47:39. [PMID: 11179760] J Postgrad Med 2001;47:274. [PMID: 11182649] Thromb Haemost 2001;85:580. [PMID: 11341489]
Huntington disease PCR + Southern blot Blood, cultured amniocytes, or buccal cells Lavender $$$	Huntington disease is an inherited neurodegenerative disorder associated with an autosomal dominant mutation on chromosome 4. The disease is highly penetrant, but symptoms (disordered movements, cognitive decline, and emotional disturbance) are often not expressed until middle age. The mutation results in the expansion of a CAG trinucleotide repeat sequence within the gene.	Normal patients have fewer than 34 CAG repeats, whereas patients with disease usually have more than 37 repeats and may have 80 or more. Occasional affected patients can be seen with "high normal" (32–34) numbers of repeats. Tests showing 34–37 repeats are indeterminate.	Huntington disease testing involves ethical dilemmas. Counseling is recommended before testing. Hum Mutat 1999;13:232. [PMID: 10090478] Clin Genet 2001;60:442. [PMID: 11846736]

Kennedy disease/spinal and bulbar muscular atrophy (KD/SBMA) PCR, Southern blot, sequencing Lavender $$$$	The disease is a degenerative neuromuscular disorder. Familial and sporadic cases are caused by expansion of a CAG trinucleotide repeat in exon 1 of the androgen receptor gene.	Normal individuals have up to 30 CAG repeats; patients with KD/SBMA have ≥ 40 CAG repeats (sensitivity >99%).	Vitam Horm 2002;65:127. [PMID 12481545]
Myotonic dystrophy (MD) PCR, Southern blot, sequencing Lavender $$$$	The most common mutation associated with DM1 is expansion of the trinucleotide repeat CTG in the *DMPK* gene, and for DM2, the expansion of the CCTG repeat in the *PROMM* gene.	Affected individuals have 50 to several thousands repeats.	Am J Hum Genet 2004;74:793. [PMID 15065017]
Neurofibromatosis (NF): von Recklinghausen disease (NF1) and Bilateral acoustic NF (NF2) PCR, Southern blot Lavender $$$$	NF1 is one of the most common genetic disorders of humans (1 in 3500). The *NF1* gene is located at chromosome region 17q11.2 and codes for the neurofibromin protein. Mutations in the *merlin* gene are responsible for NF2, which is characterized by bilateral schwannomas.	The mutations tested by the DNA analysis are laboratory-dependent. Clinical correlation is important.	Cancer Invest 2003;2:897. [PMID 14735694] Int J Clin Pract 2003;57:698. [PMID 14627181]

(continued)

TABLE 8–9. GENETIC DISEASES: MOLECULAR DIAGNOSTIC TESTING. (*CONTINUED*)

Test/Range/Collection	Physiologic Basis	Interpretation	Comments
Niemann Pick disease PCR, sequencing Lavender $$$$	Three mutations in the acid sphingomyelinase (*SMPD1*) gene account for >94% of cases of type A disease that results in severe neurologic impairment in infancy and childhood. For type C disease, mutational analysis (*NPC1* or *NPC2/HE1* gene) is also available.	The combination of DNA and biochemical (sphingomyelinase activity) analyses improves the detection rate of the disease.	Curr Opin Hematol 2000;7:48. [PMID 10608504] Prenat Diagn 2002;22:630. [PMID 12124701]
Phenylketonuria (PKU) PCR, Southern blot Lavender $$$$	The severity of the disease correlates with extent of mutations of the phenylalanine hydroxylase (*PAH*) gene. Phenylalanine hydroxylase activity determines the type of replacement therapy.	More than 400 point mutations in the PAH gene have been reported, and thus direct sequencing the entire coding regions of the gene may be necessary.	Hum Mutat 2003;21:357. [PMID 12655545]

Prader-Willi syndrome, Angelman syndrome		
Blood Lavender $$$$	Prader-Willi syndrome (PWS) and Angelman syndrome (AS) are clinically different diseases related at the molecular level. They are caused by loss of function mutations in two chromosomal regions located close to each other on chromosome 15. An interstitial deletion of 15q11-13 is found in about 70% of patients with PWS or AS. PWS results when the deletion affects the paternal chromosome, and AS occurs when it affects the maternal chromosome. A DNA probe from the affected region is used to determine the origin of the deletion by Southern blot analysis. In about 33% of patients with PWS and 20–30% with AS, no deletion can be found. Instead, uniparental disomy (UPD) may be found resulting in either two maternal or two paternal copies of chromosome 15. In 1–2% of patients with PWS and 20% of patients with AS, neither a deletion nor UPD can be found.	This test detects both the deletion and UPD defects in PWS and AS.	Brain Res Bull 2002;57:109. [PMID: 11827743] Trends Endocrinol Metab 2004;15:12. [PMID: 14693421]

(continued)

TABLE 8–9. GENETIC DISEASES: MOLECULAR DIAGNOSTIC TESTING. (*CONTINUED*)

Test/Range/Collection	Physiologic Basis	Interpretation	Comments
Tay-Sachs disease PCR, Sequencing Lavender $$$$	Tay-Sachs disease is an autosomal recessive disease caused by a deficiency of β-hexosaminidase A. Mutations in the α-subunit of hexosaminidase A are responsible for the enzyme deficiency. More than 75 mutations of the α-subunit gene have been described.	The mutations tested by the DNA analysis are laboratory-dependent. The combination of DNA and biochemical analyses improves the detection rate of the disease.	Arch Neurol 2004;61:1466. [PMID 15364698] Br J Haematol 2005;128:413. [PMID 15686451]

(continued)

α-Thalassemia	A deletion mutation in the α-globin gene region of chromosome 16 due to unequal crossing-over events can lead to defective synthesis of the α-globin chain of hemoglobin. Normally, there are two copies of the α-globin gene on each chromosome 16, and the severity of disease increases with the number of defective genes.	This assay is highly specific (approaches 100%). Sensitivity, however, can vary because detection of different mutations may require the use of different probes. α-Thalassemia due to point mutations may not be detected.	Patients with one deleted gene are usually normal or very slightly anemic; patients with two deletions usually have hypochromic microcytic anemia; patients with three deletions have elevated hemoglobin H and moderately severe hemolytic anemia; patients with four deletions generally die in utero with hydrops fetalis.
PCR + Southern blot			The most clinically significant situations arise when both parents are carriers for a deletion that encompasses both α-globin genes (cis deletion), as seen mostly in Southeast Asian and Filipino populations. Each offspring of such carriers has a 25% risk of hydrops fetalis.
Blood, cultured amniocytes, chorionic villi			
Lavender			Less deleterious effects arise from chromosomes of Mediterranean and black ancestries. These chromosomes usually carry one α-globin gene deletion per chromosome. Offspring of carriers of a two α-globin gene deletion and single α-gene deletion are at risk for Hb H disease.
$$$$			Am J Hematol 1998;58:306. [PMID: 9692395] Baillieres Clin Haematol 1998;11:215. [PMID: 10872479] Br J Haematol 2000;108:295. [PMID: 10691858]

(continued)

TABLE 8–9. GENETIC DISEASES: MOLECULAR DIAGNOSTIC TESTING. (CONTINUED)

Test/Range/Collection	Physiologic Basis	Interpretation	Comments
β-Thalassemia PCR + reverse dot blot Blood, chorionic villi, cultured amniocytes Lavender $$$$	β-Thalassemia results from a mutation in the gene encoding the β-globin subunit of hemoglobin A (which is composed of a pair of α chains and a pair of β chains). A relative excess of α-globin chains precipitates within red blood cells, causing hemolysis and anemia. Over 300 different mutations have been described; testing usually covers a panel of the more common mutations. The test can distinguish between heterozygous and homozygous individuals.	Test specificity approaches 100%, so a positive result should be considered diagnostic of a thalassemia mutation. Because of the large number of mutations, sensitivity can be poor. A panel with the 43 most common mutations has a sensitivity that approaches 95%.	β-Thalassemia is very common; about 3% of the world's population are carriers. The incidence is increased in persons of Mediterranean, African, and Asian descent. The mutations may vary from population to population, and different testing panels may be needed for patients of different ethnicities. Baillieres Clin Haematol 1998;11:215. [PMID: 10872479] Prenat Diagn 1999;19:428. [PMID: 10360511] Hum Mutat 2002;19:287. [PMID: 11857746]

PCR (polymerase chain reaction) is a method for amplifying a particular DNA sequence in a specimen, facilitating detection by hybridization-based assay (eg., Southern blot, reverse dot blot); **Southern blot** is a molecular hybridization technique whereby DNA is extracted from the sample and digested by different restriction enzymes, and the resulting fragments are separated by electrophoresis and identified by labeled probes; **reverse dot blot** is a molecular hybridization technique in which a specific oligonucleotide probe is bound to a solid membrane prior to reaction with PCR-amplified DNA.

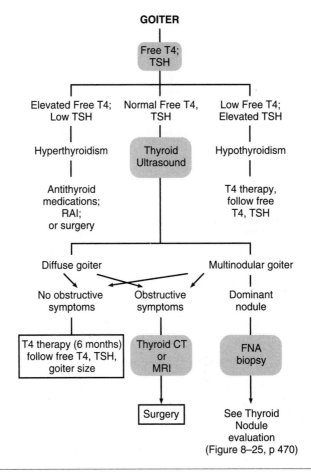

Figure 8–9. GOITER: Diagnostic evaluation and management strategy. **CT** = computed tomography; **FNA** = fine-needle aspiration; **MRI** = magnetic resonance imaging; **RAI** = radioactive iodine; **T₄** = L-thyroxine; **TSH** = thyroid-stimulating hormone. (*Modified, with permission, from Goldman L, Bennett JC [editors]. Cecil Textbook of Medicine, 21st ed. Saunders, 2000.*)

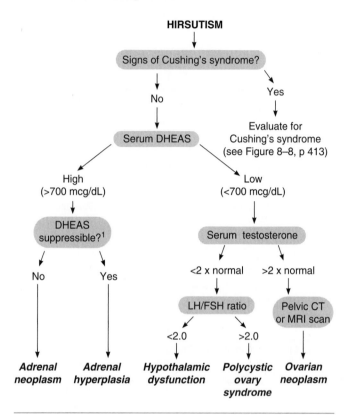

HIRSUTISM

Signs of Cushing's syndrome?

No → Serum DHEAS

Yes → Evaluate for Cushing's syndrome (see Figure 8–8, p 413)

Serum DHEAS

High (>700 mcg/dL) → DHEAS suppressible?[1]

Low (<700 mcg/dL) → Serum testosterone

DHEAS suppressible?[1]
- No → **Adrenal neoplasm**
- Yes → **Adrenal hyperplasia**

Serum testosterone
- <2 x normal → LH/FSH ratio
- >2 x normal → Pelvic CT or MRI scan

LH/FSH ratio
- <2.0 → **Hypothalamic dysfunction**
- >2.0 → **Polycystic ovary syndrome**

Pelvic CT or MRI scan → **Ovarian neoplasm**

---

[1]DHEAS <170 mcg/dL after dexamethasone 0.5 mg orally every 6 hours for 5 days, with DHEAS repeated on the fifth day.

Figure 8–10. HIRSUTISM: Evaluation of hirsutism in females. Exceptions occur that do not fit this algorithm. **CT** = computed tomography; **DHEAS** = dehydroepiandrosterone sulfate; **FSH** = follicle-stimulating hormone; **LH** = luteinizing hormone. (*Reproduced, with permission, from Fitzgerald PA [editor]: Handbook of Clinical Endocrinology, 2nd ed. Originally published by Appleton & Lange. Copyright © 1992 by The McGraw-Hill Companies, Inc.*)

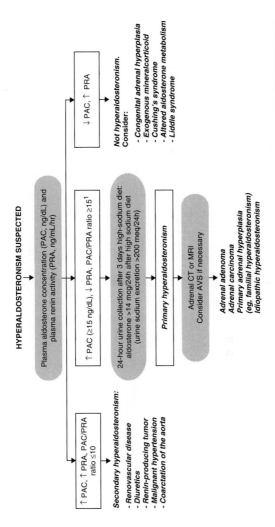

HYPERALDOSTERONISM SUSPECTED

Plasma aldosterone concentration (PAC, ng/dL) and plasma renin activity (PRA, ng/mL/hr)

↑ PAC, ↑ PRA, PAC/PRA ratio ≤10

Secondary hyperaldosteronism:
- *Renovascular disease*
- *Diuretics*
- *Renin-producing tumor*
- *Malignant hypertension*
- *Coarctation of the aorta*

↑ PAC (≥15 ng/dL), ↓ PRA, PAC/PRA ratio ≥15[1]

24-hour urine collection after 3 days high-sodium diet: aldosterone >14 mcg/24h after high sodium diet (urine sodium excretion >200 meq/24h)

Primary hyperaldosteronism

Adrenal CT or MRI
Consider AVS if necessary

Adrenal adenoma
Adrenal carcinoma
Primary adrenal hyperplasia
(eg, familial hyperaldosteronism)
Idiopathic hyperaldosteronism

↓ PAC, ↑ PRA

Not hyperaldosteronism.
Consider:
- *Congenital adrenal hyperplasia*
- *Exogenous mineralcorticoid*
- *Cushing's syndrome*
- *Altered aldosterone metabolism*
- *Liddle syndrome*

[1]The cutoff for a "high" PAC/PRA ratio is laboratory-dependent and, more specifically, PRA assay-dependent, and therefore an increased PAC is part of the diagnostic requirement.

Figure 8–11. HYPERALDOSTERONISM: Laboratory evaluation of suspected hyperaldosteronism. **AVS** = adrenal venous sampling; **CT** = computed tomography; **MRI** = magnetic resonance imaging; **PAC** = plasma aldosterone concentration; **PRA** = plasma renin activity.

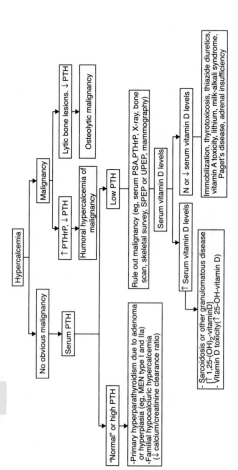

[1] "Normal" PTH in presence of hypercalcemia is inappropriate and indicative of primary hyperparathyroidism (see Figure 9–8, p 494).

[2] PTH-related protein is high in solid tumors that cause hypercalcemia.

[3] To exclude coexistent primary hyperparathyroidism.

Figure 8–12. HYPERCALCEMIA: Diagnostic approach to hypercalcemia. **PTH** = parathyroid hormone (measured by intact PTH assay), **PTHrP** = PTH related protein, **PSA** = prostate-specific antigen, **SPEP** = serum protein electrophoresis, **UPEP** = urine protein electrophoresis. (Modified, with permission, from Harvey AM et al [editors]: The Principles and Practice of Medicine, 22nd ed. Originally published by Appleton & Lange. Copyright © 1988 by The McGraw-Hill companies, Inc.)

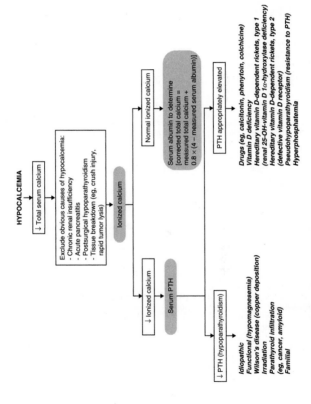

Figure 8–13. HYPOCALCEMIA: Diagnostic approach to hypocalcemia. **PTH** = parathyroid hormone.

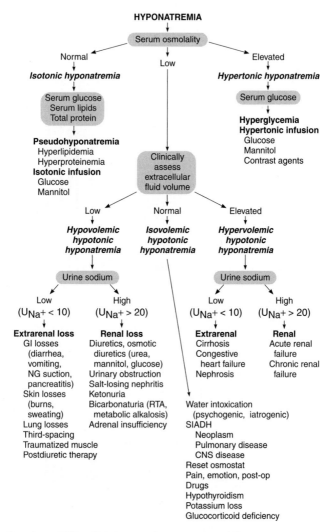

HYPONATREMIA

Serum osmolality

Normal → **Isotonic hyponatremia**
Low
Elevated → **Hypertonic hyponatremia**

Isotonic hyponatremia
Serum glucose
Serum lipids
Total protein

Pseudohyponatremia
Hyperlipidemia
Hyperproteinemia
Isotonic infusion
Glucose
Mannitol

Hypertonic hyponatremia
Serum glucose

Hyperglycemia
Hypertonic infusion
Glucose
Mannitol
Contrast agents

Clinically assess extracellular fluid volume

Low → **Hypovolemic hypotonic hyponatremia**
Normal → **Isovolemic hypotonic hyponatremia**
Elevated → **Hypervolemic hypotonic hyponatremia**

Urine sodium

Low $(U_{Na^+} < 10)$
High $(U_{Na^+} > 20)$

Extrarenal loss
GI losses (diarrhea, vomiting, NG suction, pancreatitis)
Skin losses (burns, sweating)
Lung losses
Third-spacing
Traumatized muscle
Postdiuretic therapy

Renal loss
Diuretics, osmotic diuretics (urea, mannitol, glucose)
Urinary obstruction
Salt-losing nephritis
Ketonuria
Bicarbonaturia (RTA, metabolic alkalosis)
Adrenal insufficiency

Urine sodium

Low $(U_{Na^+} < 10)$
High $(U_{Na^+} > 20)$

Extrarenal
Cirrhosis
Congestive heart failure
Nephrosis

Renal
Acute renal failure
Chronic renal failure

Water intoxication (psychogenic, iatrogenic)
SIADH
  Neoplasm
  Pulmonary disease
  CNS disease
Reset osmostat
Pain, emotion, post-op
Drugs
Hypothyroidism
Potassium loss
Glucocorticoid deficiency

Figure 8–14. HYPONATREMIA: Evaluation of hyponatremia. **SIADH** = syndrome of inappropriate antidiuretic hormone; U_{Na^+} = urinary sodium (mg/dL). *(Adapted, with permission, from Narins RG et al: Diagnostic strategies in disorders of fluid, electrolyte, and acid-base homeostasis. Am J Med 1982;72:496.)*

TABLE 8–10. HYPERLIPIDEMIA: RISK FACTOR ASSESSMENT FOR CORONARY HEART DISEASE (CHD).

Risk Score Sheet for Men[1]

Age (years)	Points
30–34	−1
35–39	0
40–44	1
45–49	2
50–54	3
55–59	4
60–64	5
65–69	6
70–74	7

Diabetes	Points
No	0
Yes	2

Smoker	Points
No	0
Yes	2

LDL-C (mg/dL)	LDL-C (mmol/L)	Points
<100	<2.59	−3
100–129	2.60–3.36	0
130–159	3.37–4.14	0
160–190	4.50–4.92	1
>190	>4.92	2

HDL-C (mg/dL)	HDL-C (mmol/L)	Points
<35	<0.9	2
35–44	0.01–1.16	1
45–49	1.17–1.29	0
50–59	1.30–1.55	0
≥60	≥1.56	−1

BP (mm Hg) Systolic	Diastolic <80	Diastolic 80–84	Diastolic 85–89	Diastolic 90–99	Diastolic ≥100
<120	0	0	0	2	3
120–129	0	0	1	2	3
130–139	1	1	1	2	3
140–159	2	2	2	2	3
≥160	3	3	3	3	3

(continued)

TABLE 8–10. HYPERLIPIDEMIA: RISK FACTOR ASSESSMENT FOR CORONARY HEART DISEASE (CHD). (*CONTINUED*)

Total CHD Risk Points	10-year CHD Risk (%)
<–3	1
–2	2
–1	2
0	3
1	4
2	5
3	6
4	7
5	9
6	11
7	14
8	18
9	22
10	27
11	33
12	40
13	47
≥14	56

Risk Score Sheet for Women[1]

Age (years)	Points	Diabetes	Points
30–34	−9	No	0
35–39	−4	Yes	4
40–44	0		
45–49	3	Smoker	Points
50–54	6	No	0
55–59	7	Yes	2
60–64	8		
65–69	8		
70–74	8		

LDL-C (mg/dL)	LDL-C (mmol/L)	Points	HDL-C (mg/dL)	HDL-C (mmol/L)	Points
<100	<2.59	−2	<35	<0.9	5
100–129	2.60–3.36	0	35–44	0.01–1.16	2
130–159	3.37–4.14	0	45–49	1.17–1.29	1
160–190	4.50–4.92	2	50–59	1.30–1.55	0
>190	>4.92	2	≥60	≥1.56	−2

(continued)

TABLE 8–10. HYPERLIPIDEMIA: RISK FACTOR ASSESSMENT FOR CORONARY HEART DISEASE (CHD). *(CONTINUED)*

	Risk Score Sheet for Women[1]				
BP (mm Hg) Systolic	Diastolic <80	Diastolic 80–84	Diastolic 85–89	Diastolic 90–99	Diastolic ≥100
<120	–3	0	0	2	3
120–129	0	0	0	2	3
130–139	0	0	0	2	3
140–159	2	2	2	2	3
≥160	3	3	3	3	3

Total CHD Risk Points	10-year CHD risk (%)
≤–2	1
–1	2
0	2
1	2
2	3
3	3
4	4
5	5

(continued)

6	6
7	7
8	8
9	9
10	11
11	13
12	15
13	17
14	20
15	24
16	27
≥17	32

The score sheet uses age, LDL-cholesterol (LDL-C), HDL-cholesterol (HDL-C), blood pressure (BP), diabetes, and smoking. To calculate the Framingham risk estimate, add points for age, presence of diabetes, smoking status, LDL-C, HDL-C, and BP. Find the total point score on the bottom table to determine the 10-year risk of CHD. The score is used to calculate the risk of developing clinical CHD in men and women who do not have known CHD.

Adapted with permission from Wilson, PW, D'Agostino, R, Levy D et al. Prediction of coronary heart disease using risk factor categories. Circulation 1998;97:1837. Copyright © 1998 Lippincott Williams & Wilkins.

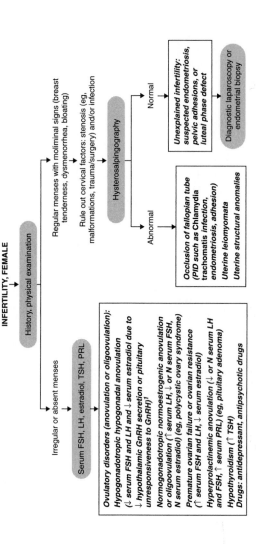

INFERTILITY, FEMALE

History, physical examination

Irregular or absent menses

Serum FSH, LH, estradiol, TSH, PRL

Ovulatory disorders (anovulation or oligoovulation):
Hypogonadotropic hypogonadal anovulation
(↓ serum FSH and LH and ↓ serum estradiol due to
↓ hypothalamic GnRH secretion or pituitary
unresponsiveness to GnRH)[1]
Normogonadotropic normoestrogenic anovulation
or oligoovulation (↑ serum LH, ↓ or N serum FSH,
N serum estradiol) (eg, polycystic ovary syndrome)
Premature ovarian failure or ovarian resistance
(↑ serum FSH and LH, ↓ serum estradiol)
Hyperprolactinemic anovulation (↓ or N serum LH
and FSH, ↑ serum PRL) (eg, pituitary adenoma)
Hypothyroidism (↑ TSH)
Drugs: antidepressant, antipsychotic drugs

Regular menses with moliminal signs (breast
tenderness, dysmenorrhea, bloating)

Rule out cervical factors: stenosis (eg,
malformations, trauma/surgery) and/or infection

Hysterosalpingography

Abnormal

Occlusion of fallopian tube
(PID such as Chlamydia
trachomatis infection,
endometriosis, adhesion)
Uterine leiomyomata
Uterine structural anomalies

Normal

Unexplained infertility:
suspected endometriosis,
pelvic adhesions, or
luteal phase defect

Diagnostic laparoscopy or
endometrial biopsy

[1]Hypogonadotropic hypogonadal anovulation (hypothalamic-pituitary amenorrhea) can be caused by Kallman syndrome, Sheehan syndrome, empty sella syndrome, autoimmune diseases (eg, lymphocytic hypophysitis), tumors/trauma/radiation of the hypothalamic or pituitary area, stress, eating disorders, and intense exercise.

Figure 8–15. INFERTILITY, FEMALE: Evaluation of female infertility. **FSH** = follicle-stimulating hormone; **GnRH** = gonadotropin-releasing hormone; **LH** = luteinizing hormone; **PID** = pelvic inflammatory disease; **PRL** = prolactin; **TSH** = thyroid-stimulating hormone.

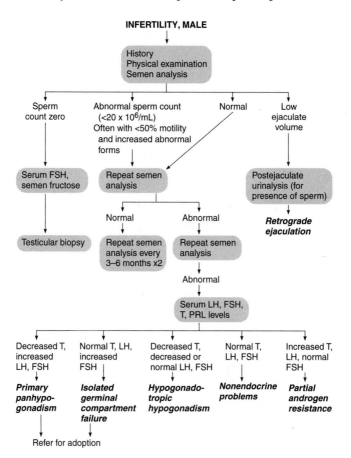

Figure 8–16. INFERTILITY, MALE: Evaluation of male factor infertility. **FSH** = follicle-stimulating hormone; **LH** = luteinizing hormone; **PRL** = prolactin; **T** = testosterone. (*Adapted, with permission, from Swerdloff RS, Boyers SM: Evaluation of the male partner of an infertile couple: An algorithmic approach. JAMA 1982;247:2418. Copyright © 1982 by The American Medical Association.*)

TABLE 8–11. LEUKEMIAS AND LYMPHOMAS: CLASSIFICATION AND IMMUNOPHENOTYPING.

Disease	Typical Immunophenotype	Comments
Acute Myeloid Leukemias (AML)		
AML with t (8;21) (q 22;q22), (*AML1/ETO*)	Blasts express CD34, HLA-DR, CD13, CD33, CD15, MPO, and CD117. CD19 is often expressed.	AML with t (8;21) is usually associated with good response to chemotherapy and high rate of complete remission with long-term disease-free survival.
AML with inv (16) (p13;q22) or t (16;16) (p13;q22), (*CBFβ/MYH11*)	Blasts express CD13, CD33, MPO, CD117, as well as CD14, CD4, CD11b, CD11c, CD64, and CD36.	AML with inv (16) or t (16;16) typically shows myeloid and monocytic differentiation and the presence of eosinophilia, referred to as AMML–Eo. The disease usually responds well to chemotherapy with high rate of complete remission.
AML with t (15;17) (q22;q12), (*PML/RARα*) and variants	Leukemic cells express CD13, CD33, MPO, and CD117, but not CD34 and HLA-DR.	AML with t (15;17), known as acute promyelocytic leukemia (APL), is sensitive to all-*trans* retinoic acid (ATRA) treatment. APL is frequently associated with DIC.
AML with 11q23 (MLL) abnormalities	Leukemic cells variably express CD13, CD33, CD117, MPO, and monocytic markers (CD4, CD14, CD11b, CD64). CD34 is often absent.	AML with 11q23 (MLL) abnormalities is usually associated with monocytic features. AML with 11q23 abnormalities has an intermediate survival.
AML with multilineage dysplasia	Blasts typically express CD34, HLA-DR, CD13, CD33, MPO, CD117.	AML with multilineage dysplasia is an acute leukemia with dysplasia present in 50% or more of the cells of at least 2 lines in a pretreatment specimen. Outcome is poor.
AML, therapy-related	Alkylating agent/radiation related: Blasts express CD34, HLA-DR, CD13, CD33, MPO, and CD117. Topoisomerase II inhibitor related: Same as AML with 11q23 abnormalities.	Alkylating agent/radiation related AML is generally refractory to chemotherapy and is associated with short survival. Topoisomerase II inhibitor-related AML often show monocytic differentiation.
AML, minimally differentiated (also known as AML-M0)	Blasts express CD13, CD33, CD117, CD34, HLA-DR, but not MPO.	Flow cytometric immunophenotyping is required for the confirmation of myeloid differentiation.

AML without maturation (also known as AML-M1)	Blasts express CD13, CD33, CD117, and MPO. CD34 is often positive.	Blasts constitute >90% of the nonerythroid nucleated cells in the marrow, and at least 3% of the blasts are positive for MPO.
AML with maturation (also known as AML-M2)	Blasts express CD13, CD33, CD15, CD117, and MPO. CD34 and HLA-DR are often positive.	Blasts constitute 20–89% of nonerythroid cells, and monocytes comprise <20% of the bone marrow cell.
Acute myelomonocytic leukemia (also known as AML-M4)	Leukemic cells variably express CD13, CD33, CD117, HLA-DR, CD14, CD4, CD11b, CD11c, and CD64. CD34 may be positive.	Monocytic component (monoblasts to monocytes) comprises 20–79% of bone marrow cells.
Acute monoblastic/monocytic leukemia (also known as AML-M5)	Leukemic cells variably express CD13, CD33, CD117, HLA-DR, CD14, CD4, CD11b, CD11c, CD64, and CD68. CD34 is typically negative.	Monocytic component (monoblasts to monocytes) comprises >80% of bone marrow cells.
Acute erythroid leukemia (also known as AML-M6) and pure erythroid leukemia	Erythroblasts generally lack myeloid markers, but are positive for CD36 and glycophorin A. Myeloblasts express CD13, CD33, CD117, and MPO with or without CD34 and HLA-DR. The erythroid cells in pure erythroid leukemia express CD36 and glycophorin A with the more immature forms expressing CD34 and HLA-DR.	The diagnostic criteria for acute erythroid leukemia: erythroblasts constitute >50% of the marrow cells, and myeloblasts comprise >20% of the nonerythroid cells. Pure erythroid leukemia is a neoplastic proliferation of erythroid precursors (>80% of nucleated marrow cells) without a significant myeloblastic component.
Acute megakaryocytic leukemia (known as AML-M7)	Blasts express one or more of the platelet glycoproteins (CD41, CD61, CD42), and variably express HLA-DR, CD34, CD117, CD13, and CD33.	Flow cytometric immunophenotyping is required for confirmation of megakaryocytic differentiation.

(continued)

TABLE 8–11. LEUKEMIAS AND LYMPHOMAS: CLASSIFICATION AND IMMUNOPHENOTYPING. (*CONTINUED*)

Disease	Typical Immunophenotype	Comments
Acute leukemia of ambiguous lineage	Undifferentiated acute leukemia: Blasts express HLA-DR, CD34, CD38, and may express TdT, but lack lineage-specific markers such as CD79a, CD22, IgM, CD3, and MPO. Bilineal acute leukemia: There is a dual population of blasts with each population expressing markers of a distinct lineaage, such as myeloid and lymphoid, or B and T. Biphenotypic acute leukemia: The blasts co-express myeloid and T or B lineage-specific antigens, or concurrent B and T antigens.	Cases of bilineal and biphenotypic acute leukemia usually present with cytogenetic abnormalities. The common abnormalities include Philadelphia chromosome, t (4;11)(q 21;q 23) or other 11q23 abnormalities. The prognosis of acute leukemia of ambiguous lineage is poor.
Acute Lymphoblastic Leukemias/Lymphomas (ALL/LBL)		
Precursor B lymphoblastic leukemia/lymphoblastic lymphoma (B-ALL/LBL) (also known as B-cell acute lymphoblastic leukemia)	Early precursor B-ALL/LBL: TdT+, HLA-DR+, CD34+/–, CD10–, CD45–/+, CD19+, cCD22+, CD20–, CD15+, clg–, slg–. Common B-ALL/LBL: TdT+, HLA-DR+, CD34+, CD10+, CD45+(weak), CD19+, CD20+, clg–, slg–. Pre–B-ALL/LBL: TdT–/+, CD34–/+, HLA-DR+, CD45+(weak), CD19+, CD20–, cIgM+, slg–.	Cytogenetic abnormalities in B-ALL/LBL include several groups: hypodiploid, low hyperdiploid (<50), high hyperdiploid (>50), translocations, and pseudodiploid. The commonly seen translocations include t (9;22), t (12;21), t (5;14), t (1;19), t (17;19), t (4;11), and other translocations involving 11q23. The cytogenetic findings are prognostically important.

Precursor T lymphoblastic leukemia/lymphoblastic lymphoma (T-ALL/LBL)	T-ALL/LBL often has an immunophenotype that corresponds to the common thymocyte stage of differentiation. The blasts are positive for TdT and often CD10, and variably express CD1a, CD2, CD3, CD4, CD5, CD7, and CD8. CD4 and CD8 are frequently co-expressed on the blasts. Some T-ALL/LBL has an immunophenotype that corresponds to prothymocyte stage of differentiation. The blasts are negative for both CD4 and CD8.	In about one-third of T-ALL/LBL translocations have been detected involving the α and δ T-cell receptor (TCR) loci at 14q11.2, the β locus at 7q35, and the γ locus at 7p14-15, with a variety of partner genes. T-ALL/LBL can be part of a unique disease entity known as the 8p11 myeloproliferative syndrome caused by constitutive activation of FGFR1. The disease is characterized by chronic myeloproliferative disorder that frequently presents with eosinophilia and associated T-cell lymphoblastic lymphoma.
Mature B-cell Neoplasms		
Chronic lymphocytic leukemia/ small lymphocytic lymphoma (CLL/SLL)	Lymphoma cells are light chain restricted and express CD5, CD19, CD20 (weak), CD22 (weak), CD79a, CD23, CD43, and are negative for CD10, Bcl-1 (cyclin D1), and FMC-7 (weak). A subset of cases expresses CD11c (weak). Cases with unmutated Ig variable region genes have been reported to be positive for CD38 and ZAP-70.	The clinical course is often indolent but incurable. The disease may progress/transform to prolymphocytic leukemia (PLL) or large B-cell lymphoma (Richter syndrome). CD38 and/or ZAP-70 positivity is associated with worse prognosis, and both have been used as prognostic markers for the disease. Trisomy 12 is reported in ~20% of cases, and deletions at 13q14 in up to 50% of cases. Trisomy 12 in CLL/SLL correlates with a worse prognosis.
B-cell prolymphocytic leukemia (B-PLL)	The cells of B-PLL strongly express surface IgM and B-cell antigens CD19, CD20, CD22, CD79a, CD79b, and FMC-7. CD5 is present in about one-third of cases and CD23 is typically negative.	B-PLL can be divided into CD5- B-PLL (arising in CLL/SLL) and CD5- B-PLL (de novo PLL). CD5+ B-PLL has a longer median survival than CD5- B-PLL.

(continued)

TABLE 8–11. LEUKEMIAS AND LYMPHOMAS: CLASSIFICATION AND IMMUNOPHENOTYPING. (*CONTINUED*)

Disease	Typical Immunophenotype	Comments
Lymphoplasmacytic lymphoma/ Waldenström macroglobulinemia (LPL)	The cells express strong surface immunoglobulin, usually of IgM type, and express B-cell antigens (CD19, CD20, CD22, CD79a) and are CD5−, CD10−, CD23−, CD43−/−, and CD38+. Lack of CD5 and strong immunoglobulin expression are useful in distinction from CLL/SLL.	Characteristic features include IgM monoclonal gammopathy; spectrum of small lymphocytes, plasmacytoid lymphocytes, and plasma cells; interstitial, nodular, or diffuse pattern of bone marrow involvement; and typical immunophenotype (sigM+, CD19,+, CD20+, CD5−, CD23−, CD10−).
Splenic marginal zone lymphoma (SMZL)	The tumor cells express surface IgM, and are positive for CD19, CD20, CD79a, and negative for CD5, CD10, CD23, CD25, CD43, CD103, and Bcl-1 (cyclin D1).	Circulating lymphoma cells are usually characterized by the presence of short polar villi (villous lymphocytes). The clinical course is indolent, but the disease is incurable.
Hairy cell leukemia (HCL)	Leukemic cells express surface immunoglobulin, B-cell markers (CD19, CD20, CD22, CD79a), and are often positive for CD11c, CD25, FMC-7, and CD103, but negative for CD5, CD10, and CD23.	Patients often present with splenomegaly, pancytopenia (monocytopenia is characteristic), and may have circulating hairy leukemic cells. Bone marrow reticulin fibers are characteristically increased, resulting in "dry tap" during aspirate procedure. Interferon-alpha, deoxycoformycin (pentostatin), or 2-chlorodeoxyadenosine (2-CdA, cladribine) can induce long-term remissions.
Plasma cell myeloma/ plasmacytoma	The malignant cells express monoclonal cytoplasmic immunoglobulin, lack CD45 and pan-B cell antigens (CD19, CD20, CD22), but CD79 is often positive. The cells are typically positive for CD38, CD138, and often express CD56, CD43, and rarely CD10. The phenotype of plasma cell leukemia is similar to that of myeloma, but CD56 is negative.	Plasma cells do not express surface immunoglobulin (or light chain restriction) determination by flow cytometry analysis, cell permeabilization procedure is necessary. The procedure gives antibodies access to intracellular structures/molecules.

Extranodal marginal zone B-cell lymphoma of mucosa-associated lymphoid tissue (MALT lymphoma)	Lymphoma cells typically express surface immunoglobulin with light chain restriction. The cells are positive for CD19, CD20, CD79a, CD43, and negative for CD5, CD10, CD23, and Bcl-1.	Trisomy 3 is found in ~60% and t (11;18) (q21;q21) has been detected in 25–50% of MALT lymphoma cases. Neither t (14;18) nor t (11;14) is present. Cases with t (11;18) appear to be resistant to *H pylori* eradication therapy.
Nodal marginal zone B-cell lymphoma (NMZL)	The immunophenotype of most cases is similar to that of extranodal MALT lymphoma.	NMZL is a primary nodal B-cell neoplasm that morphologically resembles lymph nodes involved by marginal zone lymphomas of extranodal or splenic types, but without evidence of extranodal or splenic disease.
Follicular lymphoma (FL)	Lymphoma cells are usually positive for pan–B-cell antigens (CD19, CD20), surface immunoglobulin, CD10, Bcl-2, Bcl-6, and negative for CD5. Bcl-2 is expressed in the majority of cases, ranging from nearly 100% in grade 1 to 75% in grade 3 FL.	All cases have cytogenetic abnormalities. The t (14;18) (q32;q21) translocation, involving rearrangement of the *Bcl-2* gene and *IgH* gene, is present in 80–95% of FL. FL may transform into precursor B-ALL, and c-myc (8q24) rearrangement is often associated with the transformation. Bcl-2 is useful in distinguishing reactive follicular hyperplasia (Bcl-2 negative) and FL (Bcl-2-positive).
Mantle cell lymphoma (MCL)	Lymphoma cells express surface immunoglobulin, pan–B-cell antigens (CD19, CD20), Bcl-1, FMC-7, CD5, CD43, and are typically negative for CD10, CD23, and Bcl-6.	MCL and CLL/SLL are the two common CD5-positive B-cell lymphoproliferative disorders. But unlike CLL/SLL, MCL cells express bright surface immunoglobulin, bright CD20 and FMC-7, and are CD23 negative. Virtually all cases express Bcl-1 (cyclin D1) due to gene rearrangement.
Diffuse large B-cell lymphoma (DLBCL)	DLBCL cells typically express various pan–B-cell antigens (CD19, CD20, CD22, CD79a), surface and/or cytoplasmic immunoglobulin with light chain restriction, Bcl-6, and CD10. Bcl-2 is positive in 30–50% of cases.	Morphologic variants of DLBCL include centroblastic, immunoblastic, T-cell/histiocyte rich, anaplastic, and plasmablastic DLBCL. Bcl-2 expression has been reported to be associated with an adverse disease-free survival, while expression of Bcl-6 appears to be associated with a better prognosis.

(continued)

TABLE 8–11. LEUKEMIAS AND LYMPHOMAS: CLASSIFICATION AND IMMUNOPHENOTYPING. (CONTINUED)

Disease	Typical Immunophenotype	Comments
Mediastinal (thymic) large B-cell lymphoma (Med-DLBCL)	Lymphoma cells express CD45 and B-cell antigen (CD19, CD20). Immunoglobulin and HLA-DR are often absent. The cells do not express CD5 and CD10, and lack Bcl-2, Bcl-6, and c-myc rearrangements.	Med-DLBCL is a subtype of DLBCL arising in the mediastinum of putative thymic B-cell origin with distinct clinical, immunophenotypic, and genotypic features. Tissue sections usually show diffuse lymphoid proliferation, compartmentalized into groups by fine/delicate fibrotic bands.
Intravascular large B-cell lymphoma	Lymphoma cells express pan–B-cell antigens (CD19, CD20).	The disease is a rare subtype of extranodal DLBCL characterized by the presence of lymphoma cells only in the lumina of small vessels, particularly capillaries. Brain and skin are the common sites of involvement.
Primary effusion lymphoma (PEL)	Lymphoma cells express CD45, but are usually negative for pan–B-cell markers (CD19, CD20). Surface and cytoplasmic immunoglobulin is often absent. Activation and plasma cell-related markers such as CD30, CD38, and CD138 are usually positive.	PEL is a neoplasm of large B cells usually presenting as serous effusions without detectable tumor masses. It is universally associated with human herpes virus 8 (HHV-8), most often occurring in the setting of immunodeficiency. Rare cases of PEL of T-cell origin have been reported.
Lymphomatoid granulomatosis (LYG)	Lymphoma cells express CD20, and are variably positive for CD30, but negative for CD15. The cells lack immunoglobulin expression. The background small lymphocytes are CD3–positive T cells.	LYG is an angiocentric and angiodestructive lymphoproliferative disease involving extranodal sites, composed of Epstein Barr virus (EBV)-positive B cells admixed with reactive T cells, which usually numerically predominate. LYG may progress to an EBV-positive DLBCL. The common sites of involvement are lung, kidney, brain, liver, and skin.
Burkitt lymphoma (BL)	Lymphoma cells express surface immunoglobulin with light chain restriction, pan–B-cell antigens (CD19, CD20), CD10, and Bcl-6. The cells are negative for CD5, CD23, CD34, and TdT. Nearly 100% of the cells are positive for Ki-67, a proliferation marker.	All BL cases show a translocation of c-myc gene at chromosome 8q24 to the IgH gene at 14q32 or less commonly to light chain loci at 2p12 or 22q11. Genetic abnormalities involving the c-myc gene play an essential role in BL pathogenesis. The expression of CD10 and Bcl-6 indicates a germinal center origin of the tumor cells. BL is highly aggressive but potentially curable.

Mature T-cell and NK-cell Neoplasms

T-cell prolymphocytic leukemia (T-PLL)	Leukemic cells express CD2, CD3, CD7, but not TdT and CD1a. The cells can be CD4+/CD8− (60%), CD4+/CD8+ (25%), or CD4−/CD8+ (15%).	T-PLL is an aggressive T-cell leukemia characterized by the proliferation of small to medium sized prolymphocytes with a mature post-thymic T-cell phenotype involving the blood, bone marrow, lymph nodes, spleen, and skin.
T-cell large granular lymphocyte leukemia (T-LGL)	T-LGL cells have a mature T-cell immunophenotype. Approximately 80% of cases are CD3+, TCR α β+, CD4−, and CD8+.	T-LGL is a heterogeneous disorder characterized by a persistent (>6 months) increase in peripheral blood large granular lymphocytes (LGLs), without a clearly identified cause. Severe neutropenia with or without anemia is a characteristic clinical feature. Pure red cell hypoplasia has been reported in association with T-LGL leukemia. Moderate splenomegaly, rheumatoid arthritis, and the presence of autoantibodies are commonly seen in patients with T-LGL.
Aggressive NK-cell leukemia	Leukemic cells are CD2+, surface CD3− cytoplasmic CD3ε+, CD56+, and positive for cytotoxic molecules (TIA-1, granzyme B, and/or perforin). This immunophenotype is identical to that of extranodal NK/T-cell lymphoma, nasal type.	Aggressive NK-cell leukemia is characterized by a systemic proliferation of NK cells. The disease has an aggressive clinical course. T-cell receptor (TCR) genes are in germline configuration. Clonality therefore has to be established by other methods, such as cytogenetic studies and pattern of X chromosome inactivation in female patients.
Adult T-cell leukemia/lymphoma (ATLL)	Tumor cells express T-cell antigens (CD2, CD3, CD5), but usually lack CD7. Most cases are CD4+, CD8−. Rare cases are CD4−, CD8+, or double negative for CD4 and CD8. CD25 is expressed in virtually all cases.	ATLL is a peripheral T-cell neoplasm most often composed of highly pleomorphic lymphoid cells. The disease is usually widely disseminated, and is caused by the human T-cell leukemia virus type 1 (HTLV-1). ATLL is endemic in Japan, the Caribbean basin, and parts of Central Africa.

(continued)

TABLE 8–11. LEUKEMIAS AND LYMPHOMAS: CLASSIFICATION AND IMMUNOPHENOTYPING. (CONTINUED)

Disease	Typical Immunophenotype	Comments
Extranodal NK/T-cell lymphoma, nasal type	The typical immunophenotype is CD2+, CD56+, surface CD3–, and cytoplasmic CD3 ε–. Most cases are positive for cytotoxic molecules (TIA-1, granzyme B, perforin).	The disease entity is designated NK/T (rather than NK) cell lymphoma because while most cases appear to be NK-cell neoplasms (EBV+, CD56+), rare cases show an EBV+, CD56– cytotoxic T-cell phenotype. T-cell receptor and immunoglobulin genes are in germline configuration in a majority of cases. EBV can be demonstrated in the tumor cells in nearly all cases. The prognosis is variable.
Enteropathy-type T-cell lymphoma	Tumor cells are CD3+, CD5–, CD7+, CD8–/+, CD4–, CD103+, and contain cytotoxic molecules.	The tumor occurs most commonly in the jejunum or ileum, and there is a clear association with celiac disease. The prognosis is usually poor.
Hepatosplenic T-cell lymphoma	Tumor cells are CD3+, CD4–, CD8–, CD5–, CD56+/–. The cells are usually TCR γ δ + and TCR α β–.	Hepatosplenic T-cell lymphoma is an extranodal and systemic neoplasm derived from cytotoxic T cells usually of γ δ T-cell receptor type, demonstrating marked sinusoidal infiltration of spleen, liver, and bone marrow. The clinical course is aggressive.
Subcutaneous panniculitis-like T-cell lymphoma (SPTCL)	Tumor cells are usually CD3+, TCR α β +, CD5–, CD4–, CD8–, and express cytotoxic molecules.	SPTCL is a cytotoxic T-cell lymphoma, which preferentially infiltrates subcutaneous tissue. Some patients may present with a hemophagocytic syndrome with pancytopenia. The clinical course is aggressive.
Blastic NK-cell lymphoma	Tumor cells are CD4+, CD56+, CD43+, and are usually negative for CD2, CD3, CD7, cytoplasmic CD3 ε, and cytotoxic molecules.	Blastic NK-cell lymphoma is composed of cells with a lymphoblast-like morphology and evidence of commitment to the NK lineage. TCR genes are germline in configuration. The clinical course is usually aggressive.

Mycosis fungoides and Sézary syndrome (MF/SS)	The typical phenotype is CD2+, CD3+, TCR β +, CD5+, CD4+/CD8− (rarely CD4−/CD8+). Virtually all cases are negative for CD26 (a marker for treatment monitoring). CD7 is usually negative.	MF is a mature T-cell lymphoma, presenting in the skin with patches/plaques and characterized by epidermal and dermal infiltration of small to medium-sized T cells with cerebriform nuclei. SS is a generalized mature T-cell lymphoma characterized by the presence of erythroderma, lymphadenopathy, and neoplastic T lymphocytes in the blood.
Primary cutaneous CD30–positive T-cell lymphoproliferative disorders	Primary cutaneous anaplastic large cell lymphoma (C-ALCL): Tumors cells express T-cell antigens (CD2, CD3, CD5, CD7) and are usually positive for CD4. CD30 is expressed in >75% the cells. Aberrant T-cell phenotype with loss of one or more T-cell antigens is common. Lymphomatoid papulosis (LyP): The atypical T cells are CD4+, CD8−. The cells often express aberrant phenotypes with variable loss of pan–T-cell antigens (eg, CD2, CD5, or CD7). CD30 is positive in a LyP subtype (type A).	LyP and C-ALCL constitute a spectrum of related conditions originating from transformed or activated CD30-positive T-lymphocytes. They may coexist in individual patients, they can be clonally related and they often show overlapping clinical and/or histologic features.

(continued)

TABLE 8–11. LEUKEMIAS AND LYMPHOMAS: CLASSIFICATION AND IMMUNOPHENOTYPING. (*CONTINUED*)

Disease	Typical Immunophenotype	Comments
Angioimmunoblastic T-cell lymphoma (AITL)	Neoplastic cells express T cell antigens (CD2, CD3, CD5, CD7), usually without aberrant antigen loss, and are CD4+ and CD8–. The neoplastic T cells are positive for CD10 and/or Bcl-6. CD21 stain highlights the intact or disrupted follicular dendritic meshwork.	AITL is a T-cell lymphoma characterized by systemic disease and a polymorphous infiltrate involving lymph nodes. TCR genes are rearranged in the majority (>75%) of cases. Secondary EBV-related B-cell lymphoma may occur. Almost all cases are positive for CD10 and/or Bcl-6, suggesting a germinal center derivation of the tumor cells. The clinical course is very aggressive.
Peripheral T-cell lymphoma, unspecified	Neoplastic cells express T cell antigens (CD2, CD3, CD5, CD7), but aberrant T-cell phenotypes with antigen loss are frequent. Most nodal cases are CD4+, CD8–. CD30, and CD56 may be positive.	The diseases are among the most aggressive of the non-Hodgkin lymphomas.
Anaplastic large cell lymphoma (ALCL)	The tumor cells express one or more T-cell antigens (CD2, CD3, CD5, CD7). The cells usually express CD30 (membrane and in the Golgi region), ALK (cytoplasmic and/or nuclear), EMA, cytotoxic molecules, and CD43, and CD45.	Expression of ALK in ALCL is due to genetic alteration of the ALK locus on chromosome 2. The most common alteration is t(2;5)(p23;q35), resulting in fusion of the ALK gene and nucleophosmin (NPM) gene on 5q35. ALK positivity is associated with a favorable prognosis.

For details, see Jaffe ES, Harris NL, Stein H, Vardiman JW (editors): World Health Organization Classification of Tumors: Pathology and Genetics of Tumors of Haematopoietic and Lymphoid Tissues. IARC Press: Lyon 2001.
ALK = anaplastic large cell lymphoma kinase; **CD** = cluster of differentiation; **EMA** = epithelial membrane antigen; **MPO** = myeloperoxidase.

TABLE 8–12. LIVER FUNCTION TESTS.

Clinical Condition	Direct Bilirubin (mg/dL)	Indirect Bilirubin (mg/dL)	Urine Bilirubin	Serum Albumin & Total Protein (g/dL)	Alkaline Phosphatase (IU/L)	Prothrombin Time (seconds)	ALT (SGPT) AST (SGOT) (IU/L)
Normal	0.1–0.3	0.2–0.7	None	Albumin, 3.4–4.7 Total protein, 6.0–8.0	30–115 (lab-specific)	11–15 seconds. After vitamin K, 15% increase within 24 hours.	ALT, 5–35; AST, 5–40 (lab-specific)
Hepatocellular jaundice (eg, viral, alcoholic ↑ hepatitis)	↑↑	↑	↑	↓ Albumin	N to ↑	Prolonged if damage is severe. Does not respond to parenteral vitamin K.	Increased in hepatocellular damage, viral hepatitides; AST/ALT ratio often >2:1 in alcoholic hepatitis
Uncomplicated obstructive jaundice (eg, common bile duct obstruction)	↑↑	↑	↑	N	↑	Prolonged if obstruction marked but responds to parenteral vitamin K.	N to minimally ↑
Hemolysis	N	↑	None	N	N	N	N
Gilbert syndrome	N	↑	None	N	N	N	N
Intrahepatic cholestasis (drug-induced)	↑↑	↑	↑	N	↑↑	N	AST N or ↑; ALT N or ↑
Primary biliary cirrhosis	↑↑	↑	↑	N ↑ globulin	↑↑	N or ↑	↑

AST = aspartate aminotransferase; **ALT** = alanine aminotransferase.
Modified, with permission, from Tierney LM Jr, McPhee SJ, Papadakis MA (editors): Current Medical Diagnosis & Treatment 1996. Originally published by Appleton & Lange. Copyright © 1996 by The McGraw-Hill Companies, Inc.; and from Harvey AM et al (editors): The Principles and Practice of Medicine, 22nd ed. Originally published by Appleton & Lange. Copyright © 1988 by The McGraw-Hill Companies, Inc.

TABLE 8–13. LIVER FUNCTION: MODIFIED CHILD-TURCOTTE-PUGH CLASSIFICATION FOR CIRRHOSIS.[1,2]

Parameter	Numerical Score		
	1	2	3
Ascites	None	Slight	Moderate–severe
Encephalopathy	None	Slight–moderate	Moderate–severe
Bilirubin (mg/dL)	<2.0	2.0–3.0	>3.0
Albumin (g/dL)	>3.5	2.8–3.5	<2.8
PT (seconds increased)	<4	4.0–6.0	>6.0

Total Score	Class	1-Year Survival (%)	2-Year Survival (%)
5.0–6.0	A	100	85
7.0–9.0	B	80	60
10.0–15.0	C	45	35

[1]Modified Child-Pugh classification of the severity of liver disease according to the degree of ascites, the plasma concentrations of bilirubin and albumin, the PT (prothrombin time), and the degree of encephalopathy. A total score of 5–6 is considered grade A (well-compensated disease); 7–9 is grade B (significant functional compromise); and 10–15 is grade C (decompensated disease).

[2]The MELD (model for end-stage liver disease) score, as currently used by United Network for Organ Sharing (UNOS) in prioritizing allocation of organs for liver transplantation, is calculated according to the following formula:

MELD = 3.8[Ln serum bilirubin (mg/dL)] + 11.2[Ln INR] + 9.6[Ln serum creatinine (mg/dL)] + 6.4, where Ln is the natural logarithm.

Modified, with permission, from Tierney, Jr LM, McPhee SJ, Papadakis MA (editors): Current Medical Diagnosis & Treatment *2005, Published by Appleton & Lange. Copyright © 2005 by The McGraw-Hill Companies, Inc.*

TABLE 8–14. OSMOLAL GAP: CALCULATION AND APPLICATION IN CLINICAL TOXICOLOGY.[1]

The osmolal gap (Δ osm) is determined by subtracting the calculated serum osmolality from the measured serum osmolality.

$$\begin{aligned}\text{Calculated}\\\text{osmolality (osm)}\\(\text{mosm/kg H}_2\text{O})\end{aligned} = 2\left(\text{Na}^+\left[\text{meq/L}\right]\right) + \frac{\text{Glucose (mg/dL)}}{18} + \frac{\text{BUN (mg/dL)}}{2.8}$$

$$\text{Osmolal gap}\left(\Delta\text{ osm}\right) = \text{Measured osmolality} - \text{Calculated osmolality}$$

Serum osmolality may be increased by contributions of circulating alcohols and other low-molecular-weight substances. Since these substances are not included in the calculated osmolality, there will be an osmolal gap directly proportional to their serum concentration and inversely proportional to their molecular weight:

$$\text{Serum concentration (mg/dL)} \approx \Delta\text{ osm} \times \frac{\text{Molecular weight of toxin}}{10}$$

For ethanol (the most common cause of Δ osm), a gap of 30 mosm/kg H_2O indicates an ethanol level of:

$$30 \times \frac{46}{10} = 138 \text{ mg/dL}$$

See the following for lethal concentrations of alcohols and their corresponding osmolal gaps.

LETHAL CONCENTRATIONS OF ALCOHOLS AND THEIR CORRESPONDING OSMOLAL GAPS

	Molecular Weight	Lethal Concentration (mg/dL)	Corresponding Osmolal Gap (mosm/kg H_2O)
Ethanol	46	350	75
Methanol	32	80	25
Ethylene glycol	62	200	35
Isopropanol	60	350	60

Note: Most laboratories use the freezing point method for calculating osmolality. If the vaporization point method is used, alcohols are driven off and their contribution to osmolality is lost.
Na$^+$ = sodium; **BUN** = blood urea nitrogen.
Modified, with permission, from: Tierney LM Jr, McPhee SJ, Papadakis MA (editors): Current Medical Diagnosis & Treatment 2003. *McGraw-Hill, 2003.*

TABLE 8–15. PANCREATITIS, ACUTE: RANSON CRITERIA FOR SEVERITY EVALUATION.

Criteria present at diagnosis or admission
 Age over 55 years
 White blood cell count >16,000/mcL
 Blood glucose >200 mg/dL
 Serum LDH >350 IU/L (laboratory-specific)
 AST (SGOT) >250 IU/L (laboratory-specific)

Criteria developing during first 48 hours
 Hematocrit fall >10%
 BUN rise >5 mg/dL
 Serum calcium <8 mg/dL
 Arterial PO_2 <60 mm Hg
 Base deficit >4 meq/L
 Estimated fluid sequestration >6 L

**MORTALITY RATES CORRELATE WITH THE NUMBER
OF CRITERIA PRESENT**

Number of Criteria	Mortality
0–2	1%
3–4	16%
5–6	40%
7–8	100%

AST = aspartate dehydrogenase; **BUN** = blood urea nitrogen; **LDH** = lactic dehydrogenase.
Modified from Way LW (editor): Current Surgical Diagnosis & Treatment, *10th ed. Originally published by Appleton & Lange. Copyright © 1994 by the McGraw-Hill Companies, Inc. 1994.*

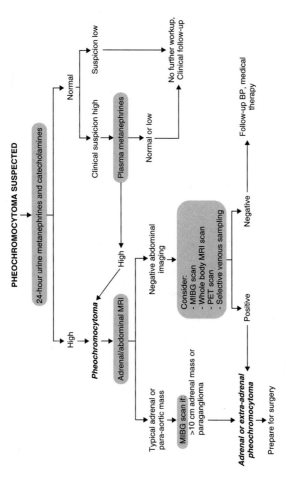

Figure 8–17. PHEOCHROMOCYTOMA: Evaluation and localization of a possible pheochromocytoma. Clinical suspicion is triggered by paroxysmal symptoms (especially hypertension); hypertension that is intermittent, unusually labile, or resistant to treatment; family history of pheochromocytoma or associated conditions; or an incidentally discovered adrenal mass. **BP** = blood pressure; **MIBG** = ^{131}I- or ^{123}I-labeled metaiodobenzylguanidine; **MRI** = magnetic resonance imaging; **PET** = positron emission tomography.

TABLE 8–16. PLEURAL EFFUSION: PLEURAL FLUID PROFILES IN VARIOUS DISEASE STATES.

Diagnosis	Gross Appearance	Protein (g/dL)	Glucose[1] (mg/dL)	WBC & Differential (per mcL)	RBC (per mcL)	Microscopic Exam	Culture	Comments
Normal	Clear	1.0–1.5	Equal to serum	≤1000, mostly MN	0 or Few	Neg	Neg	
TRANSUDATES[2]								
Congestive heart failure	Serous	<3; some-times ≥3	Equal to serum	<1000	<10,000	Neg	Neg	Most common cause of pleural effusion. Effusion right-sided in 55–70% of patients.
Nephrotic syndrome	Serous	<3	Equal to serum	<1000	<1000	Neg	Neg	Occurs in 20% of patients. Cause is low protein osmotic pressure.
Hepatic cirrhosis	Serous	<3	Equal to serum	<1000	<1000	Neg	Neg	From movement of ascites across diaphragm. Treatment of underlying ascites usually sufficient.
EXUDATES[2]								
Tuberculosis	Usually serous; can be bloody	90% ≥3; may exceed 5 g/dL	Equal to serum; Occ <60	500–10,000, mostly MN	<10,000	Concentrate Pos for AFB in <50%	May yield MTb	PPD usually positive; pleural biopsy positive; eosinophils (>10%) or mesothelial cells (>5%) make diagnosis unlikely.
Malignancy	Usually turbid, bloody; Occ serous	90% ≥3	Equal to serum; <60 in 15% of cases	1000–10,000 mostly MN	>100,000	Pos cytology in 50%	Neg	Eosinophils uncommon; fluid tends to reaccumulate after removal.

	Appearance		Glucose[1]	Cell count				Comments
Empyema	Turbid to purulent	≥3	Less than serum, often <20	25,000–100,000, mostly PMN	<5000	Pos	Pos	Drainage necessary; putrid odor suggests anaerobic infection.
Parapneumonic effusion, uncomplicated	Clear to turbid	≥3	Equal to serum	5000–25,000, mostly PMN	<5000	Neg	Neg	Tube thoracostomy unnecessary; associated infiltrate on chest x-ray; fluid pH ≥7.2.
Pulmonary embolism, infarction	Serous to grossly bloody	≥3	Equal to serum	1000–50,000, MN or PMN	100–>100,000	Neg	Neg	Variable findings; 25% are transudates.
Rheumatoid arthritis or other collagen-vascular disease	Turbid or yellow-green	≥3	Very low (<40 in most); in RA, 5–20 mg/dL	1000–20,000, mostly MN	<1000	Neg	Neg	Rapid clotting time; secondary empyema common.
Pancreatitis	Turbid to serosanguineous	≥3	Equal to serum	1000–50,000, mostly PMN	1000–10,000	Neg	Neg	Effusion usually left-sided; high amylase level.
Esophageal rupture	Turbid to purulent; red-brown	≥3	Usually low	<5000–over 50,000, mostly PMN	<5000	Pos	Pos	Effusion usually left-sided: high fluid amylase level (salivary); pneumothorax in 25% of cases; pH <6.0 strongly suggests diagnosis.

[1]Glucose of pleural fluid in comparison to serum glucose.

[2]Exudative pleural effusions meet at least one of the following criteria: (1) pleural fluid protein/serum protein ratio >0.5; (2) pleural fluid LDH/serum LDH ratio >0.6; and (3) pleural fluid LDH >2/3 upper normal limit for serum LDH. Transudative pleural effusions meet none of these criteria. Transudative pleural effusions also occur in myxedema and sarcoidosis.

MN = mononuclear cells (lymphocytes or monocytes); **PMN** = polymorphonuclear cells; **AFB** = acid-fast bacilli; **MTb** = Mycobacterium tuberculosis.

Modified, with permission, from Therapy of pleural effusion. A statement by the Committee on Therapy. Am Rev Respir Dis 1968;97:479; Tierney LM Jr., McPhee SJ, Papadakis MA (editors): Current Medical Diagnosis & Treatment 2003. McGraw-Hill, 2003, and Way LW (editor): Current Surgical Diagnosis & Treatment, 10th ed. Originally published by Appleton & Lange. Copyright © 1974 by The McGraw-Hill Companies, Inc.

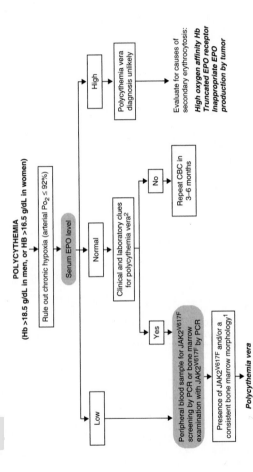

POLYCYTHEMIA
(Hb >18.5 g/dL in men, or HB >16.5 g/dL in women)

Rule out chronic hypoxia (arterial Po$_2$ ≤ 92%)

Serum EPO level

Low

Peripheral blood sample for JAK2^{V617F} screening by PCR or bone marrow examination with JAK2^{V617F} by PCR

Presence of JAK2^{V617F} and/or a consistent bone marrow morphology[1]

Polycythemia vera

Normal

Clinical and laboratory clues for polycythemia vera[2]

Yes

No

Repeat CBC in 3–6 months

High

Polycythemia vera diagnosis unlikely

Evaluate for causes of secondary erythrocytosis:
High oxygen affinity Hb
Truncated EPO receptor
Inappropriate EPO production by tumor

[1] JAK2^{V617F} mutation has been found to be present in 70–90% of patients with polycythemia vera; bone marrow biopsy showing panmyelosis with prominent erythroid and megakaryocytic proliferation.
[2] Clinical and laboratory clues for polycythemia vera include splenomegaly, platelet count >400,000/mcL, WBC>12,000/mcL, increased serum vitamin B$_{12}$ or vitamin B$_{12}$-binding capacity, and no history of familial erythrocytosis.

Figure 8–18. POLYCYTHEMIA: Diagnostic evaluation.

TABLE 8–17. PRENATAL DIAGNOSTIC METHODS: AMNIOCENTESIS AND CHORIONIC VILLUS SAMPLING.

Method	Procedure	Laboratory Analysis	Waiting Time for Results	Advantages	Disadvantages
Amniocentesis	Between the 12th and 16th weeks, and by the transabdominal approach, 10–30 mL of amniotic fluid is removed for cytologic and biochemical analysis. Preceding ultrasound locates the placenta and identifies twinning and missed abortion.	**1. Amniotic fluid** • α-Fetoprotein • Limited biochemical analysis • Virus isolation studies **2. Amniotic cell culture** • Chromosomal analysis	2–4 weeks	Over 40 years of experience.	Therapeutic abortion, if indicated, must be done in the second trimester. (RhoGam should be given to Rh-negative mothers to prevent sensitization.) Risks (approximately 1%): • Fetal: puncture or abortion. • Maternal: infection or bleeding.
Chorionic villus sampling	Between the 8th and 12th week, and with constant ultrasound guidance, the trophoblastic cells of the chorionic villi are obtained by transcervical or transabdominal endoscopic needle biopsy or aspiration.	**1. Direct cell analysis** • Chromosomal studies **2. Cell culture** • Limited biochemical analysis	1–10 days	Over 20 years of experience. Therapeutic abortion, if indicated, can be done in the first trimester.	Risks (approximately 3%): • Fetal: abortion. • Maternal: bleeding and infection (uncommon).

Modified, with permission, from Schroeder SA et al (editors): Current Medical Diagnosis & Treatment 1990. Originally published by Appleton & Lange. Copyright © 1990 by The McGraw-Hill Companies, Inc.

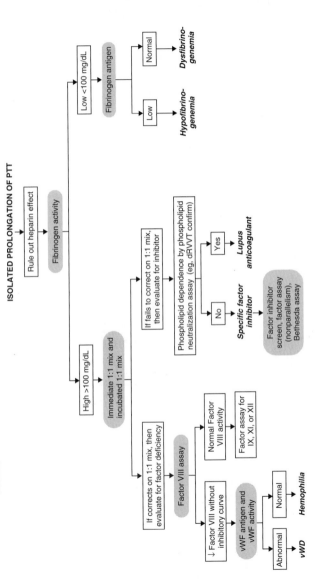

Figure 8–19. ISOLATED PROLONGATION OF PTT: Laboratory evaluation. **dRVVT** = dilute Russell viper venom time; **PTT** = activated partial thromboplastin time; **vWF** = von Willebrand factor; **vWD** = von Willebrand disease.

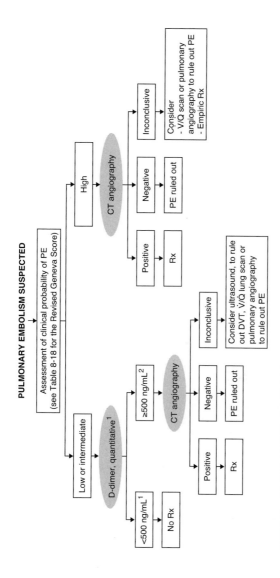

Figure 8-20. PULMONARY EMBOLISM: Diagnostic approach. **CT** = computed tomography; **DVT** = deep venous thrombosis; **PE** = pulmonary embolism; **Rx** = anticoagulant therapy; **V̇/Q̇ scan** = ventilation-perfusion scan. (*Modified from* Ann Intern Med *2006;144:165.*)

[1]D-dimer testing is typically used in emergency department setting for ruling out PE.
[2]The cut-off value is method-dependent (eg, 500 ng/mL is the cut-off for ELISA-based D-dimer assay).

TABLE 8–18. PULMONARY EMBOLISM: THE REVISED GENEVA SCORE FOR PROBABILITY ASSESSMENT.

Variable	Regression Coefficients	Points
Risk Factors		
Age >65 y	0.39	1
Previous DVT or PE	1.05	3
Surgery (under general anesthesia) or fracture (of the lower limbs) within 1 mo	0.78	2
Active malignant condition (solid or hematologic malignant condition, currently active or considered cured <1 y)	0.45	2
Symptoms		
Unilateral lower-limb pain Hemoptysis	0.97 0.74	3 2
Clinical Signs		
Heart rate 75–94 beats/min ≥95 beats/min	 1.20 0.67	 3 5
Pain on lower-limb deep venous palpation and unilateral edema	1.34	4
Clinical Probability		
Low		0–3 total
Intermediate		4–10 total
High		≥11 total

DVT = deep venous thrombosis; **PE** = pulmonary embolism.
Ann Intern Med 2006;144:165. [PMID: 16461960]

TABLE 8–19. PULMONARY FUNCTION TESTS: INTERPRETATION IN OBSTRUCTIVE AND RESTRICTIVE PULMONARY DISEASE.

Tests	Units	Definition	Obstructive Disease	Restrictive Disease
SPIROMETRY				
Forced vital capacity (FVC)	L	The volume that can be forcefully expelled from the lungs after maximal inspiration.	N or ↓	↓
Forced expiratory volume in 1 second (FEV$_1$)	L	The volume expelled in the first second of the FVC maneuver.	↓	N or ↓
FEV$_1$/FVC	%		↓	N or ↑
Forced expiratory flow from 25%–75% of the forced vital capacity (FEF 25–75%)	L/sec	The maximal midexpiratory airflow rate.	↓	N or ↓
Peak expiratory flow rate (PEFR)	L/sec	The maximal airflow rate achieved in the FVC maneuver.	↓	N or ↑
Maximum voluntary ventilation (MVV)	L/min	The maximum volume that can be breathed in 1 minute (usually measured for 15 seconds and multiplied by 4).	↓	N or ↓
LUNG VOLUMES				
Slow vital capacity (SVC)	L	The volume that can be slowly exhaled after maximal inspiration.	N or ↓	↓
Total lung capacity (TLC)	L	The volume in the lungs after a maximal inspiration.	N or ↑	↓
Functional residual capacity (FRC)	L	The volume in the lungs at the end of a normal tidal expiration.	↑	N or ↑
Expiratory reserve volume (ERV)	L	The volume representing the difference between FRC and RV.	N or ↓	N or ↓
Residual volume (RV)	L	The volume remaining in the lungs after maximal expiration.	↑	N or ↑
RV/TLC ratio	...		↑	N or ↑

N = normal; ↓ = less than predicted; ↑ = greater than predicted. Normal values vary according to subject sex, age, body size, and ethnicity.
Modified, with permission, from Tierney LM Jr, McPhee SJ, Papadakis MA (editors): Current Medical Diagnosis & Treatment 2003. *McGraw-Hill, 2003.*

TABLE 8–20. RENAL FAILURE: CLASSIFICATION AND DIFFERENTIAL DIAGNOSIS.

Classification	Prerenal Azotemia	Postrenal Azotemia	Acute Tubular Necrosis (Oliguric or Polyuric)	Intrinsic Renal Disease		
				Acute Glomerulonephritis	Acute Interstitial Nephritis	
Etiology	Poor renal perfusion	Obstruction of the urinary tract	Ischemia, nephrotoxins	Poststreptococcal infection; collagen–vascular disease	Allergic reaction; drug reaction	
Urinary indices Serum BUN: Cr ratio	>20:1	>20:1	<20:1	>20:1	<20:1	
U_{Na^+} (meq/L)	<20	Variable	>20	<20	Variable	
FE_{Na^+} (%)	<1	Variable	>1	<1	<1; >1	
Urine osmolality (mosm/kg)	>500	<400	250–300	Variable	Variable	
Urinary sediment	Benign, or hyaline casts	Normal or red cells, white cells, or crystals	Granular casts, renal tubular cells	Dysmorphic red cells and red cell casts	White cells, white cell casts, with or without eosinophils	

Reproduced, with permission, from Tierney LM Jr., McPhee SJ, Papadakis MA (editors): Current Medical Diagnosis & Treatment 2003. McGraw-Hill, 2003.

$$FE_{Na^+} = \left(\frac{Urine\,Na^+}{Plasma\,Na^+} \middle/ \frac{Urine\,Creatinine}{Plasma\,Creatinine} \right) \times 100$$

U_{Na^+} = urine sodium.

TABLE 8–21. RENAL TUBULAR ACIDOSIS (RTA): LABORATORY DIAGNOSIS.

Clinical Condition	Renal Defect	GFR	Serum [HCO_3] (meq/L)	Serum [K^+] (meq/L)	Minimal Urine pH	Associated Disease States	Treatment
Normal	None	N	24–28	3.5–5	4.8–5.2	None	None
Proximal RTA (type II)	Proximal H^+ secretion	N	15–18	↓	<5.5	Drugs, Fanconi syndrome, various genetic disorders, dysproteinemic states, secondary hyperparathyroidism, toxins (heavy metals), tubulointerstitial diseases, nephrotic syndrome, paroxysmal nocturnal hemoglobinuria.	$NaHCO_3$ or $KHCO_3$ (10–15 meq/kg/d), thiazides.
Classic distal RTA (type I)	Distal H^+ secretion	N	20–23	↓	>5.5	Various genetic diseases, autoimmune diseases, nephrocalcinosis, drugs, toxins, tubulointerstitial diseases, hepatic cirrhosis, empty sella syndrome.	$NaHCO_3$ (1–3 meq/kg/d).
Buffer deficiency distal RTA (type III)	Distal NH_3 delivery	↓	15–18	N	<5.5	Chronic renal insufficiency, renal osteodystrophy, severe hypophosphatemia.	$NaHCO_3$ (1–3 meq/kg/d).
Generalized distal RTA (type IV)	Distal Na^+ reabsorption, K^+ secretion, and H^+ secretion	↓	24–28	↑	<5.5	Primary mineralocorticoid deficiency (eg, Addison disease), hyporeninemic hypoaldosteronism (diabetes mellitus, tubulointerstitial diseases, nephrosclerosis, drugs), salt-wasting mineralocorticoid-resistant hyperkalemia.	Fludrocortisone (0.1–0.5 mg/d), dietary K^+ restriction, furosemide (40–160 mg/d), $NaHCO_3$ (1–3 meq/kg/d).

GFR = glomerular filtration rate.
Modified, with permission, from Cogan MG: *Fluid & Electrolytes: Physiology & Pathophysiology. Originally published by Appleton & Lange. Copyright © 1991 by the McGraw-Hill Companies, Inc.*

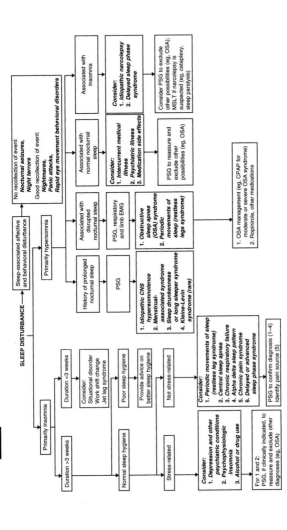

Figure 8–21. SLEEP DISTURBANCE: Diagnostic evaluation. Poor sleep hygiene refers to products or behaviors that can interfere with sleep, such as caffeine, alcohol, and tobacco, intense exercise in the evening, and irregular sleeping schedule. **CNS** = central nervous system; **CPAP** = continuous positive airway pressure; **EMG** = electromyogram; **MSLTs** = multiple sleep latency tests (note: patient must be off antidepressants and stimulants to undergo an MSLT); **PSG** = polysomnography.

TABLE 8–22. SYPHILIS: LABORATORY EVALUATION IN UNTREATED PATIENTS.

Stage	Onset After Exposure	Persistence	Clinical Findings	Sensitivity of VDRL or RPR[1] (%)	Sensitivity of FTA-ABS[2] (%)	Sensitivity of MHA-TP[3] (%)
Primary	21 days (range 10–90)	2–12 wk	Chancre	72	91	50–60
Secondary	6 wk–6 mo	1–3 mo	Rash, condylomata lata, mucous patches, fever, lymphadenopathy, patchy alopecia	100	100	100
Early latent		<1 yr	Relapses of secondary syphilis	73	97	98
Late latent		>1 yr	Clinically silent	73	97	98
Tertiary		1 yr until death	Dementia, tabes dorsalis, aortitis, aortic aneurysm, gummas	77	99	98

Late latent persistence: Lifelong unless tertiary syphilis appears

[1]VDRL is a slide flocculation test for nonspecific (anticardiolipin) antibodies, used for screening, quantitation of titer, and monitoring response to treatment; RPR is an agglutination test for nonspecific antibodies, used primarily for screening.
[2]FTA-ABS is an immunofluorescence test for treponemal antibodies utilizing serum absorbed for nonpathogenic treponemes, used for confirmation of infection, not routine screening.
[3]MHA-TP is a microhemagglutination test similar to the FTA-ABS, but one which can be quantitated and automated.
MHA-TP = microhemagglutination assay for *Treponema pallidum*; **RPR** = rapid plasma reagin test.
FTA-ABS = fluorescent treponemal antibody absorption test; **VDRL** = Venereal Disease Research Laboratories test; **RPR** = rapid plasma reagin test.
Modified, with permission, from Harvey AM et al (editors): The Principles and Practice of Medicine, 22nd ed. Originally published by Appleton & Lange. Copyright © 1988 by The McGraw-Hill Companies, Inc.

TABLE 8–23. THALASSEMIA SYNDROMES: GENETICS AND LABORATORY CHARACTERISTICS.

α-Thalassemia[1]			
Syndrome	α-Globin Genes	Hematocrit	MCV (fL)
Normal	4	N	N
Silent carrier	3	N	N
Thalassemia minor	2	32–40%	60–75
Hemoglobin H disease	1	22–32%	60–75
Hydrops fetalis	0	Fetal death occurs in utero	

[1]Alpha thalassemias are due primarily to deletion in the α globin gene on chromosome 16.

β-Thalassemia[1]				
Syndrome	β-Globin Genes	Hb A[2]	Hb A_2[3]	Hb F[4]
Normal	Homozygous beta	97–99%	1–3%	<1%
Thalassemia minor	Heterozygous beta[0,5]	80–95%	4–8%	1–5%
	Heterozygous beta[+ 6]	80–95%	4–8%	1–5%
Thalassemia intermedia	Homozygous beta[+] (mild)	0–30%	0–10%	6–100%
Thalassemia major	Homozygous beta[0]	0%	4–10%	90–96%
	Homozygous beta[+]	0–10%	4–10%	90–96%

[1]β-Thalassemias are usually caused by point mutations in the β-globin gene on chromosome 11 that result in premature chain terminations or defective RNA transcription, leading to reduced or absent β-globin chain synthesis.
[2]Hb A is composed of two α chains and two β chains: $\alpha_2\beta_2$
[3]Hb A_2 is composed of two α chains and two δ chains: $\alpha_2\delta_2$.
[4]Hb F is composed of two α chains and two γ chains: $\alpha_2\gamma_2$.
[5]β[0] refers to defects that result in absent globin chain synthesis.
[6]β[+] refers to defects that cause reduced globin chain synthesis.
Modified, with permission, from Tierney LM Jr, McPhee SJ, Papadakis MA (editors): Current Medical Diagnosis & Treatment 2003. *McGraw-Hill, 2003.*

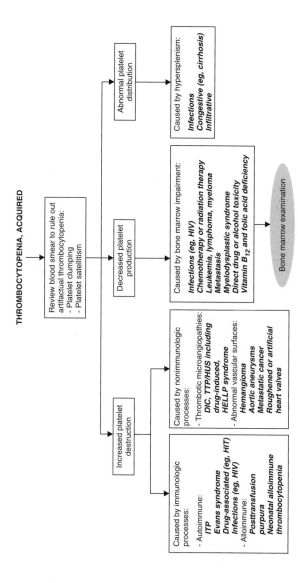

Figure 8–22. THROMBOCYTOPENIA: Causes of acquired thrombocytopenia. **DIC** = disseminated intravascular coagulation; **HELLP syndrome** = hemolysis, elevated liver enzymes, low platelets; **HIT** = heparin-induced thrombocytopenia; **HIV** = human immunodeficiency virus; **HUS** = hemolytic uremic syndrome; **ITP** = idiopathic thrombocytopenic purpura; **TTP** = thrombotic thrombocytopenic purpura.

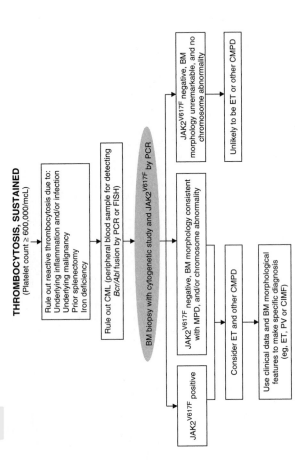

THROMBOCYTOSIS, SUSTAINED
(Platelet count ≥ 600,000/mcL)

Rule out reactive thrombocytosis due to:
Underlying inflammation and/or infection
Underlying malignancy
Prior splenectomy
Iron deficiency

↓

Rule out CML (peripheral blood sample for detecting *Bcr/Abl* fusion by PCR or FISH)

↓

BM biopsy with cytogenetic study and JAK2^{V617F} by PCR

- JAK2^{V617F} positive
- JAK2^{V617F} negative, BM morphology consistent with MPD, and/or chromosome abnormality

  ↓

  Consider ET and other CMPD

  ↓

  Use clinical data and BM morphological features to make specific diagnosis (eg, ET, PV or CIMF)

- JAK2^{V617F} negative, BM morphology unremarkable, and no chromosome abnormality

  ↓

  Unlikely to be ET or other CMPD

Figure 8–23. THROMBOCYTOSIS: Diagnostic evaluation. **BM** = bone marrow; **CML** = chronic myeloid leukemia; **CMPD** = chronic myeloproliferative disease; **CIMF** = chronic idiopathic myelofibrosis; **ET** = essential thrombocythemia; **FISH** = fluorescent in situ hybridization; **PCR** = polymerase chain reaction; **PV** = polycythemia vera.

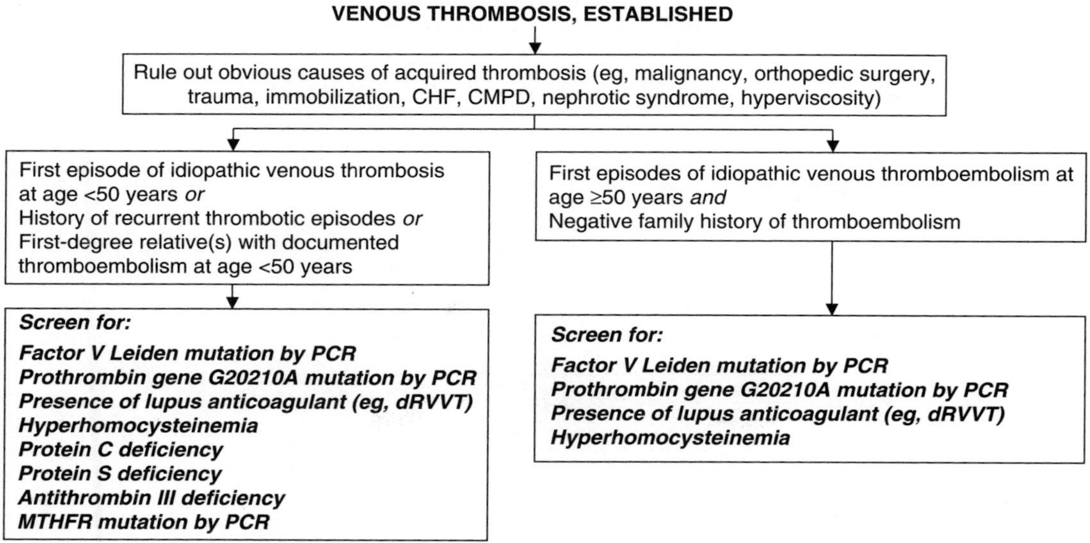

VENOUS THROMBOSIS, ESTABLISHED

Rule out obvious causes of acquired thrombosis (eg, malignancy, orthopedic surgery, trauma, immobilization, CHF, CMPD, nephrotic syndrome, hyperviscosity)

First episode of idiopathic venous thrombosis at age <50 years *or*
History of recurrent thrombotic episodes *or*
First-degree relative(s) with documented thromboembolism at age <50 years

Screen for:
Factor V Leiden mutation by PCR
Prothrombin gene G20210A mutation by PCR
Presence of lupus anticoagulant (eg, dRVVT)
Hyperhomocysteinemia
Protein C deficiency
Protein S deficiency
Antithrombin III deficiency
MTHFR mutation by PCR

First episodes of idiopathic venous thromboembolism at age ≥50 years *and*
Negative family history of thromboembolism

Screen for:
Factor V Leiden mutation by PCR
Prothrombin gene G20210A mutation by PCR
Presence of lupus anticoagulant (eg, dRVVT)
Hyperhomocysteinemia

Figure 8–24. THROMBOSIS, VENOUS: Recommended screening for causes of thrombophilia. **CHF** = congestive heart failure; **CMPD** = chronic myeloproliferative disorder; **dRVVT** = dilute Russell viper venom clotting time; **MTHFR** = methylene tetrahydrofolate reductase; **PCR** = polymerase chain reaction.

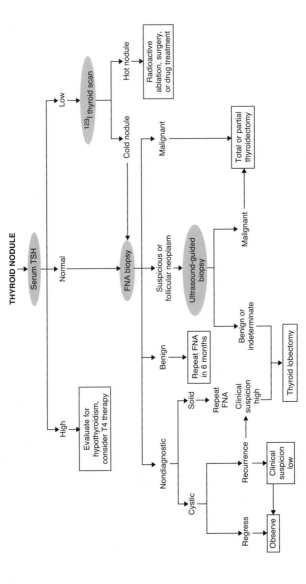

Figure 8–25. THYROID NODULE: Diagnostic evaluation. **FNA** = fine needle aspiration; **TSH** = thyroid-stimulating hormone. (*Modified with permission from Burch HB. Evaluation and management of the solid thyroid nodule.* Endocrinol Metab Clin North Am *1995;24:663–710.*)

TABLE 8–24. THYROID FUNCTION TESTING AND ITS CLINICAL APPLICATION.

Condition	TSH (mcU/mL)[1]	Free T$_4$ (ng/dL)	Total T$_4$ (mcg/dL)	Total T$_3$ (ng/dL)	Comments and Treatment
Normal[2]	0.35–5.5	Varies with method	5–12	95–190	
Hyperthyroidism	↓	↑	↑	↑	In TRH stimulation test, TSH shows no response. Thyroid scan shows increased diffuse activity (Grave's disease) versus "hot" areas (hyperfunctioning nodules). Thyroperoxidase (TPO) and thyroid-stimulating hormone receptor antibodies (TSH-R Ab [stim]) elevated in Graves disease.
Hypothyroidism	Usually ↑ (primary[3] hypothyroidism), rarely ↓ (secondary[4] hypothyroidism)	↓	↓	↓	TRH stimulation test shows exaggerated response in primary hypothyroidism. In secondary hypothyroidism, TRH test helps to differentiate pituitary from hypothalamic disorders. In pituitary lesions, TSH fails to rise after TRH; in hypothalamic lesion, TSH rises but response is delayed. Antithyroglobulin and thyroperoxidase (TPO) antibodies elevated in Hashimoto's thyroiditis.
HYPOTHYROIDISM ON REPLACEMENT					
T$_4$ replacement	N or ↓	N	N	N	TSH ↓ with 0.1–0.2 mg T$_4$ daily.
T$_3$ replacement	N or ↓	↓	↓	N	TSH ↓ with 50 mcg T$_3$ daily.
Euthyroid following injection of radiocontrast dye	N	N or ↑	N	N	Effects may persist for 2 weeks or longer.

(continued)

TABLE 8–24. THYROID FUNCTION TESTING AND ITS CLINICAL APPLICATION. (CONTINUED)

Condition	TSH (mcu/mL)[1]	Free T4 (ng/dL)	Total T4 (mcg/dL)	Total T3 (ng/dL)	Comments and Treatment
PREGNANCY					
Hyperthyroid	↓	↑	↑	↑	Effects may persist for 6–10 weeks post-partum.
Euthyroid	N	N	↑	↑	
Hypothyroid	↑	↓	N or ↓		
Oral contraceptives, estrogens, methadone, heroin	N	N	↑	↑	Increased serum thyroid-binding globulin.
Glucocorticoids, androgens, phenytoin, asparaginase, salicylates (high dose)	N	N	↓	N or ↓	Decreased serum thyroid-binding globulin.
Nephrotic syndrome	N	N	↓	N or ↓	Loss of thyroid-binding globulin accounts for serum T4 decrease.
Iodine deficiency	N	N	N	N	Extremely rare in USA.
Iodine ingestion	N	N	N	N	Excess iodine may cause hypothyroidism or hyperthyroidism in susceptible individuals.

Laboratory Test Results	Most Common Diagnosis	Other Common Diagnoses
Low TSH, Elevated free T_3 or T_4	Graves disease	Multinodular goiter Toxic nodule Transient thyroiditis
Low TSH, normal free T_3 or T_4	Subclinical hyperthyroidism	Recent thyroxine ingestion for hypothyroidism
Low or normal TSH, low free T_3 or T_4	Nonthyroidal illness[5]	Recent treatment for hyperthyroidism, Secondary (pituitary) hypothyroidism
Elevated TSH, low free T_4 or T_3	Chronic autoimmune thyroiditis (Hashimoto disease)	Hypothyroid phase of transient thyroiditis, Previous neck irradiation or thyroid surgery, Iodine deficiency Drugs (eg, amiodarone)
Elevated TSH, normal free T_4 and T_3	Subclinical autoimmune thyroiditis	Heterophile antibody Incomplete treatment for hypothyroidism
Normal or elevated TSH, elevated free T_4 or T_3	None	Interfering antibodies Intermittent T_4 therapy TSH-secreting pituitary tumor

[1] Thyroid function screening should start with TSH, and a TSH assay with ≤0.02 mcU/mL functional sensitivity is recommended.
[2] Normal values vary with laboratory.
[3] Thyroid (end-organ) failure.
[4] Pituitary or hypothalamic lesions.
[5] Commonly referred to as "euthyroid sick."
N = normal; **V** = variable.
Adapted, with permission, from Lancet 2001;357:619.

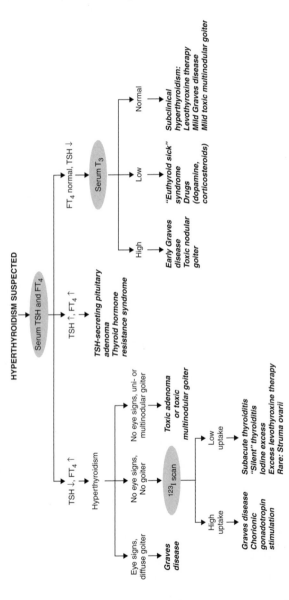

Figure 8–26. HYPERTHYROIDISM: Laboratory evaluation. **FT$_4$** = free thyroxine; **T$_3$** = 3,5,3'-triiodothyronine; **TSH** = thyroid-stimulating hormone. (Modified with permission from Gardner DG, Shoback D [editors]: Greenspan's Basic & Clinical Endocrinology, 8th ed. Published by Appleton & Lange. Copyright © 2007 by The McGraw-Hill Companies, Inc.)

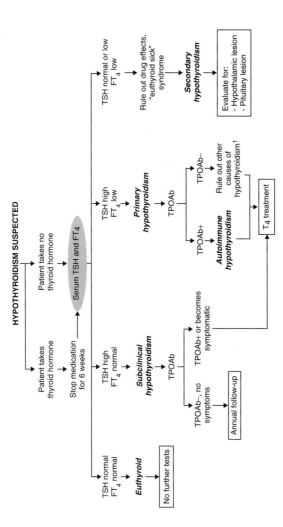

[1]Other causes of hypothyroidism include iatrogenic (eg, irradiation, thyroidectomy), drugs (eg, lithium, antithyroid drugs), congenital, iodine deficiency, and infiltrative disorders involving thyroid gland.

Figure 8–27. HYPOTHYROIDISM: Diagnostic approach. **FT4** = free thyroxine; **TPOAb+** = thyroid peroxidase antibodies positive; **TPOAb–** = thyroid peroxidase antibodies negative; **TSH** = thyroid-stimulating hormone.

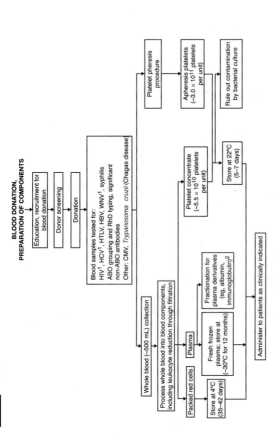

BLOOD DONATION,
PREPARATION OF COMPONENTS

Education, recruitment for
blood donation

Donor screening

Donation

Blood samples tested for:
HIV[1], HCV[1], HTLV, HBV, WNV[1], syphilis
ABO grouping and RhD typing, significant
non-ABO antibodies
Other: CMV, *Trypanosoma cruzii* (Chagas disease)

Platelet pheresis
procedure

Apheresis platelets
(~3.0 × 10[11] platelets
per unit)

Rule out contamination
by bacterial culture

Whole blood (~500 mL) collection

Process whole blood into blood components,
including leukocyte reduction through filtration

Packed red cells

Plasma

Platelet concentrate
(~5.5 × 10[10] platelets
per unit)

Store at 4°C
(35–42 days)

Fresh frozen
plasma; store at
(–30°C for 12 months)[2]

Fractionation for
plasma derivatives
(eg, albumin,
immunoglobulin)[2]

Store at 22°C
(5–7 days)

Administer to patients as clinically indicated

[1]Nucleic acid testing (NAT) should be included for HIV, HCV, and WNV screening.
[2]Plasma derivatives are also prepared through plasmapheresis.

Figure 8–28. PREPARATION OF BLOOD COMPONENTS. CMV = cytomegalovirus; **HBV** = hepatitis B virus; **HCV** = hepatitis C virus; **HIV** = human immunodeficiency virus; **HTLV** = human T-cell leukemia virus; **WNV** = West Nile virus.

TABLE 8-25. TRANSFUSION: SUMMARY CHART OF BLOOD COMPONENT THERAPY.

Component	Major Indications	Action/Benefit	Not Indicated For	Special Precautions	Hazards[1]	Rate/Time of Infusion
Whole blood	Symptomatic anemia with large volume deficit	Restoration of oxygen-carrying capacity, restoration of blood volume	Condition responsive to specific component	Must be ABO identical Labile coagulation factors deteriorate within 24 hours after collection	Infectious diseases; septic/toxic, allergic; febrile reactions; circulatory overload; GVHD	For massive loss, as fast as patient can tolerate
Red blood cells; red blood cells with adenine-saline added	Symptomatic anemia	Restoration of oxygen-carrying capacity	Pharmacologically treatable anemia Coagulation deficiency	Must be ABO-compatible	Infectious diseases; septic/toxic, allergic; febrile reactions; GVHD	As patient can tolerate, but less than 4 hours
Red blood cells, leukocyte-reduced[4]	Symptomatic anemia, febrile reactions from leukocyte antibodies or cytokines, prevention of platelet refractoriness due to alloimmunization	Restoration of oxygen-carrying capacity, reduction of risks of febrile reactions, HLA alloimmunization and CMV infection	Pharmacologically treatable anemia Coagulation deficiency	Must be ABO-compatible	Infectious diseases; septic/toxic, allergic reactions (unless plasma also removed, eg, by washing); GVHD	As patient can tolerate, but less than 4 hours
Fresh-frozen plasma[2]	Deficit of labile and stable plasma coagulation factors and TTP	Source of labile and nonlabile plasma factors	Condition responsive to volume replacement	Must be ABO-compatible	Infectious diseases, allergic reactions, circulatory overload	Less than 4 hours
Liquid plasma; plasma; and thawed plasma	Deficit of stable coagulation factors	Source of nonlabile plasma factors	Deficit of labile coagulation factors or volume replacement	Must be ABO compatible	Infectious diseases; allergic reactions	Less than 4 hours

(continued)

TABLE 8–25. TRANSFUSION: SUMMARY CHART OF BLOOD COMPONENT THERAPY. (CONTINUED)

Component	Major Indications	Action/Benefit	Not Indicated For	Special Precautions	Hazards[1]	Rate/Time of Infusion
Cryoprecipitate AHF	Hemophilia A,[3] von Willebrand[3] disease,[3] hypofibrinogenemia, factor XIII deficiency	Provides factor VIII, fibrinogen, von Willebrand factor, factor XIII	Deficit of any plasma protein other than those enriched in cryoprecipitated AHF	Frequent repeat doses may be necessary for factor VIII	Infectious diseases; allergic reactions	Less than 4 hours
Platelets; platelets from pheresis[4]	Bleeding from thrombocytopenia or platelet function abnormality	Improves hemostasis	Plasma coagulation deficits and some conditions with rapid platelet destruction (eg, ITP)	Should not use some microaggregate filters (check manufacturer's instructions)	Infectious diseases; septic/toxic, allergic, febrile reactions; GVHD	Less than 4 hours
Granulocytes from pheresis	Neutropenia with infection	Provides granulocytes	Infection responsive to antibiotics	Must be ABO-compatible; do not use depth-type microaggregate filters or leuko-depletion filters	Infectious diseases; allergic, febrile reactions; GVHD	One unit over 2–4 hours. Observe closely for reactions.

[1]For all cellular components, there is a risk the recipient may become alloimmunized.

[2]Solvent detergent pooled plasma is an alternative in which some viruses are inactivated, but clotting factor composition is changed.

[3]When virus-inactivated concentrates are not available.

[4]Red blood cells and platelets may be processed in a manner that yields leukocyte-reduced components. The main indications for leukocyte-reduced components are prevention of febrile, nonhemolytic transfusion reactions and prevention of leukocyte alloimmunization. Risks are the same as for standard components except for reduced risk of febrile reactions, HLA alloimmunization and CMV infection.

AHF = antihemophilic factor; **GVHD** = graft-versus-host disease; **ITP** = idiopathic thrombocytopenic purpura; **TTP** = thrombotic thrombocytopenic purpura. From the American Association of Blood Banks, American Red Cross, American Blood Centers. *Circular of information for the use of human blood and blood components. July 2002* (available at www.aabb.org).

TABLE 8-26. URINALYSIS: FINDINGS IN VARIOUS DISEASE STATES.

Disease	Daily Volume	Specific Gravity	Protein (mg/dL)	Esterase	Nitrite	RBC	WBC	Casts	Other Microscopic Findings
Normal	600–2500 mL	1.001–1.035	0–trace (0–15)	Neg	Neg	0 or Occ	0 or Occ	0 or Occ	Hyaline casts
Fever	↓	↑	Trace or 1+ (<30)	Neg	Neg	0	Occ	0 or Occ	Hyaline casts, tubular cells
Congestive heart failure	↓	↑ (varies)	1–2+ (30–100)	Neg	Neg	None or 1+	0	1+	Hyaline and granular casts
Eclampsia	↓	↑	3–4+ (30–2000)	Neg	Neg	None or 1+	0	3–4+	Hyaline casts
Diabetic coma	↑ or ↓	↑	1+ (30)	Neg	Neg	0	0	0 or 1+	Hyaline casts
Acute glomerulonephritis	↓	↑	2–4+ (100–2000)	Pos	Neg	1–4+	1–4+	2–4+	Blood; RBC, cellular, granular, and hyaline casts; renal tubular epithelium

(continued)

TABLE 8–26. URINALYSIS: FINDINGS IN VARIOUS DISEASE STATES. *(CONTINUED)*

Disease	Daily Volume	Specific Gravity	Protein (mg/dL)	Esterase	Nitrite	RBC	WBC	Casts	Other Microscopic Findings
Nephrotic syndrome	N or ↓	N or ↑	4+ (>2000)	Neg	Neg	1–2+	0	4+	Granular, waxy, hyaline, and fatty casts; fatty tubular cells
Chronic renal failure	↑ or ↓	Low; invariable	1–2+ (30–100)	Neg	Neg	Occ or 1+	0	1–3+	Granular, hyaline, fatty, and broad casts
Connective tissue disorders	N, ↑ or ↓	N or ↓	1–4+ (30–2000)	Neg	Neg	1–4+	0 or Occ	1–4+	Blood, cellular, granular, hyaline, waxy, fatty, and broad casts; fatty tubular cells; telescoped sediment
Pyelonephritis	N or ↓	N or ↓	1–2+ (30–100)	Pos	Pos	0 or 1+	4+	0 or 1+	WBC casts and hyaline casts; many pus cells; bacteria
Hypertension	N or ↑	N or ↓	None or 1+ (<30)	Neg	Neg	0 or Occ	0 or Occ	0 or 1+	Hyaline and granular casts

Protein concentration in mg/dL is listed in parentheses.
Modified, with permission, from Krupp MA et al (editors): Physician's Handbook, 21st ed. Originally published by The McGraw-Hill Companies, Inc.

TABLE 8–27. VAGINAL DISCHARGE: LABORATORY EVALUATION.

Diagnosis	pH	Odor With KOH (Positive "Whiff" Test)	Epithelial Cells	WBCs	Organisms	KOH Prep	Gram Stain	Comments
Normal	<4.5	No	N	Occ	Variable, large rods not adherent to epithelial cells	Neg	Gram-positive rods	
Trichomonas vaginalis vaginitis	>4.5	Yes	N	↑	Motile, flagellated organisms	Neg	Flagellated organisms	
Bacterial vaginosis (*Gardnerella vaginalis*)	>4.5	Yes	Clue cells[1]	Occ	Coccobacilli adherent to epithelial cells	Neg	Gram-negative coccobacilli	
Candida albicans vaginitis	<4.5	No	N	Occ slightly increased	Budding yeast or hyphae	Budding yeast or hyphae	Budding yeast or hyphae	Usually white "cottage cheese" curd
Mucopurulent cervicitis (*N gonorrhoeae*)	Variable, usually >4.5	No	N	↑	Variable	Neg	Intracellular gram-negative diplococci	

[1]Epithelial cells covered with bacteria to the extent that cell nuclear borders are obscured.

Modified, with permission, from Kelly KG: Tests on vaginal discharge. In: Walker HK et al (editors): Clinical Methods: The History, Physical and Laboratory Examinations, 3rd ed. Butterworths, 1990.

TABLE 8–28. VALVULAR HEART DISEASE: DIAGNOSTIC EVALUATION.

Diagnosis	Chest X-Ray	ECG	Echocardiography	Comments
MITRAL STENOSIS (MS) Rheumatic disease	Straight left heart border. Large LA sharply indenting esophagus. Elevation of left main bronchus. Calcification occ seen in MV.	Broad negative phase of biphasic P in V_1. Tall peaked P waves, right axis deviation, or RVH appear if pulmonary hypertension is present.	**M-Mode:** Thickened, immobile MV with anterior and posterior leaflets moving together. Slow early diastolic filling slope. LA enlargement. Normal to small LV. **2D:** Maximum diastolic orifice size reduced. Reduced subvalvular apparatus. Foreshortened, variable thickening of other valves. **Doppler:** Prolonged pressure half-time across MV. Indirect evidence of pulmonary hypertension.	"Critical" MS is usually defined as a valve area <1.0 cm². Balloon valvuloplasty has high initial success rates and higher patency rates than for AS. Open commissurotomy can be effective. Valve replacement is indicated when severe regurgitation is present. Catheterization can confirm echo results.
MITRAL REGURGITATION (MR) Myxomatous degeneration (MV prolapse) Infective endocarditis Subvalvular dysfunction Rheumatic disease	Enlarged LV and LA.	Left axis deviation or frank LVH. P waves broad, tall, or notched, with broad negative phase in V_1.	**M-Mode and 2D:** Thickened MV in rheumatic disease. MV prolapse; flail leaflet or vegetations may be seen. Enlarged LV. **Doppler:** Regurgitant flow mapped into LA. Indirect evidence of pulmonary hypertension.	In nonrheumatic MR, valvuloplasty without valve replacement is increasingly successful. Acute MR (endocarditis, ruptured chordae) requires emergent valve replacement. Catheterization is the best assessment of regurgitation.
AORTIC STENOSIS (AS) Calcific (especially in congenitally bicuspid valve) Rheumatic disease	Concentric LVH. Prominent ascending aorta, small knob. Calcified valve common.	LVH.	**M-Mode:** Dense persistent echoes of the AoV with poor leaflet excursion. LVH with preserved contractile function. **2D:** Poststenotic dilatation of the aorta with restricted opening of the leaflets. Bicuspid AoV in about 30%.	"Critical" AS is usually defined as a valve area <0.7 cm² or a peak systolic gradient of >50 mm Hg. Catheterization is definitive diagnostic test.

(continued)

	Radiograph	ECG	Echocardiography	Comments
			Doppler: Increased transvalvular flow velocity, yielding calculated gradient.	Prognosis without surgery is less than 50% survival at 3 years when CHF, syncope, or angina occur. Balloon valvuloplasty has a high restenosis rate.
AORTIC REGURGITATION (AR) Bicuspid valves Infective endocarditis Hypertension Rheumatic disease Aorta/aortic root disease	Moderate to severe LV enlargement. Prominent aortic knob.	LVH.	**M-Mode:** Diastolic vibrations of the anterior leaflet of the MV and septum. Early closure of the valve when severe. Dilated LV with normal or decreased contractility. **2D:** May show vegetations in endocarditis, bicuspid valve, or root dilatation. **Doppler:** Demonstrates regurgitation. Estimates severity.	Aortography at catheterization can demonstrate AR. Acute incompetence leads to LV failure and requires AoV replacement.
TRICUSPID STENOSIS (TS) Rheumatic disease	Enlarged RA only.	Tall, peaked P waves. Normal axis.	**M-Mode and 2D:** TV thickening. Decreased early diastolic filling slope of the TV. MV also usually abnormal. **Doppler:** Prolonged pressure half-time across TV.	Right heart catheterization is diagnostic. Valvulotomy may lead to success, but TV replacement is usually needed.
TRICUSPID REGURGITATION (TR) RV overload (pulmonary hypertension) Inferior infarction Infective endocarditis	Enlarged RA and RV.	Right axis deviation usual.	**M-Mode and 2D:** Enlarged RV. MV often abnormal and may prolapse. **Doppler:** Regurgitant flow mapped into RA and venae cavae. RV systolic pressure estimated.	RA and jugular pressure tracings show a prominent V wave and rapid Y descent. Replacement of TV is rarely done. Valvuloplasty is often preferred.

AoV = aortic valve; **CHF** = congestive heart failure. **LA** = left atrium; **LV** = left ventricle; **LVH** = left ventricular hypertrophy; **MV** = mitral valve; **RA** = right atrium; **RV** = right ventricle; **RVH** = right ventricular hypertrophy; **TV** = tricuspid valve.
Modified, with permission, from Tierney LM Jr, McPhee SJ, Papadakis MA (editors): Current Medical Diagnosis & Treatment 2003. McGraw Hill, 2003.

TABLE 8–29. WHITE BLOOD CELLS: INTERPRETATION OF WHITE CELL COUNT AND DIFFERENTIAL.[1]

Cells	Range (10^3/mcL)	Increased in	Decreased in
WBC count (total)	4.0–11.0	Infection, hematologic malignancy.	Decreased production (aplastic anemia, folate or B_{12} deficiency, drugs [eg, ethanol, chloramphenicol]); decreased survival (sepsis, hypersplenism, drugs).
Neutrophils	1.8–6.8	Infection (bacterial or early viral), acute stress, acute and chronic inflammation, tumors, drugs, diabetic ketoacidosis, leukemia (rare).	Aplastic anemia, drug-induced neutropenia (eg, chlor-amphenicol, phenothiazines, antithyroid drugs, sulfonamide), chemotherapy, folate or B_{12} deficiency, myelodysplasia, marrow infiltration, physiologic (in children up to age 4 years).
Lymphocytes	0.9–2.9	Viral infection (especially infectious mononucleosis, pertussis), thyrotoxicosis, adrenal insufficiency, ALL and CLL, chronic infection, drug and allergic reactions, autoimmune diseases.	Immune deficiency syndromes (HIV).
Monocytes	0.1–0.6	Inflammation, infection, malignancy, tuberculosis, myeloproliferative disorders (eg, CMML).	Depleted in overwhelming bacterial infection.
Eosinophils	0.0–0.4	Allergic states, drug sensitivity reactions, skin disorders, tissue invasion by parasites, polyarteritis nodosa, hypersensitivity response to malignancy (eg, Hodgkin disease), pulmonary infiltrative disease, disseminated eosinophilic hypersensitivity disease.	Acute and chronic inflammation, stress, drugs (corticosteroids).
Basophils	0.0–0.1	Hypersensitivity reactions, drugs, myeloproliferative disorders (eg, CML), myelofibrosis.	

[1]In the automated differential, white cells are classified as neutrophils, monocytes, lymphocytes, eosinophils or basophils based on its size and surface/internal characteristics (eg, granularity, peroxidase). Different instruments use different methodologies for the differential. The reproducibility of 100-cell manual differentials is notoriously poor. Review of blood smears is useful to visually identify rare abnormal cells (eg, imma-ture granulocytes, toxic changes, dysplastic cells, blasts, nucleated RBCs, etc).
ALL = acute lymphocytic leukemia; **CLL** = chronic lymphocytic leukemia; **CML** = chronic myeloid leukemia; **CMML** = chronic myelomonocytic leukemia.

9

Nomograms and Reference Material

Stephen J. McPhee, MD, Diana Nicoll, MD, PhD, MPA,
Michael Pignone, MD, MPH, and Chuanyi Mark Lu, MD

HOW TO USE THIS SECTION

This section contains useful nomograms and reference material. Material is
presented in alphabetical order by subject.

Contents

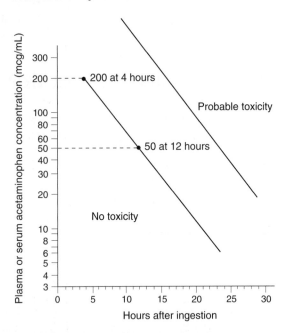

Figure 9–1. ACETAMINOPHEN TOXICITY: Nomogram for prediction of acetaminophen hepatotoxicity following acute overdosage. The upper line defines serum acetaminophen concentrations known to be associated with hepatotoxicity; the lower line defines serum levels 25% below those expected to cause hepatotoxicity. To give a margin for error, the lower line should be used as a guide to treatment. (*Modified and reproduced, with permission, from Rumack BH, Matthew H: Acetaminophen poisoning and toxicity.* Pediatrics *1975;55:871. Reproduced by permission of Pediatrics. Copyright © 1975. Permission obtained also from Saunders CE, Ho MT [editors]:* Current Emergency Diagnosis & Treatment, *4th ed. Originally published by Appleton & Lange. Copyright © 1992 by The McGraw-Hill Companies, Inc.)*

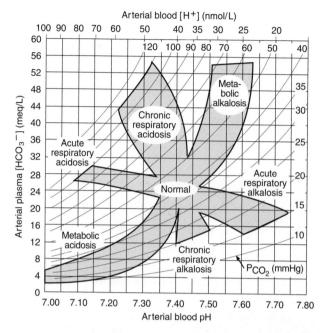

Figure 9–2. ACID–BASE NOMOGRAM: Shown are the 95% confidence limits of the normal respiratory and metabolic compensations for primary acid–base disturbances. (*Reproduced, with permission, from Cogan MG [editor]:* Fluid and Electrolytes: Physiology & Pathophysiology. *Originally published by Appleton & Lange. Copyright © 1991 by The McGraw-Hill Companies, Inc.*)

Extrinsic pathway   **Intrinsic pathway**

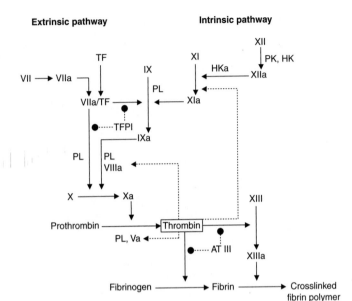

Figure 9–3. THE COAGULATION CASCADE: Schematic representation of the coagulation pathways. The central precipitating event is considered to involve tissue factor (TF), which under physiologic conditions, is not exposed to the blood. With vascular or endothelial cell injury, TF acts together with Factor VIIa and phospholipids (PL) to convert Factor IX to IXa and Factor X to Xa. The "intrinsic pathway" includes "contact" activation of Factor XI by XIIa-activated high molecular-weight kininogen complex (XIIa-HKa). Factor XIa converts Factor IX to IXa, which, in turn, converts Factor X to Xa, in concert with Factor VIIIa and PL. Factor Xa is the active ingredient of the "prothrombinase" complex, which includes Factor Va and PL, and converts prothrombin to thrombin (TH). TH cleaves fibrinopeptides from fibrinogen, allowing the resultant fibrin monomers to polymerize, and converts Factor XIII to XIIIa, which crosslinks the fibrin clot. TH also accelerates and augments the process (in dashed lines) by activating Factor V and VIII, but continued proteolytic action also dampens the process by activating protein C, which degrades Factor Va and VIIIa. TH activation of Factor XI to XIa is a proposed pathway. There are natural plasma inhibitors of the cascade: tissue factor pathway inhibitor (TFPI) blocks VIIa/TF and thus inactivates the "extrinsic pathway" after the clotting process is initiated; antithrombin III (AT III) blocks IXa and Xa and thrombin. Arrows = active enzymes; dashed lines with arrows = positive feedback reactions, which are considered important to maintain the process after the "extrinsic pathway" is shut down by TFPI; dashed lines with solid dots = inhibitory effects; **PK** = prekallikrein. It should be noted that the contact system (PK, HK, and XII) actually contributes to fibrinolysis and bradykinin formation in vivo, and its role in initiation of the intrinsic pathway in vivo is questionable.

Figure 9–4. DERMATOME CHART: Cutaneous innervation. The segmental or radicular (root) distribution is shown on the right side of the body, and the peripheral nerve distribution on the left side. **Above:** anterior view; **next page:** posterior view. (*Reproduced, with permission, from Aminoff MJ, Greenberg DA, Simon RP: Clinical Neurology, 3rd ed. Originally published by Appleton & Lange. Copyright © 1996 by The McGraw-Hill Companies, Inc.*)

Nerve root

Peripheral nerve

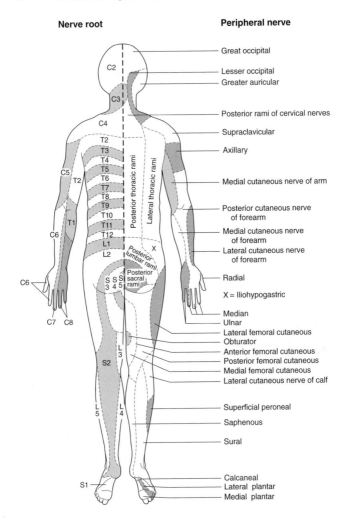

- Great occipital
- Lesser occipital
- Greater auricular
- Posterior rami of cervical nerves
- Supraclavicular
- Axillary
- Medial cutaneous nerve of arm
- Posterior cutaneous nerve of forearm
- Medial cutaneous nerve of forearm
- Lateral cutaneous nerve of forearm
- Radial
- X = Iliohypogastric
- Median
- Ulnar
- Lateral femoral cutaneous
- Obturator
- Anterior femoral cutaneous
- Posterior femoral cutaneous
- Medial femoral cutaneous
- Lateral cutaneous nerve of calf
- Superficial peroneal
- Saphenous
- Sural
- Calcaneal
- Lateral plantar
- Medial plantar

Figure 9–4. (*Continued*)

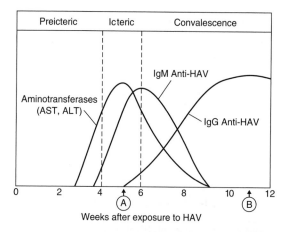

Preicteric	Icteric	Convalescence

Aminotransferases (AST, ALT)

IgM Anti-HAV

IgG Anti-HAV

0   2   4   6   8   10   12
(A)   (B)

Weeks after exposure to HAV

Patterns of Antibody Tests		
	IgM Anti-HAV	IgG Anti-HAV
A Acute HA	+	+ or −
B Convalescence (indicates previous infection)	−	+

Figure 9–5. HEPATITIS A: Usual pattern of serologic changes in hepatitis A. **HA** = hepatitis A; **AST** = aspartate aminotransferase; **ALT** = alanine aminotransferase; **Anti-HAV** = hepatitis A virus antibody; **IgM** = immunoglobulin M; **IgG** = immunoglobulin G. (*Reproduced, with permission, from Harvey AM et al [editors]: The Principles and Practice of Medicine, 22nd ed. Originally published by Appleton & Lange. Copyright © 1988 by The McGraw-Hill Companies, Inc.*)

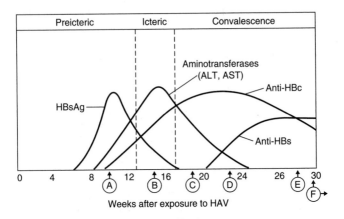

Usual Patterns of Hepatitis B Antigens and Antibodies			
	HBsAg	Anti-HBc	Anti-HBs
A Very early	+	+ or −	−
B Acute	+	+	−
C Active HB with high titer Anti-HBc ("window")	−	+	−
D Convalescence	−	+	+
E Recovery	−	+ or −	+
F Chronic carrier	+	+	−

Figure 9–6. HEPATITIS B: Usual pattern of serologic changes in hepatitis B (HB). **HBV** = hepatitis B virus; **HBsAg** = hepatitis B surface antigen; **Anti-HBc** = hepatitis B core antibody; **Anti-HBs** = hepatitis B surface antibody; **AST** = aspartate aminotransferase; **ALT** = alanine aminotransferase. (*Modified and reproduced, with permission, from Harvey AM et al [editors]: The Principles and Practice of Medicine, 22nd ed. Originally published by Appleton & Lange. Copyright © 1988 by The McGraw-Hill Companies, Inc.*)

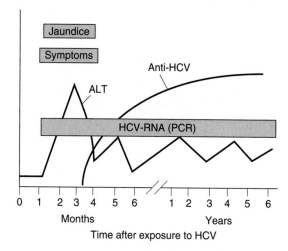

Figure 9–7. HEPATITIS C: The typical course of chronic hepatitis C. **ALT** = alanine amino-transferase; **Anti-HCV** = antibody to hepatitis C virus by enzyme immunoassay; **HCV RNA [PCR]** = hepatitis C viral RNA by polymerase chain reaction. (*Reproduced, with permission, from Tierney LM Jr, McPhee SJ, Papadakis MA [editors]:* Current Medical Diagnosis & Treatment 2003. *McGraw-Hill, 2003.*)

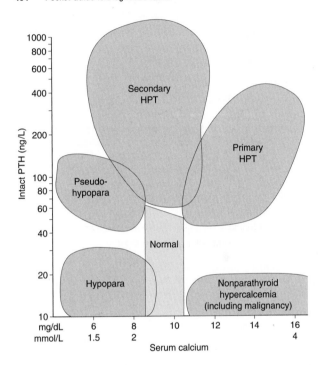

Figure 9–8. PARATHYROID HORMONE AND CALCIUM NOMOGRAM. Relationship between serum intact parathyroid hormone (PTH) and serum calcium levels in patients with hypoparathyroidism, pseudohypoparathyroidism, nonparathyroid hypercalcemia, primary hyperparathyroidism, and secondary hyperparathyroidism. **HPT** = hyperparathyroidism. (*Courtesy of GJ Strewler.*)

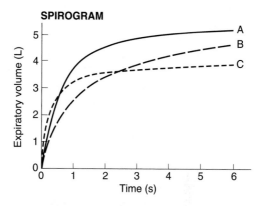

SPIROGRAM

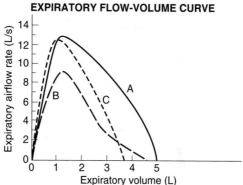

EXPIRATORY FLOW-VOLUME CURVE

Figure 9–9. PULMONARY FUNCTION TESTS: SPIROMETRY. Representative spirograms (upper panel) and expiratory flow-volume curves (lower panel) for normal **(A)**, obstructive **(B)**, and restrictive **(C)** patterns. (*Reproduced, with permission, from Tierney LM Jr, McPhee SJ, Papadakis MA [editors]:* Current Medical Diagnosis & Treatment 2003. *McGraw-Hill, 2003.*)

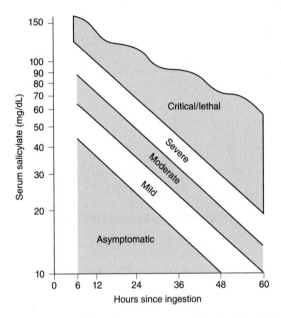

Figure 9–10. SALICYLATE TOXICITY: Nomogram for determining severity of salicylate intoxication. Absorption kinetics assumes acute ingestion of non–enteric-coated aspirin preparation. (*Modified and reproduced, with permission, from Done AK: Significance of measurements of salicylate in blood in cases of acute ingestion.* Pediatrics *1960;26:800. Permission obtained also from Saunders CE, Ho MT [editors]:* Current Emergency Diagnosis & Treatment, *4th ed. Originally published by Appleton & Lange. Copyright © 1992 by The McGraw-Hill Companies, Inc.*)

Index

NOTE: A *t* following a page number indicates tabular material, and an *f* following a page number indicates a figure.